Adventures in Food and Nutrition!

Carol Byrd-Bredbenner, Ph.D., R.D.
Extension Specialist and Professor of Nutrition
Chair, Family and Consumer Sciences Department
Rutgers, The State University of New Jersey
New Brunswick, New Jersey

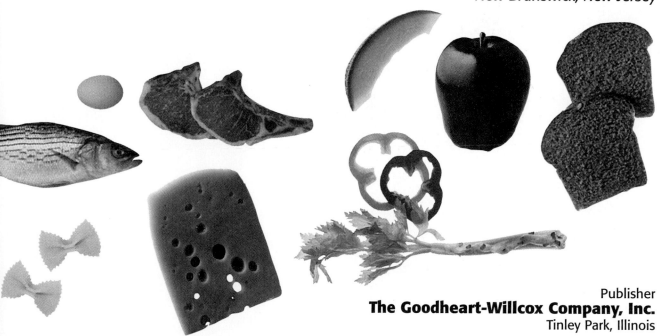

Publisher
The Goodheart-Willcox Company, Inc.
Tinley Park, Illinois

Library of Congress Catalog Card Number 96-19155
International Standard Book Number 1-56637-834-6

1 2 3 4 5 6 7 8 9 10   03   06 05 04 03 02

Library of Congress Cataloging-in-Publication Data

Byrd-Bredbenner, Carol.
Adventures in food and nutrition / Carol Byrd-Bredbenner.
p. cm.
Includes index.
ISBN 1-56637-834-6
1. Nutrition. I. Title.
QP141.B993 2003
613.2—dc20

96-19155
CIP

Introduction

Adventures in Food and Nutrition! is designed to help you explore the exciting world of food and nutrition. You will explore beyond familiar foods and preparation methods. A multicultural, multiethnic emphasis will encourage you to try new foods.

Adventures in Food and Nutrition! introduces you to food and nutrition. It will lead you to develop scientific and inquiry skills, preparing you to become nutritionally literate and able to make smart food choices. You will sharpen your critical thinking and problem-solving skills and apply math and science principles with hands-on exercises and experiments. These will help you develop the skills and knowledge you need to become an informed food consumer.

Each chapter begins with objectives and new terms you will encounter. Chapters also include a summary, review questions, application questions, and activities, plus hundreds of colorful photos and charts. Each chapter also includes special interest topics focusing on nutrition, cultures, health concerns, and technology. Math and science topics related to food and nutrition are also featured.

Adventures in Food and Nutrition! makes the study of food and nutrition a fun adventure! It will help you understand the consequences of your food choices. It will also allow you to become involved in both the science and creativity of preparing nutritious meals and snacks.

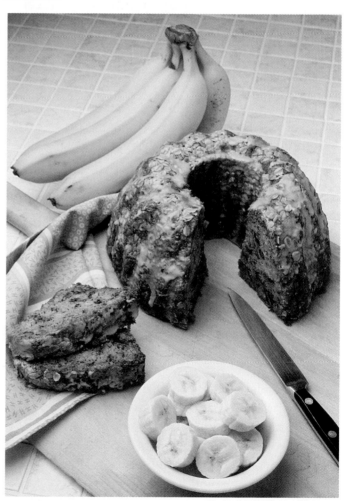

The International Banana Association

About the Author

Carol Byrd-Bredbenner, Ph.D., R.D. is a nationally recognized author and nutrition educator. Carol received her degrees in Home Economics Education and Nutrition from Florida State University and Pennsylvania State University. She is a Registered Dietitian and a member of the American Association of Family and Consumer Sciences, American Dietetics Association, and Society for Nutrition Education. In addition to being the author of *Adventures in Food and Nutrition!,* Carol has written several classroom nutrition education curriculum guides and teaching kits for preschool, elementary, middle school, and high school students. She also writes nutrition education computer software and has contributed nutrition articles to various family and consumer sciences publications as well as the *Journal of Nutrition Education.* She is actively involved in designing new methods to teach people of all ages how to improve their diets and health.

Carol has extensive teaching experience at both the secondary and university levels. As an active lecturer and consultant, she frequently conducts workshops for family and consumer sciences teachers and dietitians. She has made nutrition education presentations at national meetings of the American Association of Family and Consumer Sciences, Society for Nutrition Education, American Dietetics Association, and International Congress of Nutrition. She has served as the Director of the National Information and Resource Center at Pennsylvania State University. Currently, she is a nutrition teacher and researcher at Rutgers, The State University of New Jersey. For her expertise and significant contributions to the field of nutrition education, she has been named a Fellow of the American Dietetic Association. She also has received the Outstanding Nutrition Educator award from the Society of Nutrition Education.

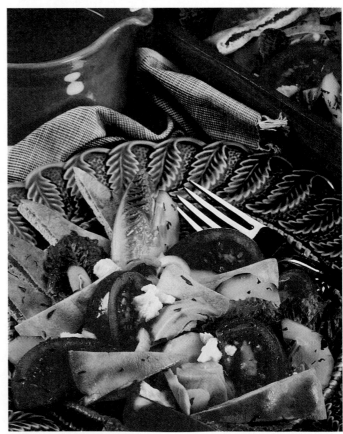

Florida Tomato Committee

Table of Contents

Chapter 12
Smart Shopping _____ 268

Chapter 13
Ready, Set, Cook _____ 293

Chapter 14
When You're on the Go _____ 317

Chapter 15
Fabulous Fruits _____ 344

Chapter 23
Delicious Desserts _____ **525**

Chapter 24
A Career to Consider _____ **547**

Appendix: Food Composition Table _____ **576**

Glossary _____ **600**

Index _____ **613**

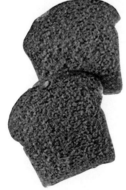
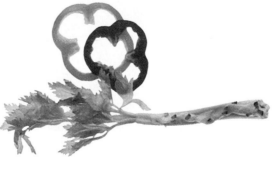

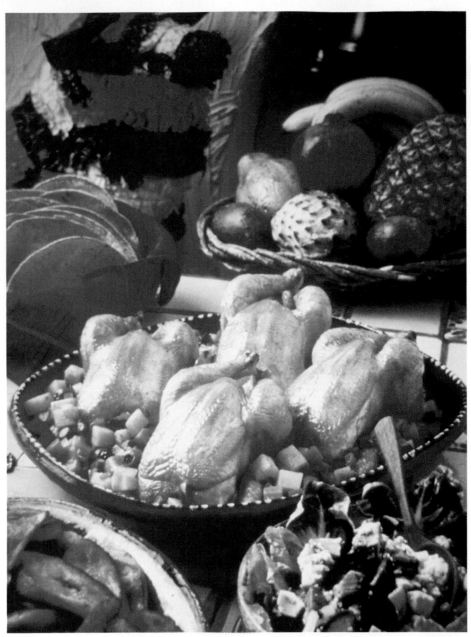

Perdue Farms

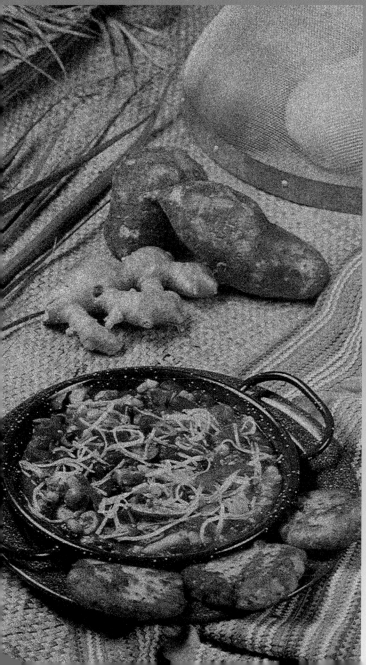

Chapter **1**
Food, Nutrition, and You

Objectives

After reading this chapter, you will be able to
- ❑ explain why a nutritious diet is important.
- ❑ describe a healthy person.
- ❑ explain how diet and health are related.
- ❑ name the needs satisfied by eating.
- ❑ list factors that affect food choices.
- ❑ explain why you eat the foods you do.

New Terms

nutrients: the materials found in foods that are needed to build and repair body tissues and provide energy.

diet: all the foods a person eats.

nutritious diet: a diet that includes energy and all the nutrients in the amounts needed.

nutrition: the study of nutrients and how the body uses them.

food science: the study of how foods change chemically through natural processes or when they are prepared or stored.

hunger: the physical need for food.

appetite: the desire to eat certain foods and reject others.

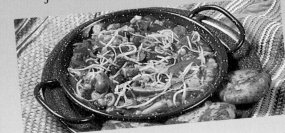

Brooks Tropicals

13

Welcome to the world of food and nutrition! This may be your first food and nutrition class, but you already know a lot about this topic. For instance, you know that every living thing needs food to survive. You have years of experience enjoying food. You know which foods you like best. You may be able to name foods that are low in fat. By now, you may have baked some cookies or cooked dinner for your family. Perhaps you have even bought groceries.

You are something of an expert already! There is still much more to learn, though. You may wonder if you are eating the right foods. Will your food choices keep you healthy? What should athletes eat? Can fast-foods be part of a healthy diet? Do foods affect the way you look? How can you keep foods safe to eat?

This book will help you answer all of these questions and more. It will help you expand your knowledge and put that knowledge to work to keep yourself strong and healthy. Let's get started with these three questions. Why is food important? Why do you eat? What affects your food choices?

Why Is Food Important?

Food affects everything about you. It influences how you look, feel, and act. It determines how well you grow. Food also affects your ability to work and play. Your physical health and mental alertness partly depend on the foods you eat, too, 1-1.

Food affects you in so many ways because it is your source of energy and nutrients. *Nutrients* are the materials needed to build and renew all parts of your body. Each day, your body uses nutrients to build a little bit of muscle, skin, and every other body part. Nutrients help you grow and replace old, worn out cells. This is how some of the food you eat today becomes part of you tomorrow. Nutrients also provide the energy you need to work and play.

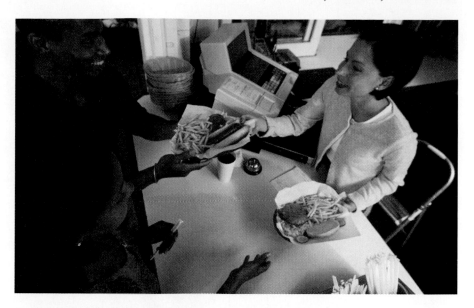

1-1 Your food choices affect how you look, act, and feel. In a lifetime, most people will eat about 60,000 pounds of food. (That's equal to the weight of six elephants!)

The best foods to eat are the ones that add up to a nutritious diet. A *diet* is all the foods and beverages you consume. A ***nutritious diet*** is a diet that provides all the energy and nutrients you need in the amounts you need. It helps you grow normally. It also helps you build strong muscles, solid bones, and healthy skin. That is, a nutritious diet provides enough energy and nutrients to richly nourish all parts of your body.

Which foods are part of a nutritious diet? You can find the answer to this question by studying nutrition and food science. ***Nutrition*** is the study of nutrients and how the body uses them. ***Food science*** is the study of how foods change chemically through natural processes or when they are prepared or stored. As you read this book, you will learn about nutrition and food science. You'll also discover how your favorite foods can be part of a nutritious diet, 1-2.

1-2 Favorite foods can add many nutrients to your diet.

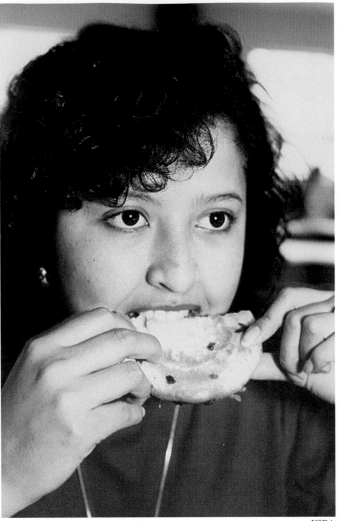

USDA

Nutrition in the Teenage Years _____

Giving good nutrition your best shot is important right now. During your teenage years, you will grow a great deal. If you don't have all the nutrients you need, you may not grow as well. Your body will not be as strong and healthy as it could be. Being healthy improves your chances of success in school. Healthy people tend to have more fun and feel good about themselves. They have the energy to do the things they like. They look their best, too. Traits of healthy people are listed in 1-3. How many of these traits describe you?

Traits of Healthy People
Shiny hair
Clear, smooth skin
Bright, clear eyes
White teeth
Firm muscles
Strong bones
Energy to work and play hard
Infection resistance
Quick recovery from illness
Ability to relax
Happy, contented outlook

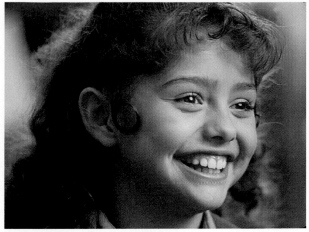

USDA

1-3 Healthy people often make wise food choices.

Good nutrition is important for your future, too. Even though you feel great now, things may be happening inside of you that you won't notice for years. For instance, the foods you select now could raise your chances of having a heart attack years from now. On the other hand, making wise food choices can help you prevent some health problems. Careful food choices today may help you avoid getting fragile bones or certain types of cancer in the future. Now is the time to make the best choices you can.

Why Do You Eat?

Does this conversation sound familiar?

Kelly: Why did I eat that pizza at Sue's house on Sunday? I wasn't even hungry. All the other kids were having pizza. So, I ate some, too.

Rachel: I wasn't hungry either when I ate that ice cream last night. I was just looking for something to do. I was so bored.

Carlos: I know why I ate dinner last night. I was starving!

Almost everyone at some time has asked "Why did I eat that?" Like Carlos, you most often eat because you are hungry. Perhaps you, like Kelly, eat when you get together with friends. Maybe you raid the refrigerator out of boredom as Rachel did. People eat to satisfy hunger, social needs, and emotional needs. See 1-4.

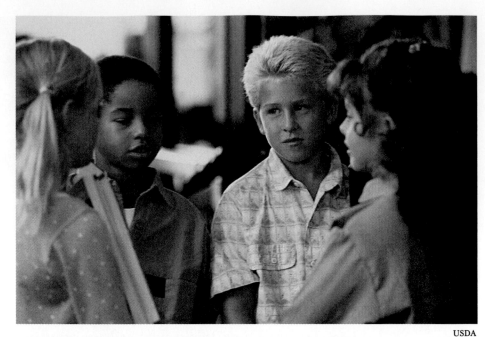

USDA

1-4 People eat for a variety of reasons. You may eat for different reasons than your friends do.

Hunger

The most obvious reason you eat is hunger. *Hunger* is a physical need for food. Your body is demanding food when your stomach growls or you feel weak or light headed. It needs a fresh supply of energy and nutrients. You eat to satisfy this demand.

Social Needs

People also eat for social reasons. Eating with others helps satisfy the need to belong and be with friends or family. People may not feel hungry at all when they eat for social reasons.

Food and get-togethers seem to go hand in hand. Offering food and drinks to guests is a common way to welcome them. When friends and family gather, they often share a snack or meal. This gives them time to talk and share their thoughts. Think about how often you eat when you are with your friends. You may offer them snacks when they visit your home. You may go with friends to restaurants to eat and talk. You might share a sandwich at lunch. See 1-5.

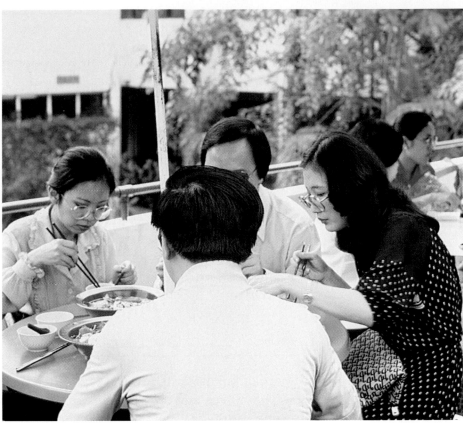

USDA

1-5 Many people enjoy eating with others.

Emotional Needs

Did you ever go out for pizza after winning a big game? If you did, you may have eaten because of your emotions. Emotions are feelings. Happiness and love are positive emotions. Negative emotions include being bored, sad, upset, tense, or angry. Both types of emotions can cause people to eat.

People may not feel hungry at all when they eat to satisfy emotional needs. Some people eat because of positive emotions. A happy event like a birthday might be celebrated with cake and ice cream. Some people eat to cope with negative emotions, too. They may try to drown their sorrows in milk shakes. Others try to use food to help them forget their troubles.

What Affects Your Food Choices?

Why do you eat some foods and not others? When people get hungry, why do some eat hot dogs? Why do others choose green snake soup? Why do still others prefer roasted termites? It is their appetites that guide them to eat certain foods to satisfy their hunger, social needs, and emotions. *Appetite* is the desire to eat certain foods and reject others.

No doubt people desire foods with flavors they like. They may prefer some foods because their cultural group and family eat them. Busy people may desire foods that are easy to prepare. People concerned about their health desire foods they think are good for them. Appetite and food choices depend on factors such as personal likes, culture, and custom. Other factors include lifestyle, environment, and knowledge.

Personal Likes

What is your favorite food? Maybe it's ice cream because you like its sweet flavor and creamy texture. Perhaps it's a certain candy bar because someone you admire eats it, too. Some people like foods that they feel give them prestige. Costly foods, such as steak and lobster, often are thought of as prestige foods.

Each person's food likes are very personal. The foods that appeal to one person may not appeal to others. For instance, you may like mushrooms and olives on your pizza. Your best friend might not like these toppings at all.

Most people like common foods more than they like exotic foods. Common foods are those they have eaten many times before. Orange juice and hamburgers are common foods in the United States. Exotic foods are new or unusual. Seaweed and snails are exotic foods to many people. Exotic foods can become common if you eat them often.

Foods that seem exotic to you may be common to someone living in another area. The reverse is true, too. Culture and family customs greatly control which foods people regard as common or exotic.

Focus on Food

Bugs for Lunch!

Insects are thought of as a delicious treat in many countries around the world. Grasshoppers are a delicacy in Japan. Grubs are popular in Zaire. Australian aborigines enjoy bogong moths. Some people even eat roasted tarantulas! Travelers to Mexico City can dine at special restaurants that serve ancient Aztec dishes such as black ants in green sauce.

Most people from the United States would be very surprised to see bugs on the menu. This is mainly because of our culture. Remember, culture teaches a person which foods are proper to eat and which are not. Our culture doesn't teach us to eat insects. So, we don't develop a liking for insects at the dinner table.

Another reason many people in the United States don't like insects is that they think insects are dirty and spread disease. It may surprise you to learn that many insects are leaf eaters and are very clean. Insects are packed with nutrients, too. Ounce for ounce, many insects provide more nutrients than meat.

Not all insects can be eaten. Some, like cockroaches, carry disease. Others, like Monarch butterflies, are poisonous. Still others, like worker bees, don't taste very good. However, many, many bugs are delicious. For example, some ants taste like lemon drops. Others have a sweet and sour flavor.

Do you remember this poem?

I know an old lady who swallowed a fly.
Why, oh why, did she swallow that fly?

Now you know the answer! She probably was hungry!

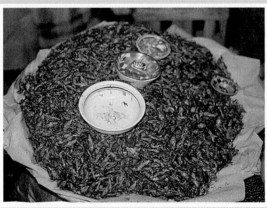

Gene R. DeFoliart

This flavorful dish is made by boiling Mexican grasshoppers with onion, garlic, and chili powder.

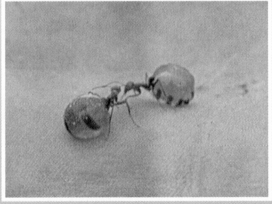

Gene R. DeFoliart

These honey pot ants taste like candy. They have different flavors, depending on what they have been eating.

Culture

    Culture is the knowledge, beliefs, religion, and traditions shared by a group of people. Culture teaches a person which foods are proper to eat and which are not.

    Foods that one cultural group feels are proper to eat may be rejected by another. For example, many people in the United States believe it is proper to eat beef. However, many cultures in India never eat beef. They believe cows are sacred. Some African cultures savor foods like blood, mice, and insects. Even though these foods are packed with nutrients and safe to eat, few other cultures feel they are proper to eat.

Family Customs

    A *custom* is a practice a group of people do often. It is the usual way of doing things. Parents pass on food customs to their children. In some families, it is a custom to serve rice at every meal. In other families, it is a custom to serve chicken for Sunday dinner. What food customs does your family have? How do the food customs of your friends' families differ from your own?

Lifestyles

    Lifestyles can affect food choices. *Lifestyle* is the type of life you lead. It includes the way you spend your time and use your energy. It is often determined partly by the amount of money you have.

    People with very busy lives have little time and energy to buy and prepare foods. They often eat foods that are quick and easy to prepare. They may grab fast-foods, vending machine foods, and snack foods when they can. People with less hectic schedules have more time to make their own meals. They don't have to always rely on quick and easy foods, 1-6.

    Food choices are partly based on what a person can afford to buy. People with more money have a wider choice of types and amounts of food than those with less money.

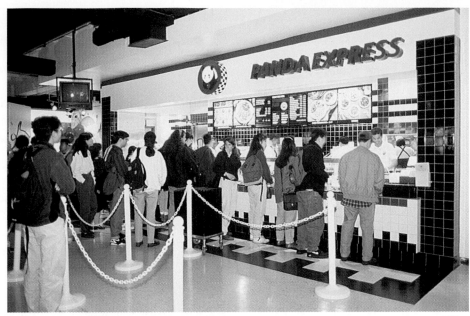

USDA

1-6 People with hectic schedules may need to eat out often.

Environment

The *environment* is your surroundings and all the experiences you have. It is filled with many sights, sounds, flavors, and textures. Seeing cupcakes at the bake sale or smelling popcorn popping can affect your appetite. Just knowing a food is there can affect your appetite, too. Have you ever wanted a slice of watermelon after seeing it in the kitchen?

Advertisements also are part of the environment. They can strongly affect your appetite. Have you ever wanted a big, juicy burger after seeing it advertised on TV?

Knowledge

What a person knows about nutrition and food can influence food choices. Did you ever eat a food just because you knew it was good for you? More and more people are learning about nutrition. They are using their knowledge to choose a healthy diet. They know that eating well can help them look and feel great.

Science in the Kitchen

The Five Senses

What is your favorite food? Is it a cold, fizzy soft drink? Perhaps it's crunchy, salty chips. Maybe your favorite food is a fragrant, red apple. Whatever your favorite food is, you may experience it through your five senses. Sight, touch, hearing, smell and taste are the senses.

Through the sense of sight you observe foods' wide array of colors. The temperatures and textures of foods are felt through the sense of touch. Even the sense of hearing is involved when you hear chewing sounds. The senses you use the most when you enjoy foods are smell and taste.

Your sense of smell works like this. When you breathe, air flows over cells inside your nose. These cells send scent messages to your brain. The message might be the aroma of bread baking. It could be the scent of fresh strawberries. It might even be burnt toast or sour milk.

Your tongue can detect four basic tastes. They are salty, sweet, sour, and bitter. Your tongue is covered with taste buds. Taste buds send taste messages to your brain. The message is sour when you bite into a lemon. It is sweet when you eat raisins. It is salty when you have a snack of green olives. A bitter message is sent when you drink grapefruit juice.

For years, scientists thought people tasted specific flavors on different parts of the tongue. For instance, they thought you tasted sweet flavors near the tip of the tongue and sour flavors on the sides. Now, they know you can taste all types of flavors almost anywhere on your tongue. Try this

experiment and see! Dip a cotton swab in salt and gently touch the 10 spots on your tongue shown in the drawing. Record where the taste was strongest. Rinse your mouth well. Try the test again with sugar, lemon juice, and coffee. Be sure to use a fresh swab with each new flavor.

Your sense of smell helps your sense of taste. Some food scientists believe that most of what you taste is really what you smell. You may have noticed that foods seem to have little flavor when you have a head cold.

You can do a simple experiment to see how the senses of smell and taste are related. While blindfolded, sample small pieces of raw potato, apple, and onion. Then, hold your nose and sample the foods again. Can you identify the foods correctly without using all of your senses?

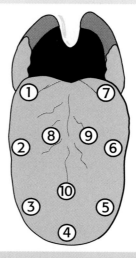

Each bump on your tongue contains hundreds of taste buds. How does the number of bumps on each part of your tongue compare with where salt, sugar, lemon juice, and coffee tasted strongest?

As you can see, many factors affect your appetite and food choices. It is sometimes hard to say why you eat a certain food. Take a look at the "Why I Eat What I Eat Diary" in 1-7. By keeping a diary like this one, you might be able to identify the factors that affect your food choices. Next time you ask yourself "Why did I eat that?", you'll have an answer!

Why I Eat What I Eat Diary		
Day/Time	**Food or Beverage**	**Reason**
Friday		
7:15 AM	Orange juice, cereal, milk	Hunger, lifestyle
10:30 AM	Chocolate chip cookies	Environment (smell of food)
1:00 PM	Burger, milk shake	Hunger, social needs, personal likes
4:15 PM	Bag of chips, soft drink	Emotional needs (boredom)
6:30 PM	Chop suey, rice, tea	Hunger, culture, knowledge
9:00 PM	Cake, ice cream	Social needs, family custom, emotional needs (celebrate)
11:30 PM	Cold pizza	Hunger

1-7 What are the most common reasons this person eats the foods he or she does?

In a Nutshell

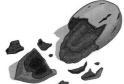

- Good nutrition is important to your health now and in the future.
- A nutritious diet includes all the energy and nutrients you need in the amounts you need.
- Food affects the way you look, feel, act, and grow.
- You eat to satisfy your hunger, social needs, and emotions.
- Personal likes, culture, custom, lifestyle, environment, and knowledge affect your food choices.

In the Know

1. List two ways a nutritious diet helps your body.
2. _____ is the study of nutrients and how your body uses them.
3. True or false? Teens who do not have all the nutrients they need may not grow well.
4. List four traits of healthy people.
5. "Why did I eat those cookies at the mall last night? They smelled good, but I wasn't even hungry," said Hans. Why do you think Hans ate the cookies?
   A. Because of his family customs.
   B. Because of his culture.
   C. Because of his environment.
   D. Because of his knowledge.
6. True or false? Appetite is the physical need for food.
7. Appetite depends on _____.
   A. personal likes
   B. lifestyle
   C. knowledge
   D. All of the above.
8. Explain how the environment can affect food choices. Give an example of how the environment has affected your food choices.

What Would You Do?

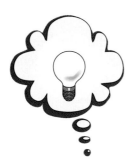

Your new friend is from a foreign country. "Will you please come to dinner at my house on Tuesday?" she asks. You are very excited and accept her invitation. When you sit down to eat you notice that there are many foods you have never seen before. What would you do?

Expanding Your Knowledge

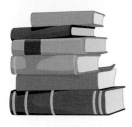

1. Make a music video on nutrition. Use the words of the song to explain how a nutritious diet is important.
2. Create a collage that shows the traits of healthy people. Make the collage with magazine pictures or drawings.
3. Brainstorm and list the words you think of when you hear the word "nutrition." Use the list of words to create a word-find puzzle. Exchange your puzzle with a classmate.
4. Discover why you eat the foods you eat. Keep a log of the foods you eat for one day. You can use a chart like the one in 1-7. Review your log. Do you eat mostly to satisfy hunger, emotions, or social needs? Which factors affect your appetite most? Write a paragraph to summarize your findings.
5. Design a bulletin board that shows magazine pictures of people eating. Write captions to explain why each person pictured is eating. Title the bulletin board "Why We Eat the Foods We Do."
6. Poll 10 people to find out how often they eat because of emotions. You could ask questions like these. "What do you do when you are bored? Do you ever eat to relieve boredom? What foods do you eat?" Make a poster to report your findings.
7. In an small group, research the food customs of one of the following religions: Islam, Judaism, or Hinduism. Share your findings with the class.
8. Interview an elderly person. Ask the person about the food customs he or she had as a child. Compare the customs to your customs. Ask the person how his or her customs have changed. Think about how food customs have changed over the years.
9. Describe a food custom you have observed in your family or a friend's family.
10. Watch three television advertisements for food. Describe how these advertisements make you want to eat the food. Research advertising techniques in the library. Find out how advertisers create a desire for their products. Write an article for your school newspaper about your discoveries.

Chapter 2

Nutrients: The Building Blocks of Health

Objectives

After reading this chapter, you will be able to
- ❏ explain what each nutrient does for your body.
- ❏ list food sources of each nutrient.
- ❏ describe ways to improve your nutrient intake.
- ❏ discuss the use of nutrient supplements.

New Terms

calorie: a measure of the energy value of food.
gram: a measure of weight.
dietitian: a nutrition expert.
Dietary Reference Intakes (DRIs): a set of guidelines for the amounts of many nutrients needed each day.

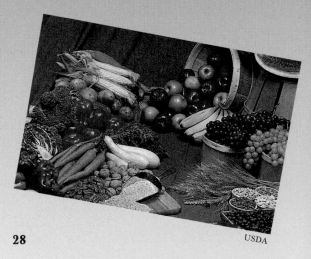

USDA

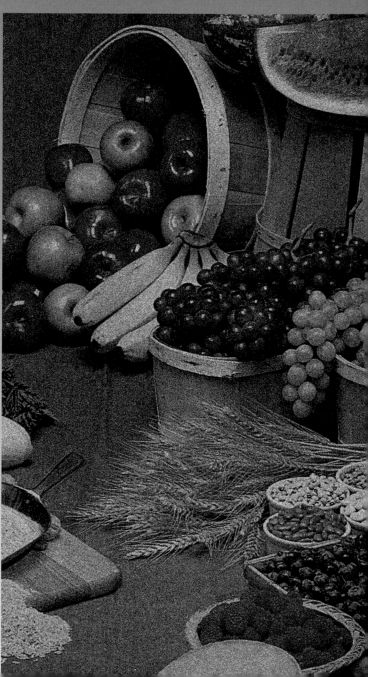

Every living thing, including plants, animals, and you, needs food to survive. Foods are as diverse as the plants and animals that eat them. Oak trees and other plants get their food from the soil and rain. Blood is food to mosquitoes. Some animals, like leopards, sharks, and snakes, eat mostly meat. Foods from plants, like berries, lettuce, and wheat, are food to many other animals. The babies of many animals consume mostly milk. Food for many humans includes a combination of plants, meat, eggs, and milk. Foods provide the calories and nutrients every living thing needs in order to grow and stay healthy.

Calories, Your Body's Fuel

Calories are the fuel that keeps your body running, 2-1. You can only get them from food. A *calorie* is a measure of the energy value of food. You burn calories, much like a car burns gasoline, to keep running. Every time you walk or when your heart beats, you burn calories. You also burn calories as your body grows, replaces worn out cells, heals wounds, digests food, and keeps itself warm.

2-1 Calories are your body's fuel. You use them every minute of the day.

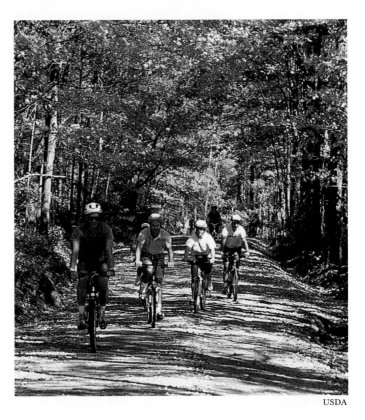

USDA

Calories are not nutrients, but some nutrients provide calories. Carbohydrate, protein, and fat are the only three nutrients that supply calories. Fat is the richest source of energy in your diet. That's because each gram of fat provides nine calories. One gram of carbohydrate or protein supplies four calories. A *gram* is a measure of weight. A small jelly bean or a raisin each weighs about one gram, 2-2.

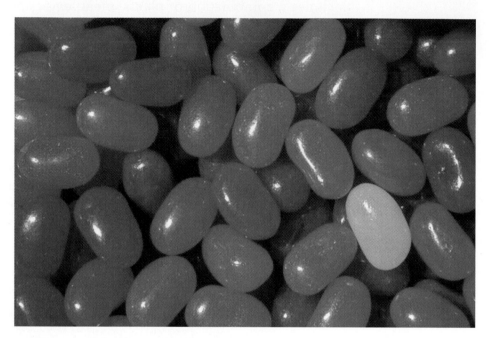

2-2 A small jelly bean weighs about one gram.

Nutrients, Your Body's Building Blocks

Nutrients are the body's building blocks. They are chemical substances found in foods. They keep your body running smoothly. Nutrients are used for growth and to build all of your body parts from teeth to toenails. Nutrients also are used to replace worn out cells and heal wounds. They provide energy, too.

There are six classes of nutrients. They are *carbohydrates*, *fats*, *proteins*, *water*, *vitamins*, and *minerals*. You need all the nutrients in the right amounts to grow normally and stay healthy. Every food provides some nutrients.

Carbohydrates _____

Carbohydrates are the most common nutrient on earth. They are found in every food of plant origin. Fruits, vegetables, breads, and cereals are rich in carbohydrates. Milk is the only food of animal origin that contains carbohydrate.

The three types of carbohydrates are *sugars, starch,* and *fiber.* Sugar and starch are the most important fuel for the brain. They should provide the largest portion of calories in your diet, 2-3. Fiber helps keep the digestive system working well. Many people in the United States eat too much sugar and not enough starch and fiber.

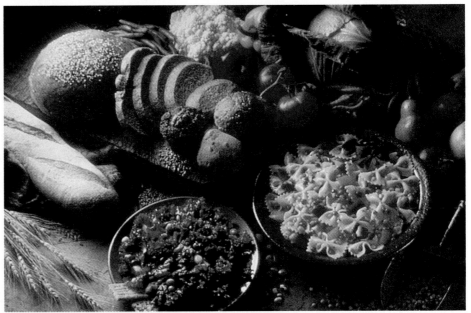

Wheat Foods Council

2-3 Carbohydrate-rich foods should be your major source of energy.

Sugar

What do you think of when you hear the word *sugar?* Many people picture pure white crystals in a sugar bowl. It may surprise you to learn there are many other types of sugar. Brown sugar, honey, corn syrup, and fructose are just a few of the sugars in foods. Sugars you might find in foods are listed in 2-4.

Other Names for Sugar		
Sugar has many aliases. Some of them are listed below.		
Brown sugar	Maltose	Dextrin
Honey	Lactose	Mannitol
Sucrose	Levulose	Syrup
Fructose	Mannose	High fructose corn syrup
Glucose	Dextrose	Maple syrup

2-4 Sugar goes by a variety of names. Some of them are listed here.

You may have heard that honey is the most nutritious sugar. Actually, no sugar is better for you than any other. However, some foods that supply sugar may be better for you than others. For instance, sugars are a natural part of fruits, milk, cereals, and dry peas and beans. These foods not only contain sugar, but they provide many other nutrients, too.

Sugars are added to pies, cakes, cookies, candies, and many breakfast cereals. Many people like the sweet taste that sugar provides, 2-5. However, adding sugar only increases calories. It does not furnish other nutrients. If you eat foods with added sugar often, you may not be getting enough of the other nutrients you need. You may get more cavities, too.

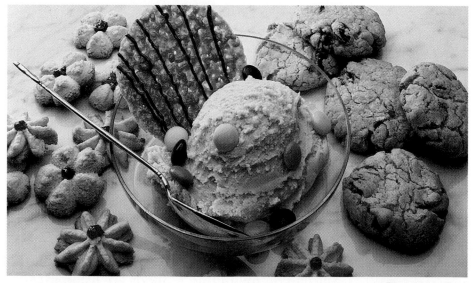

Peanut Advisory Board

2-5 Sugary foods taste sweet, but they add many calories to your diet.

Starch

Starch is a very important source of calories. Breads, cereals, and dried peas and beans are rich sources of starch. Vegetables such as potatoes and corn are other rich sources of starch. Starch and sugar supply the same number of calories per gram, but foods high in starch also supply many other nutrients. For instance, breads and cereals provide thiamin, riboflavin, niacin, folate, and iron. Dried peas and beans furnish protein. Potatoes contain vitamin C.

Some people think foods that are rich in starch are fattening. In fact, they are no more fattening than proteins or sugar. Often, though, starch-rich foods are served with fats such as butter or oil. It's the fats that pile on the calories. For example, a slice of bread has about 70 calories. If you butter it, you add 50 calories or more. A potato has only about 100 calories. If you slice it and fry it in oil to make French fries, the calories jump to 350 or higher.

Fiber

Fiber is the parts of plants that humans cannot digest. This carbohydrate does not furnish calories. It helps move waste through your digestive system and helps prevent constipation. A diet high in fiber may help prevent heart disease and certain types of cancer, too.

Breads, cereals, and dried peas and beans are the richest sources of fiber. Vegetables and fruits, especially their skins, also provide fiber. The way a food is prepared can affect the amount of fiber it contains. For instance, an unpeeled apple has more fiber than either a peeled apple or applesauce. Apple juice has even less fiber. The less the food looks like it did when harvested, the less fiber it is likely to have.

You may have seen fiber supplements for sale in stores. Foods, not supplements, are the best sources of fiber. That's because foods contain several types of fiber and each type works a little differently in the body. Also, foods contain nutrients that your body needs.

Fats

The main function of fat is to supply calories. Fat also adds flavor to food and provides some vitamins. Fat satisfies your hunger, too. That's because it takes more time to digest fat than any other nutrient. The longer it takes to digest a food, the longer it takes you to feel hungry again.

Fat is found in many foods. The richest sources are meat, poultry, eggs, milk products, nuts, seeds, and vegetable oils. Snack foods and pastries often are high in fat, too.

Fats can be put into two groups, unsaturated and saturated fat. Cholesterol is a fat-like substance. Many Americans eat more fat, saturated fat, and cholesterol than is healthy.

Health Alert

The Heart Beat

There is a vicious killer stalking the United States. Here are the clues:

- It claims the lives of nearly half the people in the United States.
  Many victims are chosen when they are teens or even younger.
  Many people don't know they will be victims until they are 40 or 50 years old.

Doctors call this killer arteriosclerosis (ar-TEER-ee-oh-scler-OH-sis). Some call it heart disease. Heart disease takes years to develop. It begins when soft deposits of fats begin to build up in the lining inside your blood vessels. These deposits look like white streaks. Many people have fatty streaks before they are 18 years old.

The fatty streaks are mostly cholesterol. As you get older, the streaks can get thicker and become hard. The more cholesterol in the blood, the faster the streaks can thicken. Over time, the fatty streaks make the opening in the blood vessel smaller. The heart has to work harder to push blood through the narrowed blood vessels. This also causes blood pressure to rise.

The blood vessels may become so narrow that blood can hardly pass through

them. Cells rely on blood to bring them oxygen and nutrients. If blood can't get through the blood vessels, the cells die in a few minutes. When blood can't reach the heart, a heart attack occurs. Part of the heart dies. A stroke occurs when blood can't reach the brain. Part of the brain dies. If too much of the heart or brain dies, the person dies.

There is some good news about this killer, though. You can do something about it. To reduce your chances of having a deadly heart attack or stroke, don't let those fatty streaks get thicker. The time to start is now. Don't wait until your blood vessels are damaged. Here are some tips to elude this killer.

- Get plenty of exercise. This helps you control your weight and gives your heart a workout. Shoot for at least 60 minutes of activity on most days.
- Control your weight. You are less likely to develop heart disease if you are not overweight. Keeping your weight down also helps reduce your chances of having high blood pressure and certain cancers.
- Have your blood pressure checked yearly. Your chances of being a victim increase when blood pressure is too high.

- Ask your doctor how often you should have your blood cholesterol checked. High blood cholesterol levels are a risk factor.
- Eat more fiber. Fiber can help remove cholesterol from your blood.
- Don't smoke. Smokers are more likely to be heart disease victims than nonsmokers. Smoking also increases your chances of developing lung cancer.
- Be extra careful if you are a male or related to a heart disease victim. Males are more likely to have heart disease than females. That doesn't let females off the hook. Anyone can be related to a heart disease victim. If a parent or grandparent had heart disease, you have a greater chance of developing it, too.

Just because you can't change your gender or family background doesn't mean you have to be a victim. It just makes it even more important for you to use your know-how to elude this killer. The sooner you get started, the better!

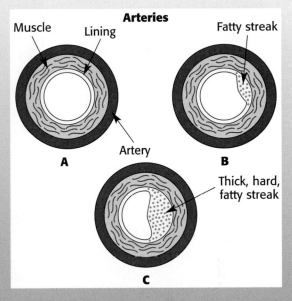

Arteries

Muscle Lining Fatty streak

Artery

A

B

Thick, hard, fatty streak

C

A: This is a normal, healthy artery.
B: Fatty streaks have begun to form in the lining of the artery. C: Fatty streaks have become thick and hard. Blood flow becomes restricted.

Saturated Fat and Unsaturated Fat

Both saturated fat and unsaturated fat provide the same number of calories per gram. They differ in the way they act in the body. *Saturated fat* causes the level of cholesterol in the blood to rise higher than normal. This increases your chances of developing heart disease. *Unsaturated fat* does not cause blood cholesterol levels to rise.

The main source of saturated fat is foods of animal origin. Butter, lard, and the fat on meat are examples. Only a few foods of plant origin contain mostly saturated fat. They are coconut oil and palm oil. Saturated fat is usually solid at room temperature.

Foods of plant origin contain mostly unsaturated fat. Corn, soybeans, sunflower seeds, olives, peanuts, and nuts are rich sources. The only food of animal origin that contains mostly unsaturated fat is fish. Unsaturated fat tends to be liquid at room temperature, 2-6.

2-6 Unsaturated fats are usually liquid at room temperature.

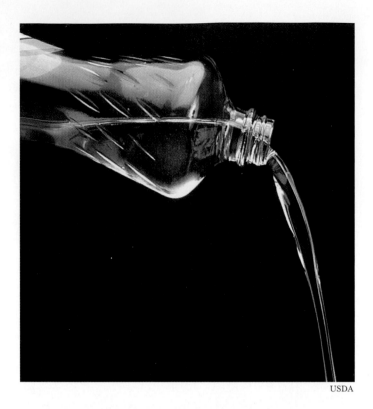

USDA

Some unsaturated fats are altered in a way that increases the amount of saturated fat they have. *Hydrogenation (hi-DRAH-gen-a-shun)* is the process that turns an unsaturated fat into a saturated one. For example, hydrogenation causes liquid, unsaturated corn oil to become a solid, saturated fat known as margarine.

Cholesterol

Cholesterol is a fatlike substance that is vital for life. Every cell in your body contains cholesterol. It forms cell walls and is used to make many body compounds. Your body can make all the cholesterol it needs. You do not need to have any cholesterol in your diet.

Cholesterol is found in all foods of animal origin. Meat, fish, poultry, eggs, and milk contain cholesterol. There is no cholesterol in fruits, vegetables, nuts, seeds, or any other foods of plant origin.

Proteins _____

Proteins are needed for growth and repair of the body. You use proteins to build new cells and to repair or replace worn out or injured cells. Foods of animal origin, such as meats, fish, poultry, eggs, and milk, are rich sources of proteins. Breads, cereals, nuts, seeds, and dried peas and beans are foods of plant origin that are rich in proteins. See 2-7.

2-7 These foods are rich sources of proteins.

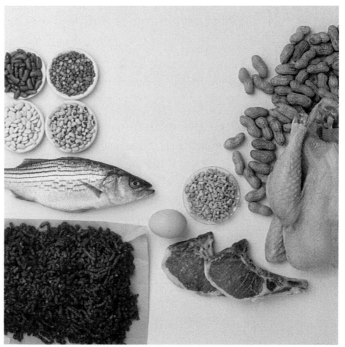

USDA

Your body digests the proteins you eat and breaks them into smaller parts called *amino acids.* Then, it reassembles the amino acids to make skin, muscles, and other body parts. This process is like taking apart a house made of bricks and then reusing the bricks to build a sidewalk.

There are 20 amino acids. Your body can make some of them out of others, but it cannot make all of them. The amino acids it cannot make must be supplied by the foods you eat. Foods of animal origin contain all the amino acids you need. These foods are called *complete proteins.* Foods of plant origin are called *incomplete proteins.*

That is because they contain most of the amino acids you need, but not all of them. You can make foods of plant origin into complete proteins by combining them with each other. To learn more about combining proteins, see "Going Vegetarian" in Chapter 22.

Many Americans eat much more protein than they need. Any protein not needed for growth and repair is used for energy, or it's stored in the body as fat. Extra protein is not stored as muscle. Many people living in other parts of the world, especially in Africa and Asia, get too little protein. A low-protein diet causes stunted growth. Also, wounds heal slowly and infections are common. A very low protein intake could even cause death.

Water

Only air is more important than water. You could only live a few minutes without air. You could only live a few days without water. Your body contains more water than anything else. Of every 10 pounds of body weight, six or seven pounds are water. Water is found in all of your cells. It makes up three-quarters of every muscle and brain cell. Half of many other cells are water. Blood is mostly water.

Water has many functions. In blood, water carries nutrients to the cells. The water in sweat cools you when you get hot. The water in urine washes harmful wastes out of your body. Water moistens the air you breathe. (Did you ever notice how the tiny water droplets in your breath condense into a fog on a cold day?) Water keeps your skin soft and elastic. It lubricates your joints and keeps them working smoothly. It protects your body by acting as a shock absorber. Water is a very important nutrient.

Each day, you lose eight cups of water in urine, sweat, and air you exhale. To replace the water lost, you need to drink eight cups of water daily. If you exercise or live in a hot climate, you will need more than eight cups, 2-8. Don't wait until you are thirsty to drink water. Thirst is a signal that the water level in your body is already too low. When you do feel thirsty, drink a cup more than your thirst tells you to drink.

2-8 Beverages are a great source of water. Be sure to drink extra water when you exercise.

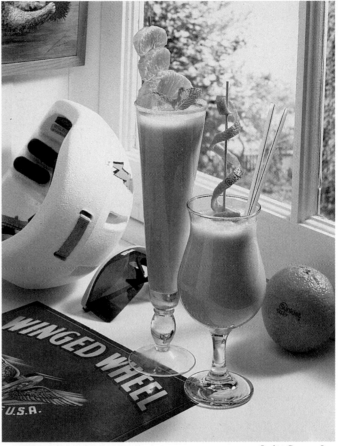

Sunkist Growers, Inc.

Soups and beverages such as juice, milk, and caffeine-free soft drinks are good sources of water. Foods supply water, too. For example, lettuce is 90 percent water and oranges are 80 percent water. Even meats are half water. Coffee, tea, colas, and other beverages that contain caffeine are not as helpful for meeting your need for water. That's because caffeine causes you to lose more water than normal in your urine.

Some people try to limit their water intake. They may think it is a good way to lose weight. Instead, they will feel weak, hot, and achy. Harmful wastes will build up in their bodies. Lost weight will be regained as soon as they drink water again. Any time people restrict water intake, they put their lives in danger.

Vitamins and Minerals

Vitamins and *minerals* are needed in tiny amounts. All the vitamins and minerals you need in a day combined weigh less than a dime. This amount seems especially small when compared to other nutrients. For instance, you need 25 times more protein and 150 times more carbohydrate each day. The amounts of vitamins and minerals you need may be small, but they are so necessary that you cannot live without them.

Vitamins and minerals are used in many of the body's chemical reactions. They help keep body processes working normally and are needed for growth and repair of the body. For example, vitamin A helps you see in dim light. The minerals calcium and sodium help keep body water in balance. Minerals also can become part of body tissues. For instance, calcium becomes part of bones and teeth. Iron is part of red blood cells. Neither vitamins nor minerals supply calories.

Vitamins and minerals are found in many different foods. Almost all foods contain some of these nutrients, 2-9. Vitamins are either water-soluble or fat-soluble. *Water-soluble vitamins* dissolve in

2-9 Vitamins and minerals are found in a wide variety of foods.

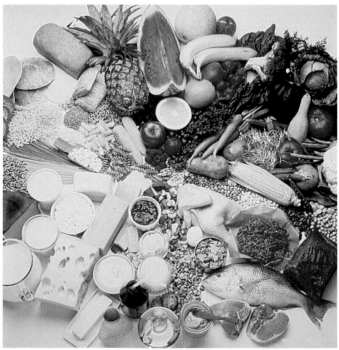

USDA

water. They include the B vitamins and vitamin C. Thiamin, riboflavin, niacin, and folate are some of the B-vitamins. *Fat-soluble vitamins* dissolve in fat. Vitamins A, D, E, and K are fat-soluble vitamins. Any fat-soluble vitamins your body does not need right away can be stored for use later. Extra water-soluble vitamins are not stored. They are washed away in body wastes. The functions and sources of each vitamin are listed in 2-10.

Vitamins		
Vitamin	**Major Functions**	**Some Rich Sources**
Vitamin A	Helps keep skin healthy Needed for normal vision	Deep yellow or orange fruits and vegetables, dark green vegetables, milk products, eggs
Thiamin, Riboflavin, and Niacin	Help release energy stored in foods Help build body tissue Help keep skin, hair, muscles, and nerves healthy	Breads, cereals, meat, fish, poultry, eggs, milk, cheese
Folate	Used to make red blood cells Helps form cells	Breads, cereals, dark green vegetables, dried beans and peas, bananas, mushrooms, oranges
Vitamin B12	Used to make red blood cells Helps keep nerves healthy	Foods of animal origin such as meat, fish, chicken, milk, cheese, eggs
Vitamin C	Helps keep gums and blood vessels healthy Helps wounds and bruises heal Used to make many body compounds	Citrus fruits, berries, melons, peppers, cabbage, potatoes, tomatoes, dark green vegetables
Vitamin D	Aids in bone and tooth formation Helps heart and nerves work normally	Fish, eggs, milk products, sunlight
Vitamin E	Protects blood and lung cells	Nuts, vegetable oils, dark green vegetables, breads, cereals
Vitamin K	Used to clot blood	Dark green vegetables, cauliflower, fruit, milk products, breads, cereals

2-10 Vitamins perform many functions in the body. Rich sources of these vitamins can be provided in a nutritious diet.

If your diet contains more minerals than your body needs, it can store many of them. Extra amounts of other minerals cannot be stored. They pass out of the body in body wastes. The functions and sources of minerals are listed in 2-11.

Minerals		
Mineral	**Major Functions**	**Some Rich Sources**
Iron	Used to build red blood cells Helps blood carry oxygen Helps cells use oxygen	Red meat, breads, cereals, dark green vegetables
Calcium	Used to build bones and teeth Helps muscles relax Balances body water	Milk products; dark green vegetables; almonds; calcium-fortified orange juice; fish with soft, tiny bones
Sodium	Helps nerves and muscles function Balances body water	Table salt, sauces, gravies, pickles, processed meat, soy sauce, many seasonings
Magnesium	Helps body make new cells Helps nerves and muscles work normally	Dark green vegetables, nuts, dried peas and beans
Phosphorus	Helps build bones and teeth Helps cells release energy from nutrients	Milk products, meat, fish, poultry, eggs, nuts, dried peas and beans
Zinc	Helps body grow and mature Helps body heal wounds and fight infections Needed for normal taste sensations	Seafood, meat, dried peas and beans, nuts

2-11 Minerals are part of bones, tissues, and body fluids. Rich sources of minerals should be included in meals and snacks.

Vitamins and Minerals of Concern in U.S. Diets

Most diseases caused by low intakes of vitamins and minerals are rare in the United States *Iron deficiency anemia* is a common disease caused by a low intake of a nutrient. Many people, especially children, teenagers, and adult women, suffer from anemia. These same people also tend to not get enough calcium, zinc, vitamin C, and folate. Sometimes, as in the case of sodium, too much of a nutrient can cause problems.

Iron

Most of the *iron* in your body is found in red blood cells. Its job is to carry oxygen to body cells and remove carbon dioxide. People with iron deficiency anemia do not get enough iron in their diets. They feel tired and run down because their cells aren't getting enough oxygen. It takes them longer to heal and fight infections.

Iron is supplied by foods of animal origin, such as meat, fish, and chicken. It also is supplied by foods of plant origin, such as breads, cereals, and dark green vegetables, 2-12. Your body absorbs more iron from animal sources than from plant sources. More iron is absorbed from plant sources if you eat these foods with meat and foods rich in vitamin C.

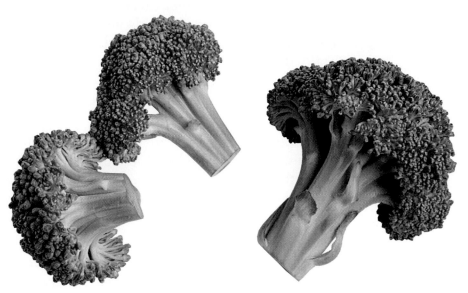

Mann Packing Company, Inc., Salinas, CA

2-12 Broccoli is a dark green vegetable. Spinach, collard greens, and kale are other dark green vegetables.

Calcium

Calcium is needed to build bones and teeth. It also is needed to transmit nerve signals and contract muscles. A diet low in calcium may lead to a painful disease called *osteoporosis*. This disease causes bones to wear away, become brittle, and break easily. Just getting out of bed or being hugged can result in broken bones. Osteoporosis takes years to develop. It cannot be cured, but you can prevent it by eating a calcium-rich diet and exercising throughout your life. This will help keep your bones strong and not let them wear away.

The best sources of calcium are milk, cheese, yogurt, and other milk products. Fish with tiny bones you can eat, such as sardines, are rich sources, too. Dark green vegetables, like spinach and broccoli, also provide some calcium.

Zinc

Zinc is a mineral needed for normal body growth and repair. Too little zinc in the diet causes stunted growth. It also delays the teenage growth spurt. Wounds heal slowly and the sense of taste is lost when zinc is lacking in the diet. The best sources of zinc are seafood and meat. Cereals and dry peas and beans supply some zinc, too.

Vitamin C

Most people have heard the claim that vitamin C helps prevent or cure the common cold. Unfortunately, scientific experiments show that vitamin C has no proven effect on the common cold. Don't give up your orange juice, though. *Vitamin C* is a vital part of several body compounds. It helps your body heal wounds and keeps your gums healthy.

Vitamin C is found mainly in fruits and vegetables. Citrus fruits, such as oranges, grapefruit, and lemons are rich sources of vitamin C. Berries and melons are other fruits rich in vitamin C. Vegetables high in vitamin C include peppers, tomatoes, cabbage, and dark green vegetables.

Folate

Folate is a B-vitamin that is used to build strong, healthy blood. Folate also is needed to fight infections. Normal growth cannot occur if folate intake is low. Too little folate in your diet can cause you to feel tired and run down. Breads, cereals, bananas, oranges, beans, and dark green vegetables are rich sources of folate.

Sodium

Sodium is a mineral that performs many vital functions. For example, sodium maintains the body's water balance. It also helps muscles to relax and nerves to transmit messages to the brain. Having enough sodium in the diet is important, but too much may cause the pressure inside your blood vessels to rise dangerously high. Many Americans tend to get too much sodium.

The main source of sodium in your diet is salt, 2-13. Sodium combines with another mineral called chloride to make salt. So, any time you sprinkle salt on your food, you increase your sodium intake. Sodium occurs naturally in some foods and is added to others. Foods with the most sodium added to them are pickled foods, processed meats like ham and bologna, snack foods, and canned vegetables. Seasonings such as soy sauce, garlic salt, and onion salt also are packed with sodium. You can reduce the sodium in your diet by eating less of these foods.

2-13 Table salt is made of two minerals: sodium and chloride.

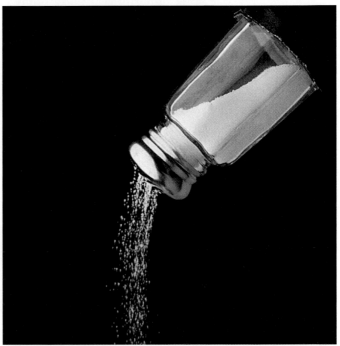

USDA

Supplements and You

Eating a nutritious diet can provide all the nutrients in the amounts most people need for good health. Usually, only people who are sick, injured, or known to have a nutrient deficiency need *nutrient supplements*. Women who are expecting a baby also need supplements. Older adults may need a supplement, too. Many people who take nutrient supplements often do not need to take them.

If you are thinking about taking a nutrient supplement, keep in mind that they are not a shortcut to good health and nutrition. No supplement can counteract a poor diet. Nutrient supplements can be costly, too. Foods usually cost less than supplements. Foods provide more nutrients that your body absorbs better than those in supplements. Foods taste better, too.

Overdosing on vitamins and minerals in food is highly unlikely. However, large doses of supplements can be wasteful and dangerous. For instance, large doses of water-soluble vitamins will be lost in your urine. Large doses of fat-soluble vitamins and certain minerals can build up, damage your body, or even kill you. You can overdose on supplements.

If you think you need a nutrient supplement, check with your doctor first, 2-14. Discuss your diet and nutrient concerns. Ask your doctor to refer you to a dietitian. A ***dietitian*** is an expert in nutrition and can help you choose a supplement that is right for you. The safest choice usually is a multi-vitamin and mineral supplement that contains no more than 100 percent of your daily need. If supplements are needed, be sure to follow the directions on the label and take them with food.

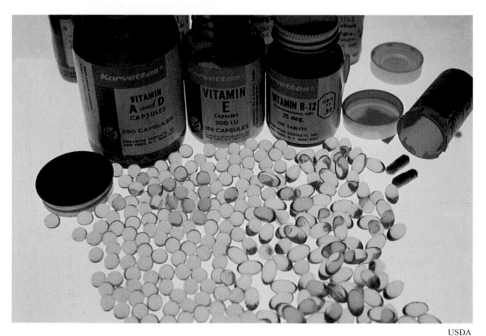

USDA

2-14 Many nutrient supplements are available. Talk to your doctor before deciding to use supplements.

Are You Getting All the Nutrients You Need?

How can you tell if you are getting enough nutrients from the foods you eat? Nutrition experts have developed tools that can help you discover the answer to that question. One tool is the ***Dietary Reference Intakes (DRIs)***. The DRIs are a set of guidelines for the amounts of many nutrients needed daily. There are many categories of DRIs, based on age and gender. The DRIs for teens are shown in 2-15.

Dietary Reference Intakes for Teens								
	Vitamin A μg*	Vitamin C mg†	Vitamin B_6 mg	Folate μg	Vitamin B_{12} mg	Calcium mg	Iron mg	Zinc mg
Females								
Ages 9-13	600	45	1.0	300	1.8	1,300	8	8
Ages 14-18	700	65	1.2	400	2.4	1,300	15	9
Males								
Ages 9-13	600	45	1.0	300	1.8	1,300	8	8
Ages 14-18	900	75	1.3	400	2.4	1,300	11	11
* 1 μg (microgram) is equal to one-millionth (⅟1,000,000) of a gram.								
† 1 mg (milligram) is equal to one-thousandth (⅟1000) of a gram.								

2-15 To make sure you are getting all the nutrients you need, it is important to meet the DRIs for your sex and age group.

To determine the amount of each nutrient you eat, you can read the nutrition labels on food packages or use the Food Composition Table in the Appendix of this text. The next chapter will tell you about two other very useful tools that can help you be sure your diet is nutritious. These tools are the Food Guide Pyramid and the Dietary Guidelines.

Science in the Kitchen

A Journey Through Your Digestive Tract

It's lunchtime and your stomach is growling. You are about to send your lunch on a trip. Every food you eat or drink travels through your digestive tract. Its journey takes it through a hollow tube that twists and turns for about 30 feet. Each bite is propelled from start to finish by gentle muscle contractions. Look at the illustration and match the numbers with the following descriptions of highlights of the journey:

1. Digestion starts in the mouth. As you chew, food is ground into smaller pieces and mixed with saliva. Chewing softens and moistens food.

2. When you swallow a bite of food, it travels through the esophagus (ee-SOF-uh-gus) and arrives at the stomach.

3. Food makes a stop in the stomach for about three hours. Here it is blended with digestive juices secreted by the stomach. When the food leaves, it has become a thick, smooth liquid called chyme (kime).

4. The journey continues as the chyme passes into the small intestine. In fact, this is the main feature of the trip. Most of the digestive process occurs here. The small intestine is a tube that is about 18 feet long and ¾-inch wide. A tiny duct connects it to the liver and pancreas. This duct delivers digestive juices to the small intestine. These juices mix with other digestive juices from the small intestine and the chyme. These juices separate the nutrients from the food particles. The nutrients are so small they can pass through the wall of the digestive tract into your blood. Once in your blood, the nutrients can be delivered to every cell in your body.

5. After the nutrients are absorbed, only water and undigested waste, such as fiber, remain. These travel on to the large intestine, which is a little wider and shorter than the small intestine. Here, most of the remaining water is removed from the waste and absorbed into the blood. At the end of the large intestine, the remaining waste passes out of the body through the anus. The amazing journey through your digestive tract has come to an end.

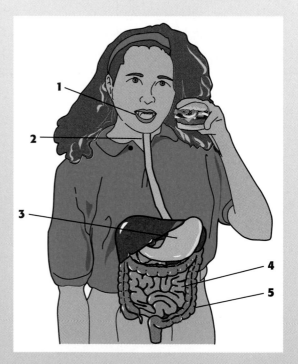

Every time you eat or drink something, you send it on a journey through your digestive tract.

In a Nutshell

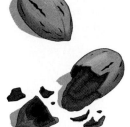

- A calorie is a measure of the energy value of food.
- Nutrients are chemical substances found in food that are used for growth, repair, and energy.
- The six classes of nutrients are carbohydrates, fats, proteins, water, vitamins, and minerals.
- All nutrients must be present in the right amounts for you to grow normally and stay healthy.
- Sugar, starch, and fiber are the three types of carbohydrates.
- The main function of fats is to supply calories.
- Proteins are needed for growth and repair of the body.
- You need eight cups or more of water every day to replace water lost in urine, sweat, and the air you exhale.
- Vitamins and minerals keep the body working normally and are used to help it grow and repair itself.

In the Know

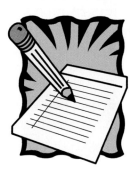

1. List three ways your body burns calories.
2. Name the three nutrients that provide calories.
3. _____ is a type of carbohydrate that keeps your digestive system working well.
4. True or false? Each gram of saturated fat provides more calories than unsaturated fat.
5. Which food does not contain cholesterol?
   A. Hamburger.
   B . Cheese.
   C. Peas.
   D. Bacon.
6. True or false? Proteins not needed for growth and repair are stored as muscle.
7. Which is a function of water?
   A. Lubricates your joints.
   B. Cools you down.
   C. Keeps your skin soft and elastic.
   D. All of the above are functions of water.
8. Name the five nutrients that are often low in the diets of teenagers.
9. True or false? Nutrient supplements can make up for a poor diet.

What Would You Do?

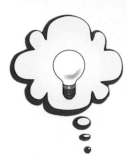

Your friend said, "I feel tired and run down. I plan to start taking six different vitamin and mineral supplements soon." Do you think this a good idea? What would you do if you were your friend? What advice would you give your friend?

Expanding Your Knowledge

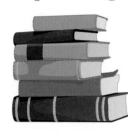

1. Make a bulletin board that describes sources of each nutrient. Use drawings or magazine pictures to illustrate the bulletin board.
2. Interview an expert on water from your community's health department. Ask the expert to describe how the water supply is kept clean. Find out if anything is added to the water supply. Also ask if any minerals are found in the local water supply.
3. Write 10 questions that could be used as a quiz for this chapter. Record the answers on a separate sheet of paper. Exchange quizzes with a classmate and answer the questions. Review the answers with your classmate.
4. Research a vitamin in your library. Write a skit that describes how the vitamin was discovered. Also include the function and sources of the vitamin. Perform your skit for younger children.
5. Clip an article on nutrition from the newspaper. Read it and report on it to your class.
6. Carbohydrates are the main source of energy around the world. Wheat is the main carbohydrate eaten in the U.S. In Asia, rice is the main carbohydrate. Find out which carbohydrates are eaten in other parts of the world. Report your findings to your class.
7. Make a set of nutrient flash cards. Write the nutrient's name on the front of the card. On the back, list its functions and some sources. Use the flash cards with a classmate.
8. Brainstorm ways to increase calcium and iron intake. Make a poster that lists your ideas. Display the poster in the school cafeteria.

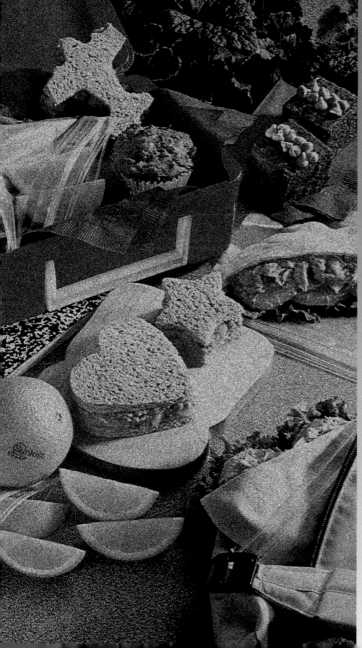

Chapter 3

Your Nutrition Toolbox

Objectives

After reading this chapter, you will be able to
- ☐ describe the Food Guide Pyramid.
- ☐ name the food groups and the nutrients they contain.
- ☐ list the Dietary Guidelines for Americans and describe how you can use them to improve your diet.
- ☐ rate your diet using the Food Guide Pyramid and the Dietary Guidelines for Americans.
- ☐ plan meals using the Food Guide Pyramid and the Dietary Guidelines for Americans.

New Terms

Food Guide Pyramid: an outline of the foods and amounts you should eat each day for a nutritious diet and good health.
Dietary Guidelines for Americans: a set of statements that can help you choose a nutritious diet.

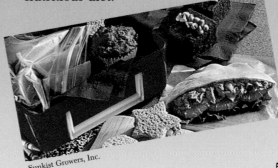

Sunkist Growers, Inc.

There are so many food choices. Which choices are best? Which will help you stay healthy? Should you select chicken nuggets and a creamy milk shake? Would crunchy celery and tangy yogurt be better choices? The Food Guide Pyramid and Dietary Guidelines for Americans are the tools you need to answer these questions. With them, you can build the most nutritious diet possible. These tools are the best, most current advice from nutrition experts.

The Food Guide Pyramid

The *Food Guide Pyramid* outlines what you should eat every day. It can help you decide what and how much to eat of each type of food. The Pyramid was developed by the United States Department of Agriculture (USDA) to help people plan nutritious diets, 3-1.

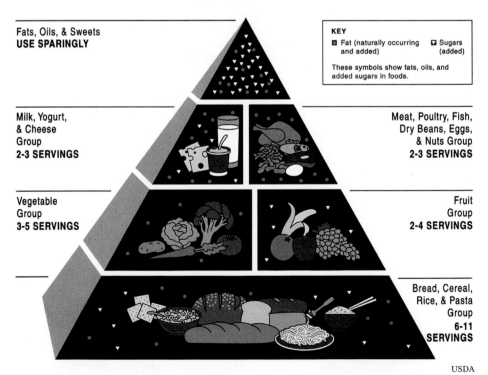

Food Guide Pyramid
A Guide to Daily Food Choices

Fats, Oils, & Sweets
USE SPARINGLY

KEY
▪ Fat (naturally occurring and added)   ☑ Sugars (added)
These symbols show fats, oils, and added sugars in foods.

Milk, Yogurt, & Cheese Group
2-3 SERVINGS

Meat, Poultry, Fish, Dry Beans, Eggs, & Nuts Group
2-3 SERVINGS

Vegetable Group
3-5 SERVINGS

Fruit Group
2-4 SERVINGS

Bread, Cereal, Rice, & Pasta Group
6-11 SERVINGS

USDA

3-1 To meet your nutrient needs, eat the recommended number of servings from each group in the Food Guide Pyramid.

As you can see, the Pyramid divides foods into six groups. The five food groups shown in the three lower sections of the Pyramid are called the *major food groups*. The foods in these groups are vital for good health. Some of the foods found in each of the groups are listed in 3-2.

Each of the major groups contains some, but not all, of the nutrients you need. You need to choose several different foods from each major food group daily. The fats, oils, and sweets group is in the small tip of the Pyramid. It is not a major food group. A nutritious diet contains mostly foods from the five major food groups and only small amounts from the Pyramid's tip.

All foods are included in the Pyramid. None are left out. That's because any food can be part of a nutritious diet. Some people think they should never have a candy bar or a soft drink. Of course, the best foods for you are in the major food groups. There is nothing wrong with eating sweets once in a while. However, if sweets add excess calories or replace more nutritious foods, your diet may be headed for trouble.

Bread, Cereal, Rice, and Pasta Group

Foods made from grains are at the base of the Pyramid. Some common grains are wheat, rice, barley, oats, rye, and corn. Grains are used to make breads such as rye bread, corn bread, biscuits, bagels, muffins, and crackers, 3-3. Grains also are used to make ready-to-eat breakfast cereals, noodles, and pasta. These foods are good sources of protein, starch, fiber, thiamin, riboflavin, niacin, folate, and iron.

Cakes, cookies, pastries, and many other desserts are made from grains, too. These foods have more calories, fat, and sugar and less fiber, vitamins, and minerals than the other foods in this group. The most nutritious diets limit the number of grain products that have added fat or sugar.

The best choices from the grains group are made from whole grains. Whole wheat bread, oatmeal, corn tortillas, popcorn, brown rice, and whole wheat pasta are examples. Foods made from whole grains have the greatest variety of nutrients and more fiber than other foods in this group.

Food Groups: Some Foods They Contain

Bread, Cereal, Rice, and Pasta Group

Whole Grain			Enriched		
Brown rice	Oatmeal	Whole wheat	Bagels	Farina	Noodles
Buckwheat	Popcorn	bread and rolls	Biscuits	French bread	Pancakes
Bulgur	Pumpernickel	Whole wheat	Corn bread	Grits	Pasta
Corn tortillas	bread	crackers	Corn muffins	Hamburger rolls	Ready-to-eat
Graham crackers	Ready-to-eat	Whole wheat	Cornmeal	Hot dog buns	cereals
Granola	cereals	Whole wheat	Crackers	Italian bread	Rice
Rye bread	Rye crackers	cereals	English muffins	Muffins	White bread

Vegetables Group

Dark Green			Deep Yellow	Starchy	
Beet greens	Dandelion	Mustard greens	Carrots	Breadfruit	Lima beans
Broccoli	greens	Romaine lettuce	Pumpkin	Corn	Potatoes
Chard	Endive	Spinach	Sweet potatoes	Green peas	Rutabaga
Chicory	Escarole	Turnip greens	Winter squash	Hominy	Taro
Collard greens	Kale	Watercress			

Other Vegetables					
Artichokes	Brussels sprouts	Chinese	Green beans	Okra	Tomatoes
Asparagus	Cabbage	cabbage	Green peppers	Onions	Turnips
Bean and alfal-	Cauliflower	Cucumbers	Lettuce	Radishes	Vegetable juices
fa sprouts	Celery	Eggplant	Mushrooms	Summer squash	Zucchini

Fruits Group

Citrus, Melons, Berries		Deep Yellow		Other Fruits	
Blueberries	Lemons	Apricots	Apples	Fruit juice	Plantains
Blackberries	Oranges	Cantaloupes	Bananas	Grapes	Plums
Citrus juices	Raspberries	Mangoes	Cherries	Guava	Pomegranates
Cranberries	Strawberries	Nectarines	Dates	Pears	Prunes
Honeydew	Watermelons	Papayas	Figs	Pineapples	Raisins
Kiwifruit		Peaches			

Milk, Yogurt, and Cheese Group

Lowfat Milk Products		Milk Products with More Fat or Added Sugar			
Buttermilk	Lowfat yogurt	American	Chocolate milk	Ice cream	Pudding
Lowfat milk	Part skim cheese	cheese	Frozen yogurt	Milk shakes	Swiss cheese
(1% and 2%)	Fat free milk	Cheddar cheese	Fruit yogurt	Process cheese	Whole milk

Meat, Poultry, Fish, Dry Beans, Eggs, and Nuts Group

Foods of Animal Origin		Foods of Plant Origin			
Beef	Lamb	Almonds	Kidney beans	Nuts	Sunflower
Chicken	Pork	Black beans	Lentils	Peanut butter	seeds
Eggs	Shrimp	Black-eyed peas	Lima beans	Pecans	Split peas
Fish	Turkey	Chickpeas (gar-	Mung beans	Pinto beans	Tofu
Ham	Veal	banzo beans)	Navy beans	Sesame seeds	Walnuts

Fats, Oils, and Sweets Group

Fats and Oils			Sweets		
Bacon, salt pork	Lard	Salad dressing	Candy	Honey	Molasses
Bologna	Luncheon meats	Shortening	Corn syrup	Jam	Ices
Butter	Margarine	Sour cream	Fruit drinks,	Jelly	Sherbets
Cream	Mayonnaise	Vegetable oil	ades, and	Maple syrup	Soft drinks
Cream cheese	Potato chips		punches	Marmalade	Sugar

3-2 These are examples of some foods within each group of the Food Guide Pyramid.

3-3 The grains group is a rich source of starch, fiber, B-vitamins, and iron.

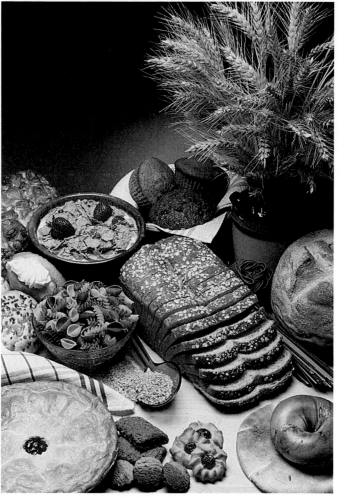

USDA

Vegetable Group

The vegetable group is on the second level of the Pyramid. Broccoli, potatoes, carrots, and peas, are just a few of the many colorful, tasty, and nutritious choices. These foods are rich sources of vitamins, such as vitamins A and C and folate. They also provide fiber and minerals, such as iron and magnesium. They are low in fat and calories, too.

It's a good idea to eat a wide variety of vegetables. That's because different types of vegetables are rich in different nutrients. For example, starchy vegetables like corn provide B-vitamins and protein. Peppers, tomatoes, and cabbage are rich in vitamin C. Other vegetables, such as beets and onions, provide small amounts of a variety of nutrients.

The color of some vegetables gives you a clue to their nutrient content. For instance, dark green vegetables are rich in iron, calcium, folate, and vitamins A and C. Collards, broccoli, spinach, and kale are dark green vegetables. Vegetables with deep yellow or orange flesh are rich in vitamin A. Carrots and sweet potatoes and some varieties of squash all have deep yellow or orange flesh and are packed with vitamin A.

Fresh or plain frozen vegetables top the list of good vegetable choices. Canned vegetables tend to be high in sodium. Vegetables in sauce often are high in sodium and fat.

Fruit Group

The fruit group is also on the second level of the Food Guide Pyramid. Cherries, bananas, and pineapple are just a few of the delicious and nutritious choices in this group. This group provides Vitamins A and C and potassium. Fruits are low in fat and sodium and provide fiber in the diet. Because different types of fruits contain different nutrients, it's a good idea to eat a wide variety of them.

3-4 Choose fruit juices that are 100 percent fruit juice.

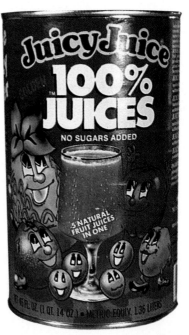

USDA

For instance, citrus fruits, melons, and berries are rich in vitamin C. Other fruits, such as pears and apples, provide small amounts of several nutrients.

Just as in vegetables, the color of some fruits gives you a clue to their nutrient content. For example, fruits with deep yellow or orange flesh are rich in vitamin A. Cantaloupe and apricots all have deep yellow or orange flesh and are rich sources of vitamin A.

Fresh fruit, plain frozen, and fruit canned in water or juice are the best fruit choices. Fruits canned or frozen in syrup contain added sugar.

To get the most nutrients, choose 100 percent fruit juice. Punches, ades, and most fruit drinks contain little or no juice and lots of added sugar. Grape and orange sodas do not belong to the fruit group. They are in the fats, oils, and sweets group, 3-4.

Milk, Yogurt, and Cheese Group

As you can tell by the name of this group, milk, yogurt, and cheese are the main foods in it, 3-5. The milk group also contains milk desserts, such as pudding, ice cream, and milk shakes. All the

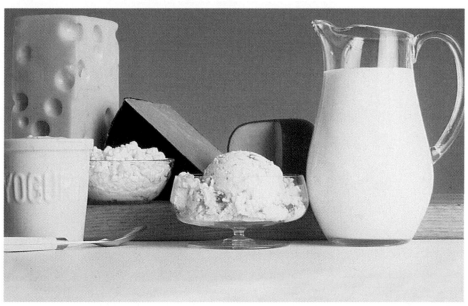

USDA

3-5 Milk and milk products are rich sources of protein, calcium, and vitamin D.

foods in this group are rich sources of protein and calcium. Many provide vitamin D, too. However, many contain large amounts of fat and cholesterol. Chocolate milk and milk desserts also contain large amounts of sugar.

It is smart to usually choose lowfat or nonfat milk products like fat free milk, part skim cheese, lowfat cottage cheese, and nonfat frozen yogurt. These foods contain all the nutrients found in other milk products except they have much less fat and cholesterol. When choosing foods from the milk group, it's also smart to go easy on milk desserts and chocolate milk because of the added sugar.

Meat, Poultry, Fish, Dry Beans, Eggs, and Nuts Group

All the foods in the meat and beans group supply protein, B-vitamins, iron, and zinc. Except for beans, most of the foods in this group contain large amounts of fat, 3-6. Keep in mind that all the foods from animals contain cholesterol. Egg yolks are high in cholesterol.

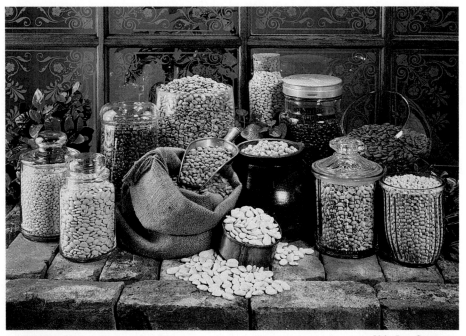

Idaho Bean Commission

3-6 Dry beans are a good source of protein. They contain no cholesterol and less fat than other foods in the meat and beans group.

When choosing foods from the meat and beans group, try to select fish, lean meat, poultry without skin, and dry beans. These foods are lower in fat and cholesterol than other choices in this group. You also can reduce fat and cholesterol intake by trimming away any fat you can see and by not frying these foods. To keep your cholesterol intake under control, experts suggest eating no more than four egg yolks each week.

Fats, Oils, and Sweets Group

Tan dots and white triangles fill the small tip of the Food Guide Pyramid. The dots stand for fats and oils, and the triangles stand for sugars added to foods. Salad dressings, vegetable oil, cream, butter, and margarine are fats and oils, 3-7. Items such as potato chips, bologna, and bacon are counted as fats, too. That's because most of their calories come from fat. Sugars, jams, jellies, soft drinks, candies, and desserts are called sweets.

3-7 For good health, it's best to keep your intake of fats and oils low.

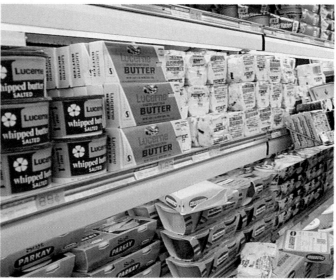

USDA

You may have noticed that dots and triangles also appear in the major food groups. They remind you that some foods in the major food groups also can be high in fat and sugar. For instance, ice cream and fruit canned in syrup are foods from the major groups that are high in sugar. Potato salad, crackers, peanut butter, and cheese are foods from the major groups that contain a great deal of fat.

The foods in the fats, oils, and sweets group provide mostly calories, fat, and sugar, 3-8. They contain limited amounts of other nutrients. Eating too many of the foods in this group makes it easy to get too many calories and gain excess weight. These foods fill you up and may keep you from eating more nutritious foods.

3-8 Sweets add calories and limited amounts of nutrients.

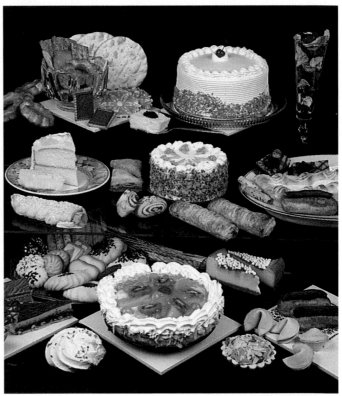

How Many Servings Do You Need? _____

The Pyramid shows a range of servings for each food group. See 3-1. The number of servings you need depends on your age, gender, and activity level. Almost everyone should eat at least the lowest number of servings in the ranges. If you eat less, it is very hard to get the calories and nutrients you need. Teen males should aim for the upper ends of the ranges. Most teen females need to aim for the middle of each range. Many teens and adults in the United States eat too few servings from the milk, fruit, and vegetable groups. They also eat too many servings from the meat and beans group and the fats, oils, and sweets group.

As you can see in 3-1, you need more servings from the grains group than any other. Six to 11 servings daily may sound like a lot, but it really is not. The menu in 3-9 is an example of how easy it is to get all the servings you need. A bowl of cereal and a slice of toast for breakfast are two servings. Two tortillas for lunch add two more servings. A cup of rice or pasta for dinner equals two more servings. A snack of four small crackers or a dish of popcorn adds yet another serving. See how quickly it adds up? This menu has seven servings from the grains group. Add another sandwich, slice of toast, and snack of crackers and you will be up to 11 servings.

Menu	
Breakfast	**Dinner**
1 ounce cereal	1 cup rice or pasta
1 slice toast	3 ounces tuna
1 teaspoon jam	6 sweet red pepper rings
¾ cup orange juice	1 small spinach salad
1 cup milk	1 tablespoon salad dressing
Lunch	1 cup cold water
2 tortillas	**Snack**
¼ cup chopped tomato	4 small crackers or a bowl of popcorn
¼ cup lettuce	1 cup yogurt topped with a sliced banana
1½ cups beans	
2 ounces cheese	
1 cup iced tea	

3-9 This sample menu shows how you can include foods from the various groups in your diet.

You need three to five servings each day from the vegetable group. Take another look at the menu in 3-9. Notice there are three servings of vegetables. The tomatoes and lettuce served for lunch equal one serving. Add the spinach salad and sweet red pepper rings and you've got three servings. To reach a total of five servings, just make the spinach salad larger and add some carrot sticks.

The menu in 3-9 also shows how you can fit two to four servings of the fruit group into your diet. Orange juice for breakfast is one serving. A banana at snack time adds a second serving. Serve a wedge of cantaloupe for lunch and peach slices for dinner and you have four servings.

Children and teens ages 9 to 18 and adults over age 50 need three daily servings from the milk group. People in other age groups need two servings daily. The menu in 3-9 shows how you can get the servings you need to supply calcium for your growing bones. The milk for breakfast, cheese for lunch, and yogurt at snack time equal three servings.

It is very easy to meet or exceed the servings you need from the meat and beans group. Notice in 3-9 that the beans served for lunch and the tuna at dinner equal two servings. To reach three servings, eat more beans or tuna or add two eggs at breakfast.

There is no suggested number of servings for the fats, oils, and sweets group. That is because these foods are "extras." If you eat the servings you need from the major food groups and still need more calories, it is fine to choose foods from this group. If not, limit the foods from this group that you eat. The jam and salad dressing listed in 3-9 are from this food group.

What Counts as One Serving?

The amount of food that counts as one serving is listed in 3-10. If you eat a larger portion, count it as more than one serving. For instance, if you eat one cup of rice, count it as two servings. If you eat a smaller portion, count it as part of a serving. For example, if you eat half an orange, count it as half a serving. Estimating the amount of food you eat can be tricky. The tips in 3-10 can help you more accurately make these estimates.

What Counts as One Serving?
Breads, Cereals, Rice, and Pasta
1 slice of bread
1 ounce of ready-to-eat cereal
½ cup of cooked cereal, rice, or pasta
Vegetables
1 cup of raw leafy vegetables
½ cup of other vegetables, cooked or chopped raw
¾ cup of vegetable juice
Fruits
1 medium apple, banana, orange
½ cup of chopped, cooked, or canned fruit
¾ cup of fruit juice
Milk, Yogurt, and Cheese
1 cup of milk or yogurt
1½ ounces of natural cheese
2 ounces of process cheese
Meat, Poultry, Fish, Dry Beans, Eggs, and Nuts
2-3 ounces of cooked lean meat, poultry, or fish
½ cup of cooked dry beans, 1 egg, or 2 tablespoons of peanut butter count as 1 ounce of lean meat
Tips for Estimating Serving Sizes
A thumb = 1 ounce of cheese
A thumb tip = 1 teaspoon
A fist = 1 cup
A handful = 1 or 2 ounces of a snack food
A deck of cards = 3 ounces

3-10 These are typical serving sizes from the Food Guide Pyramid groups.

You might wonder what to do with foods like pizza, tacos, and sandwiches. These foods are made from a mixture of other foods. They can count as a serving from more than one food group, 3-11. For instance, each slice of bread in a sandwich counts as a serving from the grains group. A sandwich made with meat or peanut butter provides a serving from the meat and beans group, too. The crust from a pizza slice provides a serving from the grains group. Its cheese topping counts as a serving from the milk group. Tomato sauce, onions, and pepper toppings are from the vegetable group. Beef stew is another example. It provides a serving from both the meat and beans and vegetable groups. What are some other foods like these that provide servings from more than one food group?

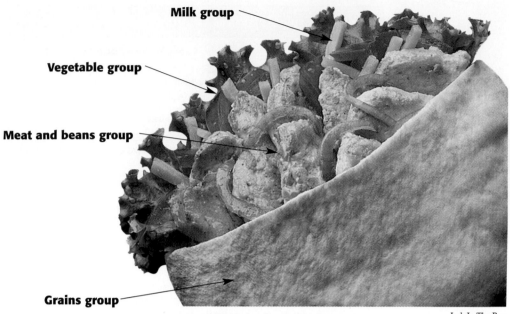

Milk group

Vegetable group

Meat and beans group

Grains group

Jack In The Box

3-11 Foods made from a mixture of other foods don't fit into just one food group. They can be divided among the food groups.

The Dietary Guidelines for Americans

The ***Dietary Guidelines for Americans*** is a set of statements that can help you choose a nutritious diet and healthful lifestyle, 3-12. A nutritious diet and healthful lifestyle can help you maintain or even improve your health. The three basic messages of the Dietary Guidelines are

- Aim for fitness.
- Build a healthy base.
- Choose sensibly.

By following the Dietary Guidelines, you can promote your health and reduce your risk for disease. The diets of many people in the United States have too many calories and too much fat, cholesterol, sugar, and salt. Many U.S. diets also contain too few grains, fruits, and vegetables. These diets are one reason so many people in the United States have too much body fat and face diet-related diseases. Tooth decay, heart disease, high blood pressure, diabetes, and some forms of cancer are known to be diet-related.

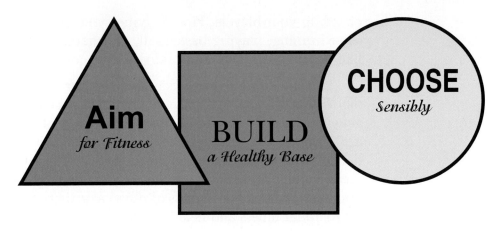

...*for good health*

3-12 You can build a nutritious diet and healthful lifestyle by following the Dietary Guidelines for Americans.

By reviewing the Dietary Guidelines, you will find out why nutrition experts give this advice. You will also discover how to use the Guidelines to select a nutritious diet.

Aim for Fitness

The first key message of the Dietary Guidelines is *aim for fitness.* Two guidelines can help you follow this advice.

Aim for a healthy weight. The goal of this guideline is to achieve a healthy weight that is just right for you. This means you do not weigh too much or too little for your age and height. Both of these conditions are linked with risks of serious health problems and can even shorten your life. For instance, having too much body fat can lead to diseases like heart disease, diabetes, and certain cancers. Weighing too little can damage bones and lead to nutrient deficiencies. Your doctor, school nurse, or a dietitian can help you determine if your weight is healthy.

Be physically active each day. The goal of the second Dietary Guideline is to move your body. Being physically active can help you use the calories you get from food so you can maintain or improve your weight. Choose activities you enjoy, such as skating or riding your bicycle. Find activities you can do with friends, such as swimming, playing basketball, and dancing. Even doing chores like mowing the lawn and raking leaves count as physical activity.

You should try to be physically active for at least 60 minutes each day. However, you don't have to do all your activity at one time. Your activities can add up throughout the day. For instance, you might take a 10-minute walk to a friend's house in the morning. You could spend half an hour playing tennis in the afternoon. You might spend 20 minutes cleaning your room before you go to bed. By the end of the day, you have built up 60 minutes of physical activity. You will be reading more about fitness and healthy weight in the next chapter.

Build a Healthy Base

The second basic message of the Dietary Guidelines is *build a healthy base*. Following four guidelines can help you meet this goal.

Let the Pyramid guide your food choices. This guideline reminds you that any food can be part of a nutritious diet. The key is to choose a variety of foods every day and eat each food in moderation. The Pyramid can help you get the variety and moderation you need. *Moderation* means not getting too little or too much of any one type of food. It means getting just the right amount. Eating too much or too little can be harmful.

You need more than 40 different nutrients to stay healthy and grow normally. Eating a variety of foods every day can help you get all the nutrients you need. Variety is important because no one food contains all the nutrients, but each food contains some. For instance, fruits and vegetables are rich sources of vitamins A and C, but they are low in protein. Foods in the meat and beans group are great sources of protein and iron, but they contain little calcium. Milk products have a lot of calcium, but they lack fiber. Breads and cereals have plenty of fiber but are low in vitamins A and C. As you can see, eating a variety of foods every day is the only way to get all the nutrients you need.

How can you be sure you are getting enough variety? Take a look at the list below. Think about how often you do each item on the list.

- Eat two or three types of foods from the grains group each day.
- Eat three kinds of vegetables daily.
- Eat a dark green vegetable every day or two.

- Eat two or more kinds of fruit or fruit juice each day.
- Eat two types of food from the milk group each day.
- Eat two types of food from the meat and beans group each day.

If you do each item on the list almost every day, you are doing fine. If you do them three times a week or less, your diet needs more variety. Using the Food Guide Pyramid as a guide can help you plan a diet that has the variety you need.

 ## Health Alert

Herbal Supplements: Healthful or Harmful?

Many people take nutrient supplements to help fill in nutrients that may be missing from their diets. In recent years, a growing number of people have started using another kind of supplement. Many people take herbal supplements to prevent or treat health conditions.

Researchers have found some herbal supplements are useful. However, others are a waste of money because they do not have health benefits. Still others are dangerous. They have caused hundreds of medical emergencies.

Herbs have been used for hundreds of years to treat aches and pains. Even so, health experts still do not know a lot about them. Scientists are busy studying herbal supplements and testing their safety. At this time, the government does not regulate herbal supplements. Therefore, if you decide to use them, it is important to keep these points in mind.

- Herbs may be natural, but natural does not mean the same thing as safe. For instance, the herb hemlock is natural and deadly.

- Some herbal supplements contain harmful bacteria or toxins.

- Herbal supplements can block the effects of medicines you are taking. Always be sure to tell your doctor about any herbal supplements you take.

- Amounts that are safe to take are not yet known for many herbal supplements.

- Herbal supplements may be fine to take for minor health problems. However, they should not be used to treat major problems like cancer or AIDS.

- Some people have adverse reactions to herbal preparations.

Choose a variety of grains daily, especially whole grains. This Dietary Guideline can help change the habits of people who overlook the wide range of foods in the grains group. These nutritious foods include much more than just bread and cereal. Tortillas, crackers, popcorn, bagels, biscuits, muffins, pasta, and rice are just some of the many foods that are part of this group. Following this guideline means choosing different types of products each day. It also means choosing foods made from different types of grains. Think about oatmeal pancakes for breakfast, corn tortillas for lunch, whole wheat crackers for a snack, and brown rice with dinner. These are all examples of foods made from whole grains. They contain more fiber and other important substances than enriched grain products.

Choose a variety of fruits and vegetables daily. Many people in the United States fail to follow this guideline. Fruits and vegetables provide vitamins, minerals, starch, and fiber. By eating more of these foods, you can reduce your chances of developing heart disease and certain cancers. The fiber in these foods helps keep your digestive system working well.

How can you be sure you are getting the variety of fruits and vegetables you need? To answer that question, name an example of each of the foods listed below. How often do you eat each of the examples you named?

- citrus fruits
- melons
- berries
- deep yellow fruits and vegetables
- dark green vegetables
- starchy vegetables
- other fruits and vegetables

If you eat several servings of these foods each day, you are on the right track. If not, you need to eat them more often. To increase your intake of these foods, try serving two or three of them at every meal. They make great snacks, too.

Keep food safe to eat. Following this guideline is vital to health. Foods that are not stored or prepared in a clean and safe manner can cause illness. Many people get sick each year from eating foods that contain harmful bacteria and other contaminants. You will learn much more about keeping food safe to eat in Chapter 9.

Choose Sensibly

The third key message of the Dietary Guidelines is *choose sensibly*. Three guidelines can help you achieve this goal.

Choose a diet that is low in saturated fat and cholesterol and moderate in total fat. A nutritious diet contains some fat. Many people in the United States eat far more total fat, saturated fat, and cholesterol than is healthful. High intakes of these substances can raise your risk of gaining excess body fat and developing certain types of cancer. High intakes can also cause the amount of cholesterol in your blood to be higher than normal. A high blood cholesterol level may damage your blood vessels and heart. It can put you in danger of having a heart attack or stroke when you are an adult.

You may think adulthood is such a long way off there is no need to worry about your diet now. However, the food choices you make now may increase your chances of developing serious diseases later. It is important to start eating a diet that meets this guideline today.

How can you tell if your diet is low in saturated fat and cholesterol and moderate in total fat? Look over the list of high-fat foods below. Think about how often you eat each one.

- fried and greasy foods
- bacon, sausage, luncheon meats, and fatty meats
- whole milk, ice cream, whipped cream, sour cream, and high-fat cheeses
- pies, cakes, and pastries
- sauces and gravies
- salad dressings and mayonnaise
- butter and margarine

If you eat fewer than four servings of these foods each week, you are doing great. Your intakes of saturated fat, cholesterol, and total fat probably are not too high. If you eat these foods more often, your intakes may be too high.

Careful food choices can help you reduce your intakes of saturated fat and cholesterol and moderate your intake of total fat. Here are some steps you can take to trim dietary fat.

- Eat the foods listed above less often or in smaller amounts.
- Use lemon juice or reduced fat dressing on salads.
- Choose lowfat or nonfat milk products, such as fat free milk or lowfat cheese.

- Trim fat off meat and remove skin from chicken, 3-13.
- Substitute dry peas and beans for meat, fish, and poultry.
- Eat lean meat, chicken, and fish and limit your intake to 6 ounces per day.
- Limit egg yolks to four per week.
- Serve fruit, fruit ices, and nonfat frozen yogurt for dessert.
- Snack on pretzels or air-popped popcorn instead of potato chips.

Some food manufacturers are selling products made with fat substitutes. *Fat substitutes* make foods moist and creamy without adding fat. Foods made with fat substitutes can help you reduce the fat and calories in your diet. However, these foods tend to cost more than similar foods that contain fat. It is not necessary to buy foods made with fat substitutes to eat a diet low in fat. You can lower your fat intake by following the steps listed in this section.

Choose beverages and foods to moderate your intake of sugars. Many people in the United States eat more sugar than is healthful. The average person eats about 142 pounds of sugar each year. At 15 calories per teaspoon, that adds up to over 600 calories from sugar each day, 3-14. In a year, that is more than 219,000 calories!

A diet high in sugar is likely to be missing vital nutrients or have too many calories. For instance, suppose you need 2,200 calories each day. If you spend 600 calories on sugar, you have only 1,600 calories left to pack in all the nutrients you need. If you eat the extra 600 calories on top of the 2,200, you will gain weight. An extra 600 calories a day can add up to a weight gain of 62 pounds a year!

Eating large amounts of sugary foods can cause tooth decay, too. The more often you eat sugary foods and the chewier the food, the more likely you are to have cavities. To learn more about sugar and tooth decay, see the *Science in the Kitchen: Sweet Tooth* feature in this chapter.

3-13 Reduce fat intake by trimming fat from meat. Too much fat in your diet can put you in danger of developing diet-related diseases.

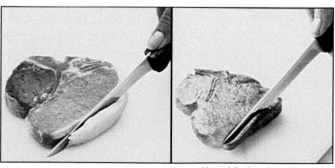

National Cattlemen's Beef Association

3-14 Sugar adds many calories to the diets of Americans.

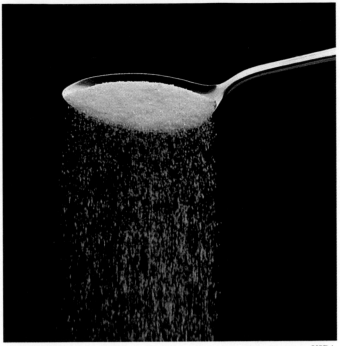

USDA

How can you tell if you eat too much sugar? The foods in the list below contain large amounts of sugar. As you examine the list, think about how often you eat each food.

- soft drinks, sweetened iced tea, fruit drinks, ades, and punches
- chocolate milk, ice cream, pudding, fruit-flavored yogurt, and frozen yogurt
- pies, cakes, cookies, candies, and other sweet desserts and snacks
- doughnuts and sweet rolls
- sugary breakfast cereals
- fruits canned or frozen in heavy syrup
- jam, jelly, and honey
- sugar added to tea, cereal, and other foods

The more often you eat any of these foods, the more sugar your diet will contain. You can control your sugar intake by cutting back on the foods listed above. Try reaching for fresh fruit or fruit canned in juice or water when you want a sweet snack or dessert. Fruits contain vitamins, minerals, and fiber. They also have fewer calories than sweet snacks and desserts.

Some people use sugar substitutes to help them cut down on sugar. Sugar substitutes sweeten foods without adding calories. *Aspartame* (AS-par-tame), *saccharin* (SACK-ah-rin), *acesulfame* K

Science in the Kitchen

Sweet Tooth

In the United States, nine million tons of sugar are sold each year. Most of it is used to prepare foods sold in supermarkets. Everyone knows sugar is added to jellies, syrups, soft drinks, cookies, and ice cream. You may be surprised to learn that some foods that do not even taste sweet have sugar added to them. For instance, sugar is added to bacon, bread, ketchup, and hamburger buns.

Cavities are one of the biggest problems caused by sugar. The bacteria that naturally live on your teeth get together with the food you eat to cause cavities. Every time you eat, some bits of food stick to your teeth. The bacteria feast on these bits and produce acid. This acid slowly eats away the hard enamel that covers your teeth. When the acid has worn a hole in a tooth, you have a cavity.

Acid + Tooth Enamel = Cavities

Sugar is the only food the bacteria can use. All sugars can cause cavities. A substance in your saliva can change starch into a type of sugar. Therefore, starch also can cause cavities, but not as easily as sugar can.

Whether or not you might get cavities depends on the answers to these questions.

- How much sugar and starch do you eat? If you eat lots of these (and they are not removed from your teeth), the bacteria in your mouth have plenty of food and can make large amounts of acid.

- How often do you eat sugar and starch? If you eat them often, the bacteria have many chances to make acid. Suppose you had 10 gum drops. You could eat them all at once or one every 20 minutes. By eating one every 20 minutes, the sticky candy is on your teeth more often than if you ate them all at once. The more often you eat sugar and starch, the more likely you are to have cavities.

- How sticky are the sugar and starch you eat? Soft or chewy foods that stick to your teeth are more likely to cause cavities than liquid or crunchy foods. That is because soft, sticky foods such as taffy and jelly beans stick to your teeth. They give bacteria more time to make acid than sugary liquids and crunchy foods such as popcorn. Sugary liquids, like soft drinks, pass through the mouth quickly. Crunchy foods do not stick to your teeth. These foods give the bacteria less time to form acid.

- How often do you brush and floss your teeth? Bacteria are removed when you brush and floss your teeth. If you brush and floss often, the bacteria you remove have less time to make acid. Plus, fewer bacteria remain in your mouth. Less time and fewer bacteria mean less acid, and less acid means fewer cavities.

An experiment with an eggshell and vinegar can show you how cavities form. Eggshells are made of some of the same substances as teeth. Vinegar is an acid like that produced by the bacteria on your teeth. Place an eggshell in a cup. Then, pour vinegar into the cup until the eggshell is covered. Cover the cup with plastic wrap. After three days, check the eggshell. How does it feel? What happens to teeth when they are exposed to acid?

(A-see-SULL-fame KAY), and *sucralose* (SOO-kra-lohs) are some of the sugar substitutes sold in the United States. They are used in over 1,500 foods, including chewing gum, pudding, diet soft drinks, and yogurt.

It is not necessary to use sugar substitutes to avoid eating too much sugar. You can reduce sugar intake by making the simple changes to your diet suggested above.

Choose and prepare foods with less salt. Many people in the United States include too much salt and sodium in their diets. This can cause some people to develop high blood pressure. High blood pressure stretches blood vessels much like air stretches a balloon. Over time, high blood pressure can damage blood vessels and the heart. It can also lead to a heart attack or stroke.

How can you know whether your diet contains too much salt and sodium? Read over the list below. All the foods in the list are high in salt and sodium. Think about how often you eat each food.

- ham, bacon, sausage, hot dogs, and luncheon meats
- canned vegetables and frozen vegetables in sauce
- foods made from packaged mixes
- sauces and gravies
- frozen dinners
- canned and dried soups
- salted nuts, popcorn, pretzels, corn chips, and potato chips
- pickles and olives
- soy sauce, steak sauce, salad dressing, catsup, and mustard

The more often you eat any of these foods, the more salt and sodium your diet will contain. If you eat more than four servings from this list weekly, your diet may contain more salt and sodium than is healthful. To cut back on salt and sodium, eat the foods listed above less often. Substitute fresh or plain frozen vegetables for canned vegetables or those served in a sauce. Also, avoid adding salt to foods or reduce the amount you add.

Some people choose *salt substitutes* to help them reduce their sodium intake. Many salt substitutes contain the mineral potassium instead of sodium. Check with your doctor before using salt substitutes that contain potassium. Some salt substitutes are a blend of herbs and spices. They add flavor to foods without adding sodium or potassium. They are safe to use anytime.

It is not necessary to use salt substitutes to lower the salt and sodium in your diet. You can reduce your salt and sodium intake by making the changes suggested above.

In a Nutshell

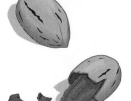

- The Food Guide Pyramid is an outline of the types and amounts of foods you should eat every day.
- The five major food groups are grains, vegetables, fruits, milk, and meat and beans.
- The grains group is a rich source of starch, fiber, thiamin, riboflavin, niacin, folate, and iron.
- The vegetable group and the fruit group provide fiber, vitamin A, vitamin C, folate, iron, calcium, and other vitamins and minerals.
- The milk group provides calcium, vitamin D, and protein.
- The meat and beans group supplies protein, B-vitamins, iron, and zinc.
- The number of servings you need from each of the food groups depends on your age, gender, and activity level.
- The Dietary Guidelines for Americans can help you choose a nutritious diet and healthful lifestyle.
- The Dietary Guidelines have three basic points: Aim for fitness, Build a healthy base, and Choose sensibly.
- Many people in the United States eat too many calories and too much fat, cholesterol, sugar, and sodium.
- Many people in the United States eat too few grains, fruits, and vegetables.

In the Know

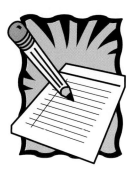

1. Draw the Food Guide Pyramid. Label each food group and list the range of servings suggested.
2. Which food is not found in the meat and beans group?
   A. Eggs.
   B. Tuna.
   C. Kidney beans.
   D. Bologna.
3. True or false? Some foods cannot be part of a nutritious diet.
4. A diet that contains few servings from the fruit and vegetable groups probably is low in _____.
   A. B-vitamins and fiber
   B. protein and calcium
   C. vitamin C and folate
   D. iron and sodium

5. Plan menus for one day that include all the food groups. The menus should have at least the lowest number of servings in the ranges for all five major food groups.
6. Explain why a high blood cholesterol level may be dangerous.
7. List four tips for decreasing the total fat, saturated fat, and cholesterol in your diet.
8. True or false? The only way to avoid having too much sugar in your diet is to use sugar substitutes.

What Would You Do?

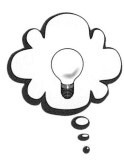

Suppose you are a newspaper columnist and you receive a letter with this comment in it. "I think I am going to go on the 'All You Can Eat Peanut Butter Diet.' For every meal and snack, you eat only peanut butter and drink water. I really like peanut butter. This must be the diet for me." Do you think this is a good diet? Why or why not? Write a reply to this letter.

Expanding Your Knowledge

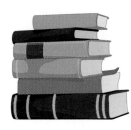

1. Assume you are a television news reporter and the Dietary Guidelines for Americans have just been released. Write and videotape a one-minute news story for the six o'clock news.
2. Take a milk poll. Find out which milk products the students in your class eat or drink. Which is the most popular milk product? How many students get three servings each day?
3. Produce a puppet show about the Food Guide Pyramid. Perform the puppet show for children in your neighborhood.
4. List all the foods you ate yesterday. Compare your list to the Pyramid. Did you get the recommended number of servings of all the major food groups? If not, how could you improve your diet?
5. Think about all the foods served in fast-food restaurants. Use the Pyramid and Dietary Guidelines to plan a fast-food meal. What foods would you need to eat at other meals to balance the meal?
6. Make a poster about one of the Dietary Guidelines for Americans. Explain why the Guideline is important and how teens can follow it. Display the poster in your classroom.

7. Create a display for your classroom that shows how much fat or sugar is in foods. Collect empty food packages. Use the Nutrition Facts panel on the packages to determine how much fat or sugar is in each food. Measure the equivalent of the amount of fat or sugar in each food. You can use ¼ teaspoon of vegetable shortening or margarine to represent about 1 gram of fat. Measure the fat onto small pieces of waxed paper. You can use a sugar cube to represent 2 grams of sugar. Place the fat or sugar cubes beside the food packages.

8. Show how much sugar is in soft drinks. Mix a 12-ounce bottle of seltzer water with 10 teaspoons of corn syrup or sugar. (Sugar won't dissolve as easily as corn syrup.) Add ¼ teaspoon of your favorite flavoring. Orange, lime, lemon, or grape flavorings make good choices. Then, add a few drops of food coloring. Did you know soft drinks contained so much sugar? How could you trade off the sugar in soft drinks?

9. Do some sodium sleuthing. Examine the list of ingredients found on food packages. Which ones have sodium listed? Do any list sodium more than one time? Make a poster that lists ways to decrease the sodium in your diet. You could title your list "How to Shake the Sodium Habit" and hang it on your refrigerator as a reminder.

10. Put on a good nutrition campaign at school. Write slogans, make mobiles, and create advertisements for eating a varied diet.

Chapter 4

Weighing Your Choices

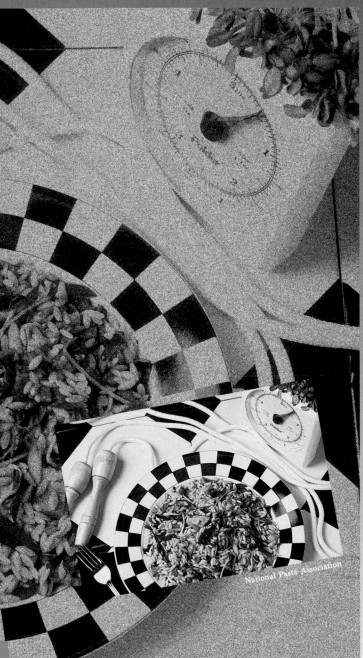

National Pasta Association

Objectives

After reading this chapter, you will be able to
- ❑ explain how your body uses energy.
- ❑ discuss how calories affect growth and weight.
- ❑ list the advantages of a healthy weight.
- ❑ describe the dangers of being underweight or obese.
- ❑ describe binge eating, bulimia nervosa, and anorexia nervosa.

New Terms

healthy weight: the weight that is right for your age and height.
underweight: a weight that is much lower than a healthy weight.
obese: having an excessive amount of body fat.
weight control: keeping your body at a healthy weight.
fad diet: a quick weight loss diet that doesn't usually work and can harm your health.
binge eating: an eating disorder that involves the rapid eating (or chewing and spitting out) of thousands of calories in a short time.
bulimia nervosa: an eating disorder that causes people to binge and purge themselves.
anorexia nervosa: an eating disorder that causes people to starve themselves.

Everyone seems to be talking about calories. Some people worry that they eat too few. Most worry that they eat too many. This chapter explores how calories affect growth and body weight. It explains why being underweight or obese is dangerous and what to do about it. It also shows why fad diets don't work and describes eating disorders.

The Calories You Burn

When does your body burn calories? Does it burn them when you sleep? Are calories used when you watch TV? How about swimming? Does that require calories? The answer is yes to all of these questions. In fact, your body uses calories every second of every day. Calories are the fuel for vital functions and physical activities, 4-1.

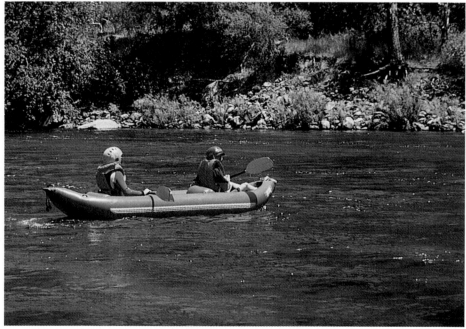

USDA

4-1 Every move you make burns calories.

Vital Functions

Vital functions are body processes that keep you alive. Your breathing and your heartbeat are vital functions. Other vital functions include keeping your body warm, repairing wounds, digesting food, and growing.

Some people burn more calories for vital functions than others do. The number of calories used for vital functions depends mostly on age, gender, and body size.

- Younger people use more energy for vital functions than older people. The main reason for this difference is that young people are still growing. Many calories are needed for normal growth to occur.
- After age 14 or so, males tend to use more energy for vital functions than females. This is because most adult males have more muscle and are larger than females.
- Larger people burn more energy for vital functions than people who are smaller.

Physical Activities

Biking, writing, and playing video games are examples of physical activities. Any time you move your body or exercise, you are doing a physical activity. The number of calories burned in physical activity is affected by body size. The amount of calories used also is affected by time spent doing the activity and how hard you work.

- Larger people burn more calories than smaller people doing the same activity for the same length of time.
- The longer you spend doing an activity, the more energy you will use. Playing ball for an hour burns more calories than playing ball for 10 minutes.
- The harder you work, the more calories you will burn. Which burns more energy–running, walking, or sitting? If you said running, you're right! Take a look at 4-2. You'll see that it takes only 14 minutes to burn 200 calories running. It takes more than two hours to burn this amount just by sitting!

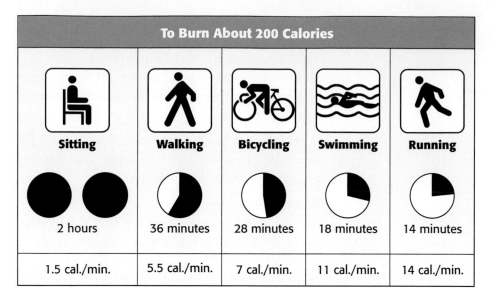

To Burn About 200 Calories				
Sitting	**Walking**	**Bicycling**	**Swimming**	**Running**
2 hours	36 minutes	28 minutes	18 minutes	14 minutes
1.5 cal./min.	5.5 cal./min.	7 cal./min.	11 cal./min.	14 cal./min.

4-2 This is how long it takes to burn about 200 calories. You can see that the harder you work, the more quickly calories are burned. How many calories would you burn if you ran for two hours instead of sitting?

The Calories You Eat

All foods supply energy, but some foods supply more than others. The energy found in a food depends on the amount of fats, carbohydrates, and proteins it contains. Foods high in fats usually have more calories than foods high in carbohydrates or proteins. This is because every gram of fat you eat provides nine calories. One gram of carbohydrate or one gram of protein each supply only four calories.

You can find out how many calories a food has. If the food comes in a package, you can check the nutrition label. You also can find this information in a calorie chart like the one in 4-3. You'll find more foods and their calorie content in the Food Composition Table in Appendix A.

4-3 A calorie chart can help you to determine how many calories are in certain foods.

Sample Calorie Chart	
Food	**Calories**
1 hamburger	250
1 cheeseburger	300
1 enchilada	235
1 slice of cheese pizza	300
12-ounce soft drink	175
1 milk shake	335
8 ounces orange juice	110
1 small bag of potato chips	210
15 pretzel sticks	15
10 carrot sticks	30
1 apple	80
1 dip of ice cream	125
1 dip of non-fat frozen yogurt	95
4 medium chocolate chip cookies	180
2 graham crackers	60

The most healthy diets contain carbohydrates, fats, and proteins in the following amounts:

- About 58 percent of the calories you eat should come from carbohydrates.
- No more than 30 percent of the calories you eat should come from fats. Most of these fats should be unsaturated fats instead of saturated fats.
- Only about 12 percent of the calories you eat should come from proteins.

The *Math in the Kitchen* feature in this chapter will help you see how your diet compares to the amounts given above.

How many calories does a person need? The answer depends on your age, weight, and how much you exercise. A fairly active teen burns about 20 to 22 calories per pound of body weight each day. Very active teens will use more calories. Less active ones will use fewer calories.

÷ Math in the Kitchen

Fat Math

Eating too much fat can damage your health. Diets that are high in fat can cause you to gain excess weight. They also can increase your chances of having heart disease.

Is your fat intake on target? Are more than 30 percent of your calories coming from fat? Here's how to find out.

1. List everything you ate and drank since this time yesterday. Estimate the amount you ate or drank of each food.
2. Look up each food in the Food Composition Table in Appendix A. Write down the calories and grams of fat. You can use a chart like the example below to record your data.
3. Add up the total number of calories you ate.
4. Add up the grams of fat you ate.
5. Compute the number of calories that came from fat. To do this, multiply the total grams of fat you ate by nine. (There are nine calories in each gram of fat.)

   calories from fat = grams of fat x 9

6. Compute the percent of calories that came from fat. Do this by dividing the calories from fat by the total calories you ate. Then, multiply this number by 100.

   percent of calories from fat = (calories from fat ÷ total calories) x 100

7. Your fat intake is fine if it is equal to or lower than 30 percent of your calories. If it is higher, you need to make some changes.

Questions

1. How many calories did you eat?
2. How many grams of fat did you eat?
3. Which food in your diet had the most fat?
4. How many calories came from fat?
5. What percent of calories came from fat?
6. Is your fat intake lower, equal to, or higher than 30 percent of your calories?
7. If your fat intake is higher than 30 percent of your calories, what changes could you make to eat less fat?

Food	Amount	Calories	Grams of Fat
Cheese Pizza	2 slices	600	19
Soft Drink	12 ounces	150	0
		TOTAL=_____	TOTAL=_____

Balancing Calories

Why are calories so important? One reason is that the number of calories you eat and burn determine how well you grow. Another reason is that calories affect your weight. The number of calories you eat compared to the number you burn determines your calorie balance. See 4-4.

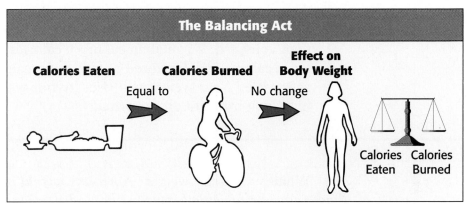

You are in calorie balance when calories eaten equal calories burned.

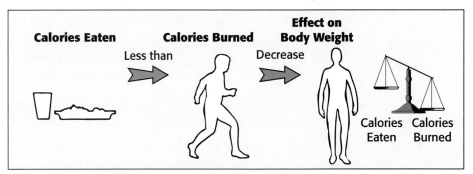

Weight declines when fewer calories are eaten than are burned.

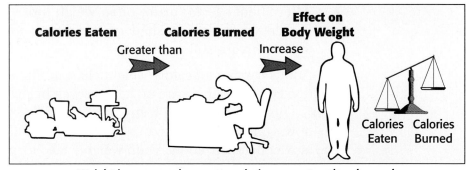

Weight increases when more calories are eaten than burned.

4-4 The calories you eat and the calories you burn affect your body weight.

- You are in *calorie balance* when you eat the same number of calories as you burn. Babies, children, and teens who are in calorie balance can grow normally. Once they are finished growing, their weight will stay the same if they are in calorie balance.
- You are out of calorie balance when you eat fewer calories than you burn. You will lose weight and may not grow normally if you often eat fewer calories than you burn. Your weight drops because some stored body fat and muscle must be broken down to supply needed calories. You cannot grow if your body lacks the calories it needs to develop normally.
- You also are out of calorie balance when you eat more calories than you burn. If you often eat more calories than you burn, the extra calories will be stored as fat. (Extra calories are not stored as muscle.) Your weight will rise. If your weight becomes very high, you may not grow normally.

Healthy Weight

What is a healthy weight? A ***healthy weight*** is one that is neither too high nor too low for your age and height. You feel good and move freely when you're at a healthy weight. A healthy weight also includes an average amount of body fat. You need this fat to keep your body warm and protect your organs. You also need it to pad your bones and give your body shape. This body fat serves as an energy reserve for times when you don't eat enough.

The weight that is healthy for you is a personal matter. It depends on your body type, gender, and where you are in your growth.

- Body type depends mostly on the size of your bones and muscles. People with large bones or muscles will weigh more than those with smaller bones and muscles.
- After about age 14, males often weigh more than females.
- People who have finished growing tend to weigh more than those who are still growing.

Adults can use a healthy weight chart to find out if their weight is healthy. However, there are no healthy weight charts designed just for teens. This is because each teen grows at a different rate. If you wonder how your weight compares to other teens, take a look at 4-5. If you are concerned about your weight, talk to your doctor, school nurse, or a dietitian. They can help you decide whether your weight is healthy. If it's not, they will help you figure out why it isn't healthy. They can help you plan a safe way to improve your weight, too.

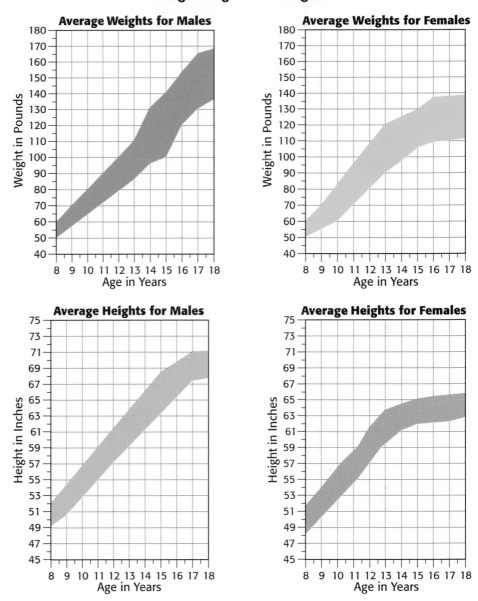

Average Weights and Heights

4-5 These charts show the average weight and height ranges for males and females.

Being Out of Calorie Balance

Being out of calorie balance can cause you to grow poorly. It also can cause your weight and body fat to drop or rise. Having too much or too little body fat can put your health and your life in danger.

Underweight

Anyone who often eats fewer calories than he or she burns will become ***underweight***. Underweight people have little body fat and weigh much less than they would at their healthy weight. Being too thin is not a common problem in the United States, but it is a problem in many other countries.

Why are some people underweight? In many cases, they simply can't get the food they need, 4-6. They may not be able to afford to buy it. In some parts of the world, crops may be so damaged that there is little food to eat. People who have plenty to eat may become underweight, too. They may eat too little because they are too busy to eat. Others may stay on weight loss diets too long. Some might have an eating disorder. No matter what causes people to be underweight, they face serious health risks.

4-6 Many people around the world are underweight because they have too little to eat.

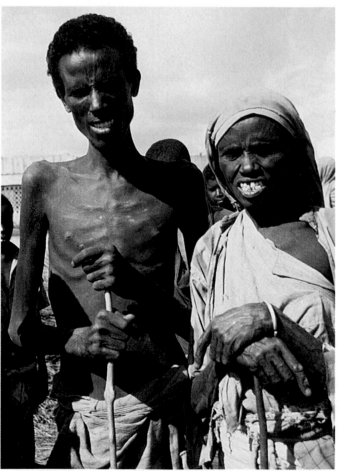

Dangers of Being Underweight

Underweight babies, children, and teens seldom grow normally. They may never be as tall as they could be. Their muscles and bones may not be as strong as those who eat enough. Their brains may be smaller than normal. Their skin may look dry, pale, and sickly. They may not feel well. Limiting calorie intake can cause them to have permanent physical damage and lifelong problems.

Underweight people often have many other health problems. For instance, they are more prone to getting colds and infections than people who weigh more. They also tire faster. People who are underweight may lose some of their hair. Many find it painful to sit and lie down because they lack the padding that body fat provides. They feel cold even on warm days because they have too little fat to insulate their bodies. If an underweight person loses even more weight, he or she could die.

Those who are underweight also often must deal with psychological burdens. For example, many feel depressed and sad. Some feel embarrassed about being "scrawny."

Many teens go through a short period when they feel too tall and skinny. Sometimes they are growing so fast that all their calories are used for growth and not body fat. When their growth slows down, their bodies can store some fat and fill out. Then, most find they are no longer too thin.

Gaining Weight

Underweight people often find gaining weight to be hard work. The safest way to put on extra pounds is to eat more servings from each of the major food groups. It is not healthy to try to gain weight by eating only sweets or fatty foods or cutting down on physical activity. There is no medicine that will safely increase weight.

Those who are underweight can follow these tips to obtain more calories.

- Eat several small meals instead of a few large ones. This makes it easier to eat extra calories.
- Try not to skip meals.
- Eat larger servings than normal.
- Have second helpings.
- Eat extra snacks.

- Drink beverages at the end of the meal because beverages fill up the stomach fast.
- Replace diet soft drinks and water with juice or milk.
- If lack of time for eating is a problem, pack a sandwich and piece of fruit to eat on the run. Better still, slow down and make time to eat.

Overweight

People who often eat more calories than they burn will store the extra calories as fat. Having excess body fat creates health concerns. People who have an excessive amount of body fat and weigh much more than their healthy weight are ***obese***.

Having too much body fat is a common problem in the United States. Nearly one of every three Americans has too much body fat. Why do so many people have excess fat? Lack of physical activity is the main reason. Less than half of all teens spend 60 minutes or more being physically active each day.

Instead of being active, many people sit in front of a computer or TV. Some children and teens spend nearly 30 hours a week viewing TV! Researchers have found the chances of becoming obese rise with every hour of sitting in front of a computer or TV. Being more physically active can help people control weight and enjoy other health benefits, 4-7.

Another reason some people have too much body fat is they have a habit of eating too much. They may take large helpings at meals. Large portions at restaurants may tempt them to eat more than they need or want. Personal problems, such as sadness, boredom, or stress, cause some people to overeat. Failing to realize that eating too much and being inactive can lead to excess body fat is the reason behind some people's habits.

Dangers of Being Overweight

Obese children and teens may have problems growing normally. They often do not grow as tall as their more slender peers. Excess fat strains the heart and lungs. Excess fat also puts great pressure on hip and leg joints. Teens who enter adulthood obese find it more difficult to lose weight than people who become obese in adulthood. As adults, obese teens also are more likely to develop health problems than slim teens.

4-7 Being physically active has many advantages for your health.

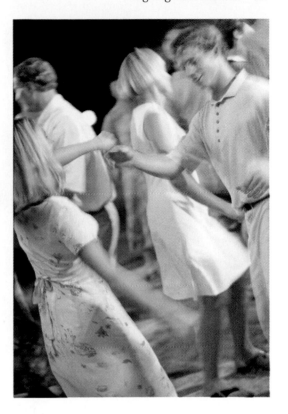

Health Benefits of Regular Physical Activity

- Helps manage weight
- Increases physical fitness
- Helps build and maintain healthy bones, muscles, and joints
- Builds endurance and muscular strength
- Lowers risk factors for cardiovascular disease, colon cancer, and Type 2 diabetes
- Helps control blood pressure
- Promotes psychological well-being and self-esteem
- Reduces feelings of depression and anxiety

Obese people face many other health risk. Many obese people find it hard to breathe. Also, too much body fat can lead to high blood pressure. Obese people have a greater chance of developing heart disease, one type of diabetes, and certain types of cancer.

Some obese people have more health problems than others. Those having apple shapes seem to have more health problems than those who have pear shapes. See 4-8. People with *apple shapes* store fat mostly in their stomach. Those with *pear shapes* store fat mainly in their thighs and hips. The place a person stores body fat is set by his or her heredity and cannot be changed. It is possible, though, to control the amount of fat stored.

Having too much body fat not only damages a person's physical health. It can affect mental health, too. Many who are obese say they often feel embarrassed, sad, or angry. They feel hurt when others reject or tease them. Some have trouble making new friends.

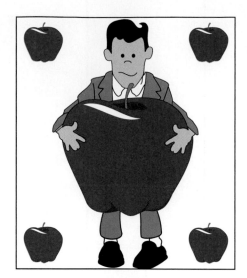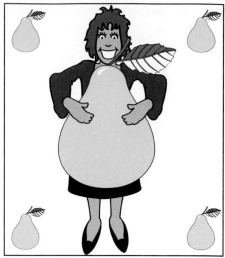

4-8 People with apple shapes store fat in the stomach area. Those with pear shapes store fat in the thighs and hips.

Who Should Lose Weight?

Many people go on weight loss diets every day. At least half of these dieters don't need to lose weight at all. For instance, many females think they have too much fat when they really do not. Just before the adolescent growth spurt begins, many teens worry that they are getting pudgy and want to diet. It is normal to put on a little extra weight at this time. This fat helps supply the thousands of calories needed for this very rapid growth.

It seldom is a good idea for babies, children, or teens to go on weight loss diets. This is because these diets could slow or even stop their growth. If they are athletes, weight loss diets can impair their skills. If you think you have excess body fat, talk to your doctor, school nurse, or a dietitian before trying to lose weight. If you have too much body fat, they can help you plan a safe weight control program.

Losing Weight Through Weight Control

Weight control means to get your body to a healthy weight and keep it there. If an obese teen is still growing taller, the goal of a safe weight control program is not to lose weight. The goal is to provide enough calories for normal growth, but not so many calories that excess fat is stored. This approach lets young teens hold their weight steady while they grow into it. As they grow taller, they will redistribute their body fat and become slimmer.

The goal of safe weight control programs for older teens and adults is to slowly shrink body fat stores. When a healthy weight is reached, the goal is to keep off the excess fat.

The safest weight control programs for people of all ages include foods from each of the major food groups and exercise. It is not healthy to try to lose weight by omitting one or more of the major food groups. Increasing physical activity should also be part of a weight control program.

These tips can help you keep your weight under control.

- Avoid skipping meals. You may get so hungry that you overeat.
- Take smaller portions.
- Skip second helpings.
- Eat slowly and take small bites. People who gulp their food eat so fast that they may overeat before their bodies can tell them they are full.
- Eat more fruits and vegetables. They fill you up and are low in calories.
- Trade high-fat foods for lowfat foods. For instance, you could select fat free milk instead of whole milk.
- Trade foods high in sugar for foods lower in sugar. For example, you could have a peach instead of peach cobbler.
- Pack a sandwich, fruit, or carrot sticks for a snack instead of buying fast foods.
- Buy air-popped popcorn and pretzels from vending machines instead of chips, crackers, cookies, and cupcakes.
- Try baked, grilled, and broiled foods instead of fried foods.
- Drink plenty of water. It is calorie-free. (Don't drink fewer beverages to lose weight because you could become dehydrated. Being dehydrated causes you to feel tired and weak. It could even kill you.)
- Be physically active for at least 60 minutes five or more days a week.
- Work physical activity into your daily routine. You could walk or skate to a friend's house instead of getting a ride. Shoot hoops rather than watch TV. Try using the stairs instead of an elevator.
- When you are angry, sad, or lonesome, do something besides eat. You could call a friend, play a game, or go for a bike ride.
- Choose physical activities you enjoy and will do often. You could play basketball, swim, ski, or go dancing. These activities will help strengthen your heart and lungs. Lifting weights and stretching help increase your strength and flexibility.

There is no fad diet, pill, or device that will safely decrease body fat. ***Fad diets*** promise quick weight loss. Most don't work because people can't stay on them long enough to lose more than a few pounds. People may lose weight fast, but they'll quickly regain it. If they stay on a fad diet for more than a week or so, they may get sick. Diet pills are a risky way to lose weight. They can disrupt normal body functions and hurt you. Gadgets that promise to melt away fat don't work. The only way to lose weight is to eat fewer calories than you burn.

Eating Disorders

Society puts a lot of pressure on people to be thin. Slender fashion models appear in most magazines. TV shows include mostly slim actors and actresses. Newspapers advertise weight loss treatments. This pressure makes some people want to be thin so much that they diet all the time.

The problem with this pressure is that it causes some people to live in constant fear of getting fat. Even when they are at a healthy weight, they still want to be thinner. The pressure to be thin may cause some people to develop eating disorders such as binge eating, bulimia nervosa, and anorexia nervosa.

Eating disorder victims usually have severe personal problems. They try to solve these problems through extreme and bizarre eating habits. Some of these eating habits are described in 4-9. Of course these habits can't solve their problems. Instead these habits can damage their health and, perhaps, even kill them.

Binge Eaters

Binge eaters are out of control when they eat. ***Binge eating*** is the rapid eating (or chewing and spitting out) of thousands of calories in a short time. Binge eaters tend to consume high-calorie foods that are easy to eat. Pies, cakes, cookies, ice cream, doughnuts, and pastries are common choices.

When binge eating, a person eats about 3,400 calories in an hour or so. Sometimes a binge eater may continue eating for eight hours and eat as many as 20,000 calories! A binge eater often doesn't stop until he or she is in great pain, falls asleep, or is interrupted.

Warning Signs of Eating Disorders

All eating disorders share these warning signs:

- Using body weight and lack of fat as a measure of your worth. Those with eating disorders think they are bad or ugly if they are not thin. Neither thinness nor fatness has anything to do with your value as a person.
- Seeing your body much differently than others see it. Most people with eating disorders think they look fat, even if they are thin.
- Constantly thinking and talking about food (or refusing to discuss it). Many people with eating disorders are always planning menus, clipping recipes from magazines, buying food, and cooking it.
- Having bizarre thoughts, feelings, and behaviors when food is present. Most people with eating disorders are afraid of eating. They fear they won't be able to stop once they start eating.
- Making and following strict food rules. Rules might include "no sweets with any meals" or "no eating after dark."
- Binge eating to cope with negative emotions. Many people with eating disorders don't know how to manage emotions in a healthy manner.
- Going on weight loss diets often. Eating disorders may develop after going on many weight loss diets.
- Nonstop exercising. A daily workout might include swimming 96 laps, running five miles, and doing two hours of aerobic exercises.
- Having problems getting along with your family and friends.

4-9 If any of these warning signs describes you or someone you know, get help right away.

Many factors can cause people to become binge eaters. Some become binge eaters because they use food to cope with emotions. They eat instead of finding healthy ways to deal with their emotions. Others become binge eaters after going on and off fad diets a few times. Fad diets often restrict calories so much that dieters get very, very hungry. In fact, dieters can become so hungry that they begin to binge. After dieting and binge eating a few times, these people may become binge eaters.

Effect on Health

Binge eating can lead to obesity and all the health problems obesity causes. Bingeing can stretch the stomach so much that it bursts. If the stomach bursts, the binge eater is likely to die. Many binge eaters cut themselves off from their friends because they don't want others to know they binge. This makes them feel lonely.

Treatment

Most binge eaters need the help of health professionals to stop binge eating. Treatment includes helping binge eaters learn to eat normal amounts of food. Treatment also teaches them healthy ways to manage their emotions and help them build friendships. Treatment may include a weight loss program if they are obese.

Bulimia Nervosa

People with ***bulimia nervosa*** (called bulimics) binge eat and then purge themselves. Bulimics *purge* (get rid of the food) by vomiting or abusing laxatives. They may binge and purge from twice a week to five times daily. Bulimics are very secretive and embarrassed about bingeing and purging. They don't want others to know about it.

Bulimia nervosa may develop after people try to lose weight. They mistakenly think that they can eat anything and lose weight if they purge themselves. It seems easy at first, then they realize they can't stop bingeing and purging. They are caught in a vicious cycle. That is, after a binge and purge event they feel guilty and never want to do it again. They decide to stay away from food so they won't be tempted to binge. Then, they get so hungry that they binge again. Sometimes just being upset, sad, or lonely can cause the person to binge. The binge is followed by purging. Then, the whole process starts all over again, 4-10.

4-10 Bulimics feel caught in a never ending cycle of bingeing and purging.

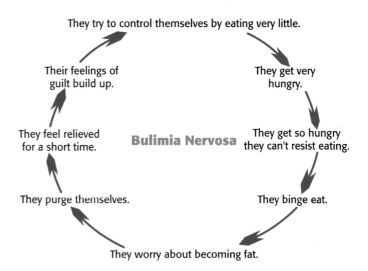

They try to control themselves by eating very little.

They get very hungry.

Their feelings of guilt build up.

Bulimia Nervosa

They get so hungry they can't resist eating.

They feel relieved for a short time.

They purge themselves.

They binge eat.

They worry about becoming fat.

Effect on Health

Bulimia nervosa can cause many health problems. People with this eating disorder often have dry skin and brittle hair. Their weight can vary 10 pounds or more in a few days. Bulimics often feel tired, sleep poorly, and have nightmares. Many feel very sad, ashamed, and guilty. They often end friendships because they fear their friends will find out about their bingeing and purging.

Constant vomiting causes many problems. It irritates the glands in the throat and causes them to swell. The swollen glands make a bulimic's face look puffy. The stomach acid in the vomit burns the throat and makes it sore. The acid also weakens the teeth and causes cavities. Vomit can get into the lungs. If this happens, bulimics can develop a deadly lung disease. Vomiting also can cause skin rashes and swelling around the eyes. It can even break blood vessels in the face.

Frequent vomiting and laxative abuse both cause bulimics to lose large amounts of water and minerals. These losses can cause muscle cramps. They also can cause the heart, nerves, and brain to malfunction. Losing large amounts of water or minerals or eating so much that the stomach bursts can kill the bulimic.

Treatment

Bulimics know that what they are doing is harmful. Many feel very guilty about their behavior. They want to stop bingeing and purging, but few can stop on their own. They need medical care. Treatment for bulimia nervosa includes helping the bulimic break the binge-purge cycle. Treatment also helps the bulimic eat normal amounts again. It teaches the bulimic how to build friendships and cope with emotions in healthy ways. Treatment also may include medication that helps bulimics feel less sad.

Anorexia Nervosa

People with *anorexia nervosa* (called anorexics) have an abnormal fear of being fat. This fear is so great that they eat only tiny amounts of food or even starve themselves. They skip most meals, exercise constantly, and become thinner and thinner. Anorexics are always thinking about food. When they do eat, they have strange rituals such as crumbling their food or cutting it into tiny pieces. Some also purge themselves.

Many anorexics develop this disorder after going on a weight loss diet. When friends notice they have lost weight, they keep on dieting to get more praise. Soon, they become so caught up in losing weight that they don't want to stop dieting. When others tell them they are too thin, anorexics argue that they look good. They believe that they still look and feel fat even when they are very underweight. Many wear baggy clothes to hide their slimness from people who tell them they are too thin, 4-11.

4-11 Some people who are at a healthy weight may see themselves as fat. This distorted body image may lead to eating disorders.

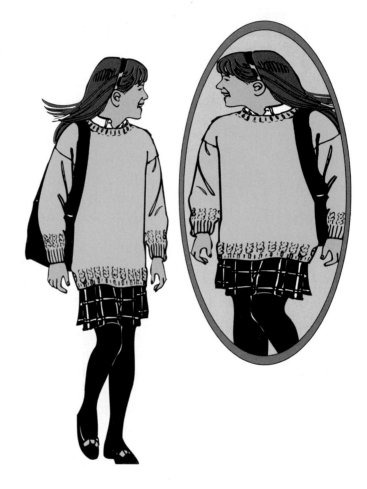

Effect on Health

As anorexics lose enough weight to become underweight, their health begins to decline. The skin becomes rough, dry, and scaly. Nails become brittle and hair looks dull and gets thinner. The muscles of anorexics waste away and body organs shrink and weaken. A thick coat of fine hair begins growing all over the body. Anorexics become unable to sleep and have nightmares. They feel cold all the time, even on hot days. Anorexics also tire quickly and feel faint and dizzy often. They become hostile and grouchy and often lose their friends.

Treatment

Anorexia nervosa can be fatal. Without treatment, anorexics may die from suicide or starvation. Treatment includes learning how to cope with problems. It also includes learning how to eat and exercise normally. Treatment helps anorexics accept their bodies as they are.

Eating Disorder Prevention

You can prevent eating disorders by having a good attitude about eating and your body. Here are some tips that can help you and your friends.

- Eat nutritious meals.
- Eat enough calories. Don't skip meals or eat very low-calorie diets.
- Find healthy ways to deal with emotions. Don't use food to cope with them.
- Give food and eating the right amount of attention. Don't let them be the most important things in your life.
- Accept the body type with which you were born. All body types are attractive. No amount of dieting or exercise can change your body type.
- Admire people for who they are, not what they look like.
- Try to avoid making either positive or negative comments about a person's weight or appearance.

If you think you have an eating disorder or know someone who does, get help right away. Early treatment is important. Your doctor or school nurse can assist you in finding professionals who are specially trained to treat eating disorders.

Focus on Food

Making Changes for the Better

Eating better doesn't mean you have to give up favorite foods or eat foods you don't like. It means taking a close look at your diet, deciding how to improve it, and then making the improvements. Making improvements is easy if you start with small changes. Over time, small changes add up to big improvements.

You can find ways to improve your diet. Here's how you can change your diet for the better.

1. Think about the foods you ate yesterday and today. Compare the foods you ate with the Food Guide Pyramid and the Dietary Guidelines for Americans. Identify any problem areas. For instance, do you eat candy, cookies, chips, pretzels, or ice cream instead of a meal? Do you eat fast-food meals more than three times a week? Is your only vegetable French fries? Do you eat enough servings from each of the major food groups? Do you skip meals often? Are there more soft drinks in your diet than milk? Do you eat to cope with emotions?

2. Set goals to overcome your problem areas. Some sample goals are listed here.

    • I will eat a carton of yogurt instead of eating candy for a meal.

    • I will put a few apples in my backpack to snack on instead of buying corn chips from the vending machine.

    • I will include breads, cereals, rice, or pasta in every meal.

    • I will choose fruit juice instead of soft drinks.

    • I'll take a walk instead of eating when I'm upset.

3. Decide which goal you want to achieve first. Then, make a plan for reaching it. For example, think about how you can avoid skipping breakfast. You could wrap up a sandwich before you go to bed. If you aren't hungry when you wake up, take the sandwich to school and eat it later. Another plan might be to buy a frozen fruit bar or milk at school. Be sure your plan is realistic. If you eat a fast-food meal daily, it might be hard to totally give it up. Your goal might be to make better choices at the fast-food restaurant. For instance, you could order a taco instead of a fried burrito. You could decide to order a small regular burger instead of the super deluxe one. If you eat at a chicken place, you could pass up the mashed potatoes and gravy and order corn-on-the-cob. To get more vegetables, try ordering a pizza with vegetable toppings. You could pack a lunch of carrot sticks, cheese chunks, and crackers to eat instead of a fast-food meal.

4. Once your plan is made, stick to it. At the end of each week, make other changes. In three or four weeks, you can make a lot of progress toward your goal. You may even reach your goal in that time and be ready to work on another goal. It's important to work on only one or two goals at a time. If you try to reach all your goals overnight you're likely to become frustrated and give up! Keep in mind that your food habits have been forming since you were born. So, it isn't realistic to expect them to change right away.

5. Each time you reach a goal, reward yourself. Be sure not to use food as a reward. Instead, go to a movie, visit a friend, or go swimming.

6. Every few weeks, review your goals. It's easy to slip back into old habits. Don't feel bad if you do, just make plans to try again. The key is to keep working to reach your goals.

In a Nutshell

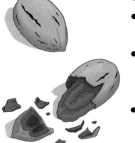

- Your body uses energy for vital functions and physical activities.
- The amount of energy burned for vital functions depends on age, gender, and body size.
- The number of calories used for physical activities depends on body size, time spent doing the activity, and how hard you work doing the activity.
- The most healthy diets obtain about 58 percent of their calories from carbohydrate, 12 percent from protein, and no more than 30 percent from fat.
- Eating too many or too few calories can affect growth and can cause body weight and body fat to rise or drop.
- Being underweight or obese can endanger your health and shorten your life.
- The goal of safe weight control programs for young teens is to hold weight steady and grow into it.
- People with eating disorders live in constant fear of food and becoming fat.
- Binge eaters eat thousands of calories in a short time.
- Bulimics binge and purge themselves.
- Anorexics starve themselves.

In the Know

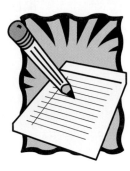

1. Maria is 16 years old. She is five feet tall and weighs 115 pounds. Rolanda is 16 years old, too. She is six feet tall and weighs 175 pounds. Who uses more energy for vital functions?
   A. Maria.
   B. Rolanda.
   C. Maria and Rolanda both use the same amount of energy for vital functions.
2. Which activity will burn the most calories?
   A. Watching TV.
   B. Sleeping.
   C. Biking.
   D. Eating dinner.
3. What happens when a teen eats fewer calories than his or her body uses?
4. Explain the meaning of the term "healthy weight."
5. True or false? Having too much body fat can damage a person's physical and mental health.
6. List three tips for keeping weight under control.
7. True or false? People with eating disorders usually have severe personal problems.
8. A puffy face, sore throat, dry skin, and guilty feelings best describe a _____.
   A. binge eater
   B. person with bulimia nervosa
   C. person with anorexia nervosa
   D. any person with an eating disorder

What Would You Do?

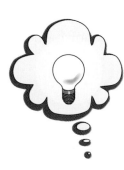

Tom is on the wrestling team. He tells you, "I need to lose 10 pounds by next week because I want to wrestle in a lower weight class. I guess I'll stop eating and drinking water. I know I'll lose weight, but it makes me feel tired and weak." Is Tom's plan safe? What could happen if he goes through with his plan? What advice would you give him?

Expanding Your Knowledge

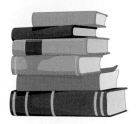

1. Examine a weight loss diet printed in a magazine. Why might a person try this diet? Compare the diet to the Food Guide Pyramid. Does it contain all the major food groups in the amounts recommended? Do you think the diet is safe? Write a paragraph to defend your answer.

2. Request nutrition information from a fast-food restaurant. Determine the number of calories you usually eat when you visit that restaurant. Think of ways you can trim the calories you eat there.

3. Find out what it feels like to gain excess weight. Place 20 pounds of books in a backpack. Spend a few minutes wearing the backpack. How did you feel? Imagine that your body weight increased by 20 pounds. How do you think you would feel? What problems might you have?

4. Make a poster that shows 10 ways to put more physical activity in daily routines. Use magazine pictures or drawings to illustrate the poster.

5. Interview a dietitian about weight control. You could ask questions like the following: What's the best way to control body weight? How can fad diets hurt you? What role does physical activity play in weight control?

6. Brainstorm with a partner to create a list of weight control tips. Create a bulletin board that features the tips you listed.

7. Invite an eating disorders expert to speak to your class. You could ask the expert to describe eating disorders, their treatment, and how to prevent them.

8. Visit the library and find out more about eating disorders. Use the information to make a video on eating disorders.

Chapter 5
A Look at the Kitchen

Objectives

After reading this chapter, you will be able to
- ❏ describe the types of major appliances available.
- ❏ explain how to clean and care for appliances.
- ❏ describe the work centers in a kitchen.
- ❏ identify the kitchen equipment needed in each work center.
- ❏ list ways to save energy in the kitchen.

New Terms

warranty: the seller's guarantee that a product will perform as specified and will be replaced or repaired if it fails within a certain time.

work center: area in the kitchen where a certain type of task is done and the equipment needed for the task is stored.

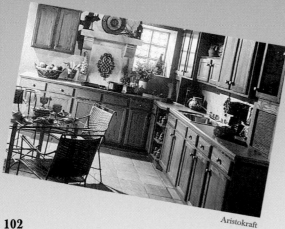

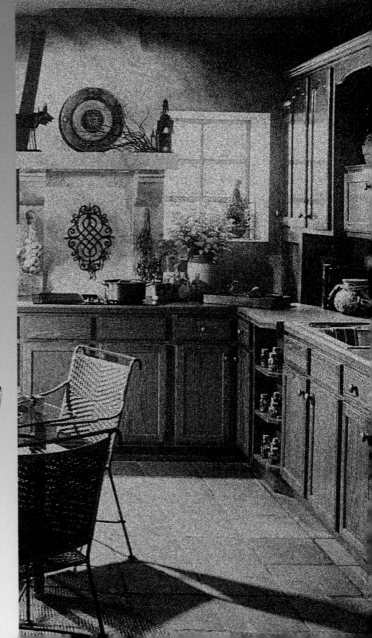

102

Aristokraft

The kitchen is the center of activity in many homes. Food is prepared and stored there. The family may gather in the kitchen to eat and talk. The kitchen may also serve as a family's message center. With all these activities going on in one room, the kitchen can be a busy place. Since the kitchen is such a busy place, it needs to operate efficiently. In this chapter, you will explore how kitchen appliances and work centers can help accomplish this.

Major Kitchen Appliances

How many items in 5-1 can you identify? Here's a hint. They all are kitchen appliances. Do you have any of these appliances in your home?

Your answer would be different if you lived 100 years ago. Then, your family's stove might have looked like photo A in 5-1. If you lived in Europe 70 years ago, you might have had a dishwasher like the one in photo B in 5-1.

If you work in a restaurant, you might use an oven like the one in photo C in 5-1. In the future, you might have a free-standing burner like the one in photo D in 5-1. It uses an ultra-hot light to cook food.

A refrigerator of the future is shown in photo E in 5-1. It has no doors! How does it keep foods cold? A cool air tornado swirls around the interior to keep the inside cool. A vertical curtain of air is created by forcing air through jets in the top of the openings. The forced air moves down over each opening to keep warm air out. Just reach through the air curtain and grab your favorite snack!

Whenever or wherever you live, appliances can make your work easier and safer. For instance, it is easier to cook food in an oven than it is to roast it over an open fire. It is safer to store meats in a refrigerator or freezer than to leave them at room temperature. Cold temperatures help prevent the growth of harmful bacteria.

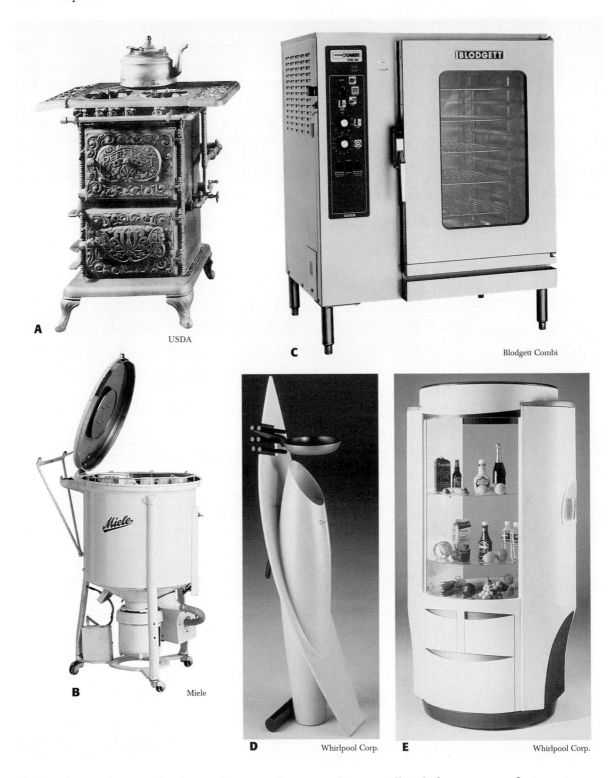

A USDA

B Miele

C Blodgett Combi

D Whirlpool Corp.

E Whirlpool Corp.

5-1 Appliances have evolved over the years. Future appliances will include even more features to make working in the kitchen more efficient.

Major appliances not only make work easier and safer. They help you save time, too. You can wash many dishes quickly in a dishwasher. You can easily cook a meal on a range. If you didn't have a refrigerator, meats and milk products would spoil quickly. You would need to buy them every day. With a refrigerator, you can shop less often.

The major appliances found in most U.S. kitchens are ranges, ovens, refrigerators, freezers, and dishwashers. These large, costly pieces of equipment are designed to last many years.

Ranges

A range is an appliance that provides heat for cooking food. Cooking helps to make foods tasty and appealing. Heat also kills harmful bacteria.

Ranges are sometimes called stoves. One of the first stoves was invented in China in the 700s. It was made of baked clay. Over 1,000 years later, Benjamin Franklin made a stove out of cast iron. All of these early stoves were used mainly to warm rooms. People cooked foods over a fire outside or in a fireplace.

It wasn't until 1790 that a stove was designed that could heat rooms and also cook foods. This stove was invented by Count Rumford. He might be surprised to see how his idea has changed. Today's ranges look quite different than the early stoves. The ranges today are used only to cook food. They should not be used to heat rooms.

A range often has two parts. These parts are *surface units* and an *oven*. Pots containing food are placed on surface units. The heat from the surface unit warms the pot and cooks the food inside. You might prepare vegetables, soup, and sauces on the cooktop. An *exhaust fan* is often used with a cooktop. The exhaust fan helps to remove smoke, odors, steam, and grease from the air.

Ovens can be used to bake bread and roast meat. Pans containing food are placed on the oven's shelves. When the oven is on, the air inside the oven gets hot. The hot air cooks the food. This type of oven is sometimes called a *conventional oven*. A *convection oven*, which is described later in this chapter, cooks food with circulating hot air. (*Microwave ovens* will be described in Chapter 6.)

Types of Fuels Used

The first stoves used wood or coal for fuel. Today, they use gas or electricity. A *gas range* produces heat when the gas combines with oxygen in the air and burns. A device that makes sparks or a pilot light causes the gas to burn. A pilot light is a small flame that burns all the time. Robert Bunsen helped design the first gas range. He is famous for the Bunsen burners used in chemistry labs.

The amount of heat produced depends on the amount of gas used. The more gas used, the hotter the surface unit or oven becomes. You can adjust the amount of gas used with the range controls. When the surface unit is on, you see flames. See 5-2.

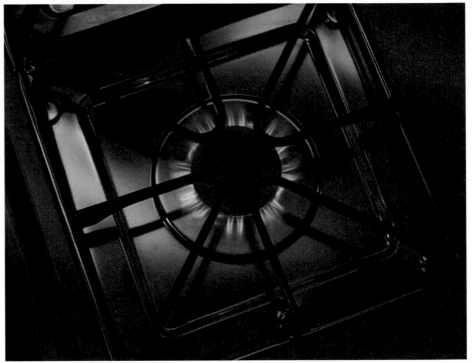

Whirlpool Corp.

5-2 Small flames appear when a gas range's surface unit is on.

Electric ranges produce heat when electricity flows through coils of wire. The surface unit coils often are round. Most electric ovens have two rectangular coils. One is located in the top of the oven. The other is in the bottom.

The more electricity that flows through the coils, the hotter the surface unit or oven will be. You can adjust the flow of electricity with the controls. The most electricity flows through the coil when the control is set on high. When the surface unit or oven coils are very hot, they glow orange.

When you buy appliances, look for labels from respected safety organizations. Many appliances have a UL seal from *Underwriters Laboratories (UL)*. Appliances with these and other safety seals meet the latest safety requirements. See 5-3.

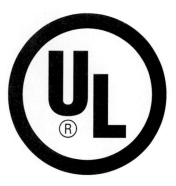

5-3 This Underwriters Laboratories (UL) seal on an appliance means the appliance meets the latest safety requirements.

Range Styles

There are three basic range styles. They are free-standing, slide-in, and drop-in. *Free-standing ranges* have surface units on the top and an oven below. Some also have a second oven that is above the surface units. These ranges can be placed almost anywhere in the kitchen. They can stand alone. They also can be placed next to a counter or between two counters. See 5-4.

5-4 Free-standing ranges can be placed in almost any location in the kitchen.

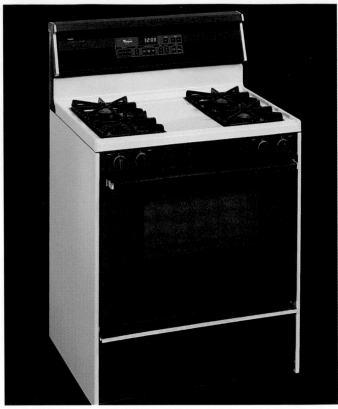

Whirlpool Corp.

Slide-in and drop-in ranges are designed to fit between two counters. They are like free-standing ranges, except their sides are not finished. See 5-5.

Surface units and ovens are also available separately. The surface units are built into countertops. The ovens are built into walls and may take the place of cabinets.

Care and Cleaning

The best way to care for a range is described in its care manual. The manual explains how to safely clean the range.

The cooktop should be cleaned after every use. Wait until the surface units are cool before cleaning. Without cleaning, spills bake on and are hard to remove. Spills may cause bacteria to grow and may attract insects and mice. Most cleaning can be done by wiping the cooktop with a sponge, 5-6. A plastic scrubber can help you remove spills. Steel wool pads and scouring powder should not be used. They can scratch the range surface areas.

5-5 Slide-in ranges are built to fit between two kitchen cabinets.

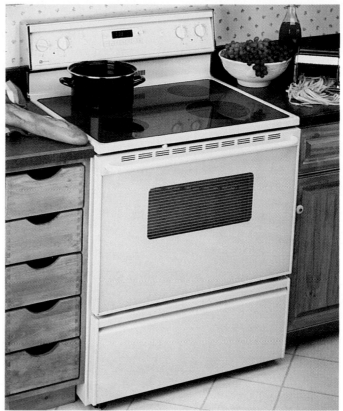

Maytag Company

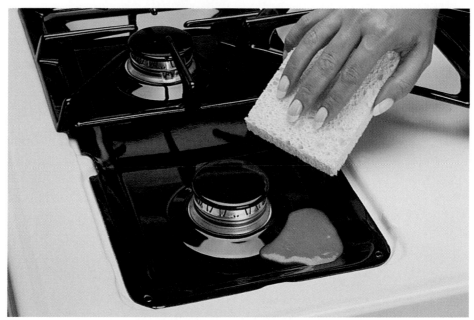

GE Appliances

5-6 Wipe up spills on the cooktop as soon as the range is cool.

To clean the surface units, remove the drip bowls that are below the surface units. If you are using a gas range, remove the metal grates from the surface units. Wash the drip bowls and metal grates in warm, soapy water. Electric surface units are self-cleaning; do not wash them. Spills will burn off when the electric surface unit gets hot.

You can clean the outside of the oven with a damp cloth. To keep the inside of your oven clean, wipe up spills and spatters as soon as the oven cools. If you leave the spills and spatters in the oven, they will bake on the next time you use the oven. Soon, they will become very hard to remove. You can use oven cleaner to dissolve burned-on food.

Some ovens have self-cleaning or continuous cleaning features. These ovens clean themselves. You do not need to use oven cleaner. There are two types of ovens that clean themselves. The walls on *continuous cleaning ovens* have a special coating. This coating causes spatters and spills to burn away during cooking. A *self-cleaning oven* has a special setting marked "clean." When this oven is set to clean, it becomes very hot (up to 1,000° F (540° C)). Food spills burn to ashes. After the cleaning, you will need to wipe a few ashes out of the bottom of the oven. Self-cleaning and continuous cleaning ovens both cost more than ovens without these features.

Convection Ovens

A *convection oven* is a conventional oven with a fan inside. The fan blows hot air around the food. See 5-7. Convection ovens may be gas or electric. They also are called hot air ovens. The hot blowing air causes convection ovens to cook food faster and more evenly than conventional ovens. Conventional ovens also cook foods at a lower temperature. Quick cooking and low temperatures mean you save energy. Convection ovens are cleaned in the same way as a conventional oven.

In a few years, consumers will be able to buy a new type of convection oven called an *injection oven*. Instead of using a fan to blow hot air around food, this oven blasts hot air over the food. Nozzles spray hot air at a speed of 100 miles per hour, causing foods to cook very rapidly.

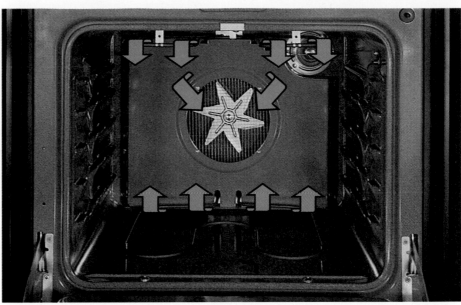

GE Appliances

5-7 A convection oven has a fan inside that blows hot air around the oven.

Refrigerators and Freezers

Refrigerators and freezers keep food cold. The cold temperatures slow the growth of harmful bacteria. These appliances also keep foods fresh longer than if they were stored at room temperature. Refrigerators and freezers enable you to buy some foods a week or more before you plan to serve them.

Few homes had refrigerators until the 1920s. Before then, people had to rely on ice or snow to cool foods. Many families had an ice box. Blocks of ice were delivered two or three times a week to homes having ice boxes. Today, more than 98 percent of all the homes in the United States have a refrigerator.

Refrigerator Styles

Refrigerators come in two styles. One style has one outside door. The other style has two or more outside doors. Almost all refrigerator styles include a freezer.

Most one-door refrigerators have a small freezer compartment. A door inside the refrigerator closes off the freezer. The temperature of the freezer compartment is colder than in the refrigerator. It often can't get as cold as a freezer that has a separate outside door.

Refrigerators with two outside doors have a separate refrigerator and freezer. The freezer may be above, below, or to the side of the refrigerator. Some refrigerators have more than two doors. Extra doors may allow you to remove ice without opening the entire freezer. They may allow you to remove cold beverages without opening the whole refrigerator. These smaller doors help the refrigerator and freezer stay much cooler. This is because less cold air escapes through the small door than when you open the large door.

Refrigerators come in many sizes. Large models are found in many kitchens. They have enough room to store foods needed for a week or more. Compact refrigerators are small. Most have only one door. They are often used in college dorm rooms, mobile homes, and offices. The freezer compartment is only large enough to hold two ice trays.

Large refrigerators may have added features. See 5-8. Many have special food drawers. For instance, a vegetable drawer keeps vegetables crisp and moist. A meat drawer keeps meats very cold.

5-8 There are many features to consider when choosing a refrigerator. Which would be the most important features for your family?

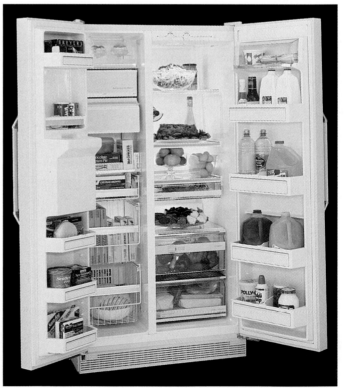

An ice maker and dispenser make it easy to get the ice you need. Water dispensers, located on the outside of the refrigerator, provide ice-cold water.

Freezer Styles

Freezers are also sold as separate units. They come in chest and upright styles. Both have one large door. An *upright freezer* looks like a one-door refrigerator. Its door swings outward. A *chest freezer* is low with the door on top. You open it by lifting its door upward. See 5-9. Chest freezers take more floor space than upright freezers. Chest freezers stay colder than upright freezers because less cold air escapes when they are opened. Chest freezers are best for storing large, bulky packages. Upright freezers are best for storing smaller packages.

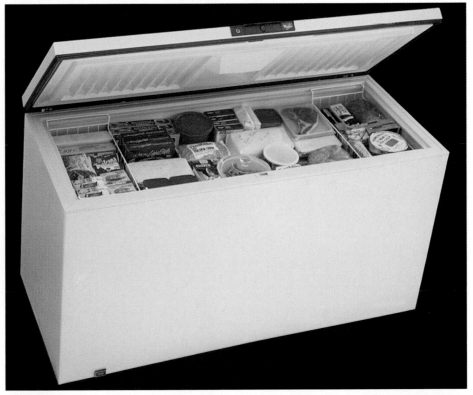

Whirlpool Corp.

5-9 Chest freezers are ideal for storing large packages.

Frost forms when water vapor settles on the freezer walls and shelves and freezes. Frost needs to be removed when it gets over 1/2 inch thick. You will need to remove the frost if you have a manual defrost freezer. The frost is removed automatically if you have an automatic defrost or frostless freezer. Manual defrost freezers cost the least to buy and operate. However, they require the most time to maintain.

Care and Cleaning

The care manuals that come with refrigerators and freezers describe how to care for them. They will tell you the best and safest way to clean these appliances.

Here's what you can do to keep your refrigerator and freezer clean.

- Wipe up spills right away. Bacteria grow in spilled foods, 5-10.
- Check for spoiled foods every week and throw them away.

5-10 Prevent bacterial growth by wiping up spills as soon as they happen.

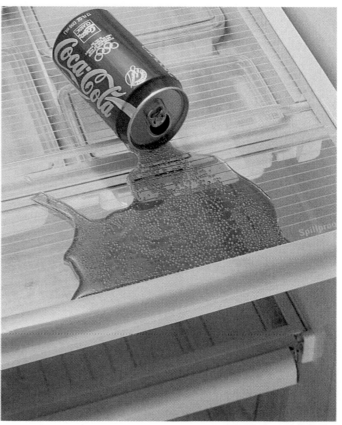

GE Appliances

- Wipe shelves, drawers, and the outside with a damp cloth every month. You can wash removable parts in the sink with warm, soapy water. Steel wool pads and scouring powder will scratch refrigerator and freezer surfaces.
- Keep an open box of baking soda in the refrigerator. It will absorb odors and keep the refrigerator smelling fresh.
- Vacuum or wash the grill at the bottom of the refrigerator every few months.
- Empty the drip pan below the refrigerator and wash it twice a year. The drip pan is behind the grill.
- Dust or vacuum the coils on the back of the refrigerator twice a year. Dust build-up causes refrigerators and freezers to work less efficiently.
- Don't let freezer ice get to be more than 1/2 inch thick. Thick ice build-up may cause the freezer to stop working. Read the care manual to learn how to defrost your freezer.

 ## Science in the Kitchen

Protecting Stored Foods

Cold air circulates through refrigerators and freezers. The cold air chills the foods. It also can dry out foods.

An experiment can help you see how well different wrapping materials help frozen foods retain moisture. You'll need four dry sponges that are the same size and shape. Label the sponges 1, 2, 3, and 4 and weigh each sponge separately. Record the weight of each sponge.

Next, tear off a piece of aluminum foil, plastic wrap, and freezer paper large enough to wrap one sponge. Weigh these wrappings separately and record their weights.

Thoroughly soak the sponges. Wrap sponge #1 tightly in aluminum foil. Wrap sponge #2 tightly in plastic wrap. Wrap sponge #3 tightly in freezer paper. Place sponge #4 unwrapped on a plastic dish. Weigh each sponge with its wrapping or dish and record the weights.

Place the sponges in the freezer for one week. Then, weigh each sponge and its wrapper or dish and record its weight. Compare the weights before and after storing the sponges. Which sponge retained the most water? Which retained the least? How can you use this information when you store foods?

Storing Foods in the Refrigerator or Freezer

Refrigerated and frozen foods can be stored in glass, metal, or plastic containers. The containers should be covered with a lid, aluminum foil, or plastic wrap. The cover will keep the food from drying out. It also will prevent food odors from escaping.

Frozen foods also can be wrapped in freezer paper. Be sure to put a date on every food you freeze. The date will let you know how long a food has been frozen. Over time, the quality of frozen food decreases. Chart 5-11 shows how long frozen foods are expected to maintain their quality. Foods stored longer than the time given in the chart will likely be safe to eat, but they may not taste or look as good.

5-11 This chart tells you how long foods stored in a freezer will likely maintain their quality.

Frozen Food Storage	
Food	**Maximum Storage Time**
Frozen fruits	9 to 12 months
Vegetables	6 to 8 months
Juice	6 to 8 months
Ice cream, sherbet	1 month
Meat	6 to 9 months
Ground meat	1 to 3 months
Sausage	1 to 2 months
Chicken and turkey	6 months
Fish	3 to 6 months
Breads, cakes, pies	3 to 6 months
Cookies	9 to 12 months
Stews, pot pies, and other meat and vegetable mixtures	3 to 6 months

Food quality is maintained longer if refrigerators and freezers are kept at the correct temperature. To keep foods fresh and safe, set refrigerator thermostats to between 32° F and 40° F (0° C to 5° C). Keep freezer thermostats at 0° F (-18° C).

Dishwashers

Dishwashers save clean-up time. Dishes washed in a dishwasher also have fewer bacteria than hand-washed dishes. Dirty dishes, pots, and pans are loaded into the dishwasher. Special dishwasher detergent is added and the door is closed. A tight seal keeps water from leaking out the dishwasher door. After the washing cycle ends, the dishwasher dries the dishes with hot air. The dried dishes will be very hot. It's a good idea to wait until the dishes are cool to unload them. You will be less likely to burn yourself or drop the dishes when they are cool.

Here's what you need to get the cleanest dishes.

- Hot water 140° -160° F (60° -70° C)
- Good water pressure
- Dishwasher detergent

Only use detergent made for dishwashers. Other detergents do not work well. They produce excess bubbles and cause the dishwasher to leak. Also, the dishes won't get clean. They may be covered with a film of soap. It's also important not to overload the dishwasher. If dishes are crowded together, they won't get completely clean.

Types of Dishwashers

There are two basic dishwasher styles. They are built-in and portable. *Built-in dishwashers* are built into cabinets. They have a permanent connection to hot water, a drain, and electricity. A *portable dishwasher* can be stored anyplace. When you plan to wash dishes, it's rolled to the sink. See 5-12. Each time it is used, you will need to attach its hoses to the faucet and plug it into an outlet. After the dishes are washed and put away, the dishwasher is rolled to its storage place.

Care and Cleaning

Always follow the directions in the care manual. Dishwashers are self-cleaning. They wash themselves as they wash the dishes. You may need to remove the drain screen and rinse it. Small bits of food may build up on it. The outside can be cleaned with a damp cloth.

5-12 Portable dishwashers are rolled to the sink when you want to wash dishes. They can be stored anywhere when not in use.

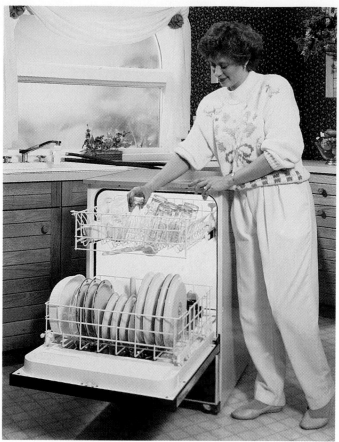

Whirlpool Corp.

Appliance Know-How

When you get a new appliance, always read the care manual before using it. See 5-13. It may work differently from your old appliance. The care manual will tell you how the appliance works. It also tells you how to clean it and use it safely.

If an appliance doesn't work, check for the following:

- Is it plugged into an outlet?
- Has the circuit breaker tripped?
- Are the controls set correctly?

If the appliance still doesn't work, write down the model and serial number. Then call the store where you bought the appliance or the company that made it. Explain your problem and ask how to get the appliance repaired or replaced.

5-13 Use and care manuals describe how to care for and clean appliances. Always read them before using a new appliance.

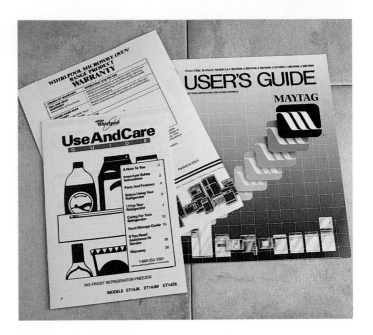

A ***warranty*** is the seller's guarantee that a product will perform as specified and will be replaced or repaired if it fails within a certain time. It will cost you little or nothing to replace or repair it. A *full warranty* covers the entire appliance. A *limited warranty* states conditions under which an appliance will be serviced, repaired, or replaced. For instance, you may be charged for labor costs or only certain parts may be covered. Read the warranties when shopping for appliances. Look for the appliance that offers the best warranty.

At Work in the Kitchen

You can save time and energy in the kitchen if it is set up in work centers. A ***work center*** is an area where a certain type of task is done. All the equipment, appliances, counter space, and storage space needed for the task are found there. Work centers save you time and energy because everything you need for a task is handy.

Most kitchens have three work centers. They are a preparation and storage center, cooking and serving center, and clean-up center. See 5-14. Large kitchens may include an eating center and a planning and message center, too.

Kitchen Basics

Saving Energy in the Kitchen

Major appliances use energy in the form of gas or electricity. Many people are concerned that the world's supplies of energy are becoming scarce. You can reduce the amount of gas or electricity used in many ways. This will lower your gas or electric bill. It also will conserve these valuable fuels. Here are some energy-saving tips to keep in mind.

Ranges
- Put a lid on pans heated on surface units whenever you can. The lid keeps the heat in the pan. Less heat escapes into the room.
- Match the size of pan you are using to the surface unit. Heat escapes if the pan is smaller than the surface unit.
- Contact your gas company if your gas stove's flames are yellow instead of blue. Yellow flames mean the gas is not burning efficiently.
- Preheat the oven only if your recipe tells you to do so.
- Open the oven door only when you need to do so. Every time you open the door, the temperature drops. More energy is needed to heat the oven again.
- Turn surface units or the oven off as soon as you finish cooking.

Refrigerators and Freezers
- Arrange foods so you can find them quickly. Decide what you need before you open the door. Less cold air will escape if you don't keep the door open long.
- Open the door as few times as possible.
- Check the door seal to be sure the door shuts tightly. Replace the seal if it is torn. Use the dollar bill test. Insert a dollar bill between the door and the refrigerator. If the dollar pulls out easily, the seal is not tight. It should be replaced.
- Keep the coils dusted. It takes more energy to cool a refrigerator or freezer if the coils are dusty.
- Defrost freezers before ice builds up to 1/2 inch thick. It takes more energy to keep a freezer cold if it has a thick ice coating.

Dishwashers
- Run dishwashers only when they are full.
- Arrange dishes so they will get completely clean. Dishes crowded into the dishwasher won't get clean. You will have to wash them again. This uses extra energy.
- Select a short wash cycle and the air-dry option. Dishes will get clean using less energy.

You can see from these energy-saving tips that saving fuels is simple. Ranges, refrigerators, freezers, and dishwashers can make your work easier and safer and use fuel efficiently. Microwave ovens are another appliance that conserves fuels. You will learn about these ovens in the next chapter.

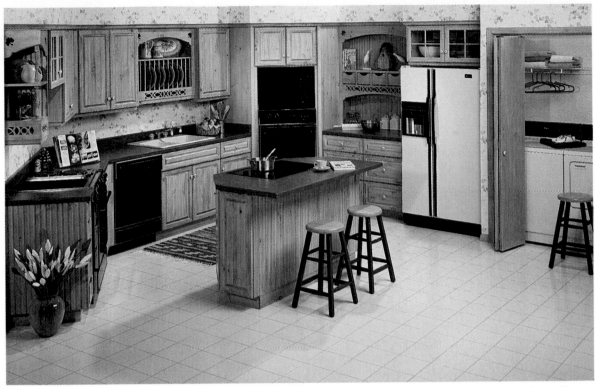

5-14 Can you identify the work centers in this kitchen?

Preparation and Storage Center

Foods are prepared and stored in the *preparation and storage center*. In many kitchens, the preparation and storage center is between the refrigerator and range.

The refrigerator and freezer are used to store foods that need to be kept cold. Cabinet space in this center is used to store foods that can be kept at room temperature. For instance, canned foods and dried food can be stored in cabinets.

Some kitchen equipment is stored in the cabinets in this center, too. Can openers, mixing bowls, measuring cups, and mixers are some of the equipment found here. This equipment is used to prepare foods for cooking. Storage containers, aluminum foil, plastic wrap, and freezer paper are kept here, too.

Counter space in this center is used to unpack grocery bags. It also is used to prepare ingredients. For instance, you may need to measure or blend ingredients.

Cooking and Serving Center

Food is cooked and placed in serving dishes in the *cooking and serving center*. The cooking and serving center includes the appliances that cook foods. It can include a range, microwave oven, and convection oven. This center is often near the eating center.

The storage space in this center is used for cooking and serving equipment. Cooking equipment includes pots, pans, pot holders, and wooden spoons. Serving equipment includes serving bowls, spoons, and tongs.

The counter space in this center provides a place to set ingredients. It is also a place to set hot pots and pans. Serving dishes are set on the counter and filled, too.

Clean-up Center

The clean-up center provides the water needed for cooking and cleaning. The clean-up center includes the sink. The dishwasher and nearby counter space are part of this center, too.

Foods are cleaned in this center. For instance, you could wash and trim fresh fruits and vegetables. Dishes, pots, and pans are washed here, too.

The kitchen equipment stored in this center includes knives, cutting boards, sponges, and dish towels. Detergent, scouring powder, and other cleaning supplies are also stored here. Some families store dishes and glasses in this center.

Eating Center

The *eating center* may be in the kitchen itself or in another room. Some kitchens have a counter or table where food is served. The eating center needs to provide space where people can sit to eat a meal or snack.

Planning and Message Center

Some kitchens have a *planning and message center*. This center includes counter space for writing menus and making shopping lists. It has a storage space for cookbooks.

A telephone and bulletin board may be found here, too. Family members can leave messages for each other on the bulletin board. This center also may include a computer.

In a Nutshell

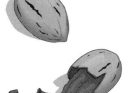

- Appliances make your work easier and safer.
- Foods are cooked on the surface units or in the oven of a range.
- Safety seals on appliances indicate the appliances have met safety standards.
- A convection oven blows hot air over foods to bake them.
- Refrigerators and freezers keep foods cold, slow the growth of harmful bacteria, and keep foods fresh longer.
- Cover foods stored in a refrigerator or freezer to keep them from drying out.
- Dishwashers quickly wash dirty dishes, pots, and pans.
- The best way to care for an appliance is described in its care manual.
- Work centers are where a certain type of task is done.
- Foods are prepared and stored in the preparation and storage center.
- Foods are cooked and put into serving dishes in the cooking and serving center.
- Foods are cleaned and dishes are washed in the clean-up center.
- There are many ways to conserve the use of gas and electricity in the kitchen.

In the Know

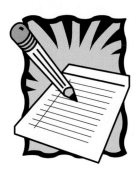

1. The two fuels used by ranges are _____ and _____.
2. True or false? A slide-in range has unfinished sides.
3. Explain why the cooktop should be cleaned after every use.
4. Describe how a convection oven differs from a conventional oven.
5. Give five tips for keeping your refrigerator clean.
6. True or false? Dishes washed in a dishwasher often have fewer bacteria than dishes washed by hand.
7. What is the advantage of setting up work centers in the kitchen?

8. Which would you expect to find in the cooking and serving center?
   A. Sink.
   B. Oven.
   C. Dishwasher.
   D. Refrigerator.
9. Which would you NOT expect to find in the clean-up center?
   A. Detergent.
   B. Cutting board.
   C. Range.
   D. Dish towel.
10. True or false? To save energy when using a range, avoid putting a lid on pans whenever possible.

What Would You Do?

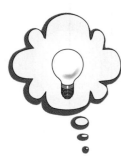

Your cousin is moving into her first apartment. She has asked you to help her unpack. She isn't sure which cabinets to use to store her kitchen equipment. Where should she put her kitchen equipment? What advice would you give her?

Expanding Your Knowledge

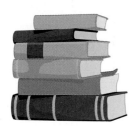

1. Visit an appliance store. Examine at least five different dishwasher models. Make a list of the features each offers. Also make a note of the prices. Which model do you think would be best for the school food labs? Why? Report your findings to the class.
2. Interview a kitchen designer. Ask the designer to show you pictures of a kitchen he or she designed. See if you can find each of the work areas. Find out how the person became a designer. You could ask the designer these questions. How did you decide to become a kitchen designer? What education do you need for this job? What information do you need before you design a kitchen? What is the most important thing to remember when designing a kitchen? What advice would you give someone who would like to be a kitchen designer?

3. Diagram a school foods lab or your kitchen at home. Make a list of all the items stored in each cabinet and drawer. Identify each work center. If this were your kitchen, how might you rearrange it? Why?

4. Read the care booklet that comes with a major appliance. Examine the appliance as you read the booklet. Make a poster that describes how a care booklet can help you.

5. Review a warranty for a major appliance. What does the warranty cover? When would you use a warranty? Why is a warranty important?

6. Design a bulletin board on energy-saving tips. Include as many ideas for saving energy in the kitchen as you can.

7. Keep a log of all the activities that take place in your kitchen. Also, list the people who participate in each activity. After keeping the log for a week, analyze it. How many hours is the kitchen used each day? Who uses it the most? Do you think the kitchen should be changed to make it more useful? What changes would you suggest? Why?

8. Research appliances and kitchens of the future. Create a bulletin board for your classroom.

9. Find out how Underwriters Laboratories tests appliances. Report your findings to the class.

Chapter 6

Cooking with Microwaves

Objectives

After reading this chapter, you will be able to
- ❏ explain how a microwave oven works.
- ❏ prepare foods in a microwave oven.
- ❏ describe microwave oven cookware.
- ❏ list safety tips for using a microwave oven.

New Terms

microwaves: a type of electromagnetic energy.

magnetron: a device that converts electricity into microwaves.

standing time: the period of time that occurs right after cooking time is up. During this time, the heat inside the food causes it to finish cooking. It also helps to evenly distribute heat inside the food.

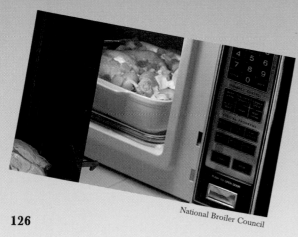

National Broiler Council

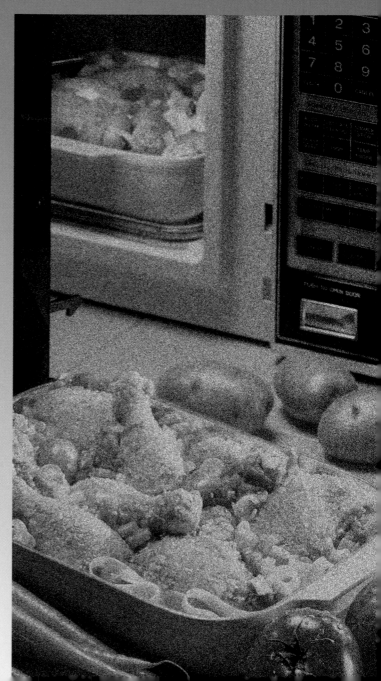

In a hurry? Need to make a meal in minutes? Maybe you need to make some waves. Microwaves, that is.

Many busy people with hectic schedules depend on this super time-saver. Microwaves help them make nutritious, delicious meals and snacks fast. People are using microwave ovens morning, noon, and night! These ovens are so popular that almost everyone eats food warmed, cooked, or thawed in this appliance at least once a day.

The use of microwave cooking has caught on fast. In the late 1960s, very few American homes had microwave ovens. Today, microwave ovens can be found in over 80 percent of American homes. Some even have two! More homes have microwave ovens than dishwashers! Many people rate microwave ovens second only to smoke alarms in importance.

How Microwave Ovens Work

Microwaves are a kind of electromagnetic energy. They are like the radio waves that carry your favorite songs. The ability of microwaves to cook food was discovered over 50 years ago. A scientist working with radar noticed that microwaves melted his candy bar. He began to study microwaves. This study led to the development of the microwave oven.

When a microwave oven is on, a *magnetron* converts electricity into microwaves. A fan scatters the microwaves around the oven. See 6-1. The microwaves cannot pass through metal. They bounce off

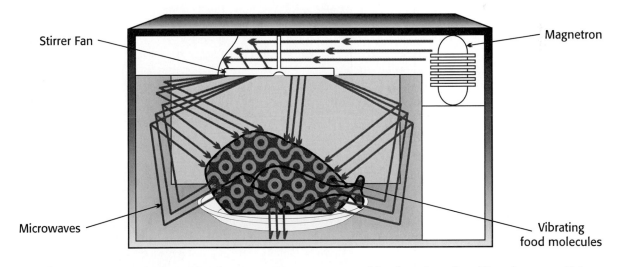

Stirrer Fan

Magnetron

Microwaves

Vibrating food molecules

6-1 The microwaves produced by the magnetron are scattered by the stirrer fan. They bounce off the oven's walls and are absorbed by food.

the oven's metal walls. They also bounce off the metal screen in the door. Foods inside the oven absorb the microwaves.

Microwaves make a food's molecules vibrate more than two billion times per second. The vibration causes friction. The friction produces heat. (If you rub your hands together, you will feel heat produced by friction.) The heat develops throughout the food and cooks it.

The number of microwaves produced by the magnetron is adjusted by the oven's controls. The most are produced when the microwave oven is set to "high." Microwave ovens are not set to a certain temperature like conventional ovens. They have power settings. See 6-2. Some microwave ovens have many power settings. Others have only one or two. The power setting you should use depends on the food you are preparing. The chart in 6-3 tells you which power setting is usually used for certain foods.

6-2 Microwave ovens have power settings that control the speed of cooking.

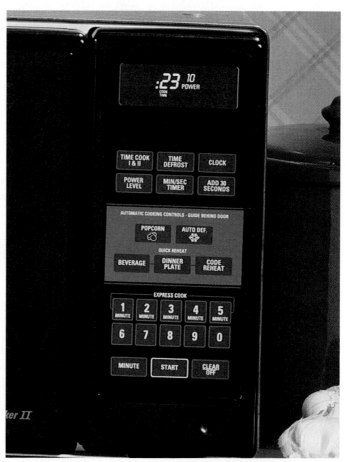

GE Appliances

6-3 Follow these general guidelines when trying to decide which power setting to use.

Power Settings Commonly Used to Prepare Specific Foods	
Power Setting	**Foods/Functions**
High	Fruits and vegetables Popcorn Sauces Soup Using a browning dish
Medium High	Some cakes Hot dogs Muffins Eggs Fish Tender meat Reheating leftovers
Medium Low	Melting chocolate Less tender meat
Defrost/Low	Defrosting frozen foods

Which Foods Can You Prepare in a Microwave Oven?

Almost anything you eat—from breakfast pancakes to a midnight snack—can be prepared in a microwave oven, 6-4. You can thaw frozen foods, heat leftovers, cook fresh foods, or heat packaged foods. Many food manufacturers package foods especially for microwave cooking. They call these foods *microwaveable foods*. See 6-5. Popcorn, puddings, pot pies, pizza, pasta, pretzels, and potatoes are just some of the microwaveable products. These foods come in containers that can be safely used in a microwave oven. Their packages also give directions for cooking the food in a microwave oven.

Some foods are more suited than others to microwave cooking. For instance, meats stay juicy. Many people think leftovers taste better when heated in a microwave oven than when heated on a range. Microwave cooking is a good way to prepare fruits and vegetables. They are tasty and retain the bright color they have when raw.

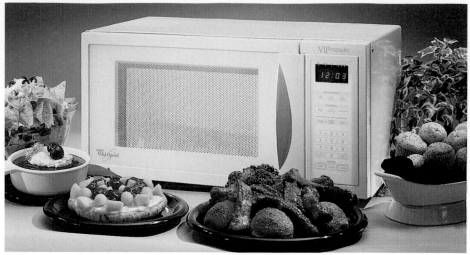

Whirlpool Corporation

6-4 Many delicious foods can be prepared in a microwave oven.

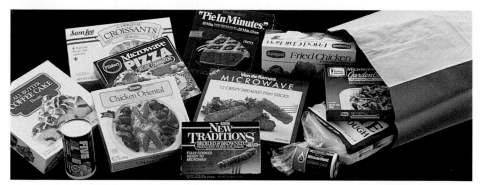

Sharp Electronics Corporation

6-5 These food packages include directions for microwaving the food.

Microwave ovens are great for many foods, but not all. Some foods, especially breads, turn out better in a conventional oven. Cakes, biscuits, bread, and muffins cooked in a microwave oven will be pale, not golden brown. They may look raw even when they are fully cooked. The hot air in a conventional oven causes foods to brown. The air in a microwave oven doesn't get hot enough to brown foods the way a conventional oven does. Foods also don't get crisp in a microwave oven the same way they do in a conventional oven. You could make a microwaved cake more appealing by frosting it. You could top a microwaved muffin with brown sugar. How do you feel about eating a biscuit that looks raw and doesn't have a crisp crust? What about a pizza with a moist (and soggy) crust?

To help microwave oven users make brown, crisp foods, food scientists have created browning pans and heat susceptors. *Browning pans* and *heat susceptors* are made of materials that absorb microwave energy. This causes them to get so hot that foods become brown and crisp. Browning pans may be sold with some microwave ovens. They also can be bought separately. Some microwaveable foods are sold in heat susceptor packages. A heat susceptor is a cooking tray or cover that works like a browning pan.

Microwave Oven Cookware

Microwave cooking is a lot like cooking in a conventional oven. There are some differences, though. One of the biggest differences is in cooking containers.

Microwaves must be able to pass through the cookware in order to cook the food. Microwaves can pass through glass, paper, and plastic. They cannot pass through metal.

Foods placed in metal cooking containers will not cook. The metal will reflect the microwaves away from the food. The reflected microwaves can damage the magnetron. Metal containers may cause sparks, flames, or a fire inside the oven. In some microwave ovens, you can use small amounts of aluminum foil. See 6-6.

6-6 Small amounts of aluminum foil can be used in some microwave ovens. The aluminum foil helps to protect areas of the food that might get overcooked.

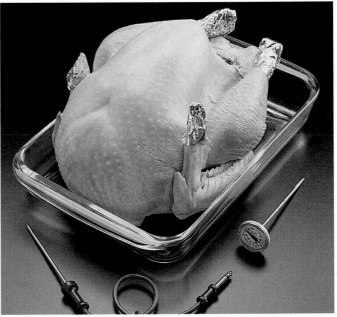

Sharp Electronics Corporation

You should check the appliance's care manual before using any metal or aluminum foil.

Microwave cooking containers are made of paper, glass, and plastic. See 6-7. You can buy special microwave cookware. See 6-8. You also can use paper towels, paper plates, waxed paper, plastic wrap, glass dishes, and some plastic dishes. Wooden skewers, straw baskets, and wooden dishes should not be used. These materials may dry out and burn in a microwave oven. Wooden dishes may warp and crack.

It's safest to use paper products that are labeled *microwave safe*. For instance, some paper plates are made of very thin paper. They aren't microwave safe because during cooking the paper may get soggy. Hot food might leak through the paper plate and burn you.

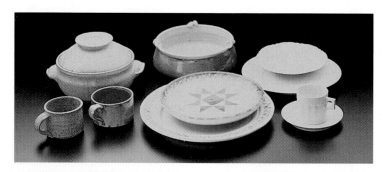

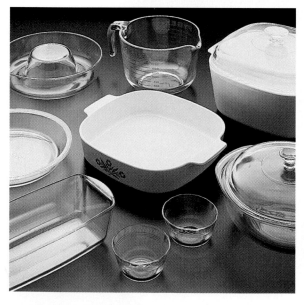
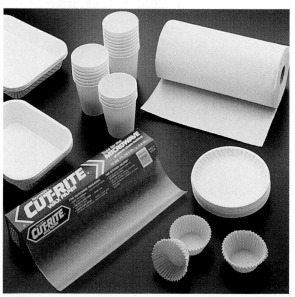

Sharp Electronics Corporation

6-7 These glass dishes and paper products can be used in microwave ovens.

6-8 You can buy special cookware and plastic wrap to use in microwave ovens.

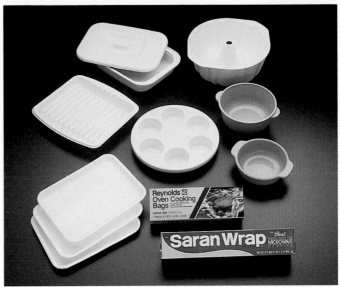

Some paper towels aren't microwave safe because they contain plastic threads that melt in a microwave oven. Brown paper bags and recycled paper products may contain tiny bits of metal or chemicals that burn in a microwave oven.

Some glass and plastic containers may not be safe to use in a microwave oven. Some plastics melt in microwave ovens. Dishes that have gold or silver trim shouldn't be used. The gold or silver is metal and will get very hot.

You can use this test to find out if a container is microwave oven safe.

1. Place the container in the microwave oven. Place a cup of water on top of the container.
2. Set the microwave on "high" and cook for one minute.
3. Carefully touch the container. If it feels cool, it is safe to use in a microwave oven. If it feels warm or hot, it is not safe to use.

Remember, browning pans and heat susceptors will get hot. Other safe containers should not get hot in this test.

Cooking with Microwaves

Microwave ovens are time and energy savers. See 6-9. Many foods cook in a fraction of the time they take to cook in a conventional oven or on a cooktop. Quick cooking means you save electrical energy, too. It also means that there is less time for heat to destroy nutrients.

Cooking Time

The amount of time and energy you save depends on the type of food being cooked. Most foods cook faster in a microwave oven than in a conventional oven or range. Fruits, vegetables, leftovers, bacon, and frozen dinners are examples. Some foods take about the same amount of time to cook in a microwave oven as on a range. Pasta and rice are examples.

6-9 Microwave ovens are a popular time-saving appliance.

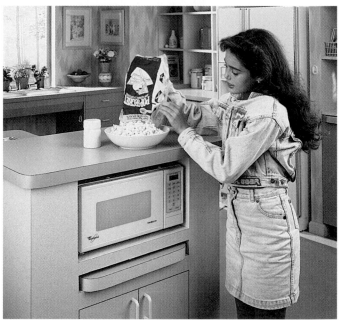

Whirlpool Corporation

Four factors affect cooking time. One factor is the type of the food. Foods that are spongy and dry cook faster than solid, moist foods. For instance, a muffin is a spongy, dry food. It heats faster than a solid, moist food like potatoes. Foods that contain large amounts of sugar and fat heat much more quickly than foods with small amounts of these ingredients.

The second factor that affects cooking time is the amount of food being cooked. Microwave ovens save the most time and energy when you prepare small to medium amounts of foods. For example, it takes about four minutes to cook one potato in a microwave or 15 minutes to cook four. It takes 50 minutes to cook eight potatoes. That's the same amount of time it takes in a conventional oven!

The third factor that affects cooking time is the size of the food pieces. Small pieces of food cook faster than large pieces. Long, narrow pieces cook faster than square chunks.

The fourth factor that affects cooking time is the location where foods are placed inside the oven. Foods placed toward the sides of the oven cook faster than foods placed in the center of the oven. This is because there are more microwaves near the sides of the oven and less in the center. Foods near the sides will get hotter than foods in other parts of the oven. A bowl of soup may feel warm in the middle and be burning hot on the edge.

Cooking time in a microwave oven is critical. A food can overcook in just a few seconds. Also keep in mind that the heat of the food will cause it to continue cooking for a short time after the oven is off. **Standing time** is the period of time that occurs right after cooking time is up. During this time, the heat inside the food causes it to finish cooking. Standing time also helps to evenly distribute heat inside the food. For instance, the cooking time for one slice of bacon is two to four minutes. Its standing time is the one to two minutes right after the cooking time.

A microwave cookbook can help you decide how long to cook a food. Cooking times and standing times mostly are listed as a range of minutes. It's a good idea to start out with the least amount of cooking time listed. It is easy to add cooking time to an undercooked food. Once a food is overcooked, cooking time cannot be reversed.

Science in the Kitchen

Investigating Microwaves

The size of the food pieces affects how quickly they cook in the microwave. Their location in the oven also affects cooking time. This is because more microwaves are found in some parts of the oven than others. This experiment will help you see how the size of food pieces affects cooking time in a microwave oven. It will also show you how location in a microwave oven affects cooking time.

Here's what you need to do. Wash two potatoes. Pierce the skin of one potato several times with a fork. Cut the second potato in half crosswise. Cut one half of the second potato into slices that are 1-inch thick. Cut the other half into slices that are ¼-inch thick.

Arrange the ¼-inch thick slices in a single layer on one side of a microwave-safe dish and the 1-inch thick slices on the other side. Put the potato slices and the whole potato in a microwave oven and cook on high power for 1 minute. Test for doneness by piercing the potatoes with a fork. Remove any potatoes that are done. Cook on high power for 1 minute and test for doneness four more times. Which potatoes cooked the fastest? Which cooked the slowest? Did the potato slices near the center of the cooking container cook faster or slower than the potatoes near the edge? How can you put these observations to work?

Cooking Evenly

Foods in some parts of a microwave oven get hotter than others. This uneven heating pattern causes part of the food to get hot while other parts stay cool. Food cooks more evenly in round or oval shaped cooking containers than in square ones. Foods in the corners of square containers overcook before the other parts get done. In a round or oval shaped container, the edges will cook before the center. To help the center get done at the same time as the edges, you could stir liquids. If it's a solid food such as a meatloaf, you could put it in a ring shape. See 6-10. If several small dishes are used, arrange them in a circle. See 6-11. You could turn large pieces of food such as potatoes or rotate the dish to help foods cook evenly. Some microwave ovens have a turntable to help foods cook evenly. The turntable rotates when the oven is on and rotates the food.

6-10 This glazed turkey loaf was shaped into a ring before it was cooked in a microwave oven. The ring shape helps the food cook more evenly.

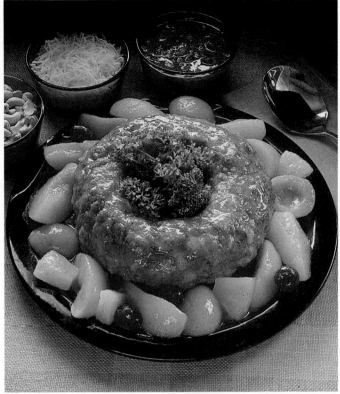

Whirlpool Corporation

6-11 Arranging cooking containers in a ring helps the food cook more evenly.

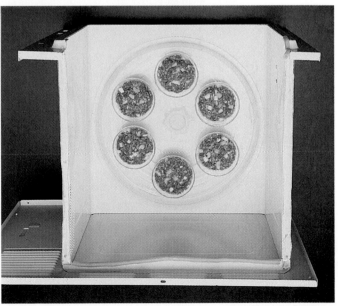

Sharp Electronics Corporation

Covering Foods

Foods that you want to stay moist need to be wrapped while they cook in a microwave oven. If you want moisture to be absorbed, such as when you cook bacon or hamburger, line the cooking container with paper towels. The paper towels will absorb the moisture produced during cooking.

Covering foods cooked in a microwave oven also helps food to cook evenly and reduces cooking time. Glass or plastic lids, paper towels, waxed paper, and plastic wrap can be used to cover foods. All covers should fit loosely so that steam can escape. Steam cannot escape when foods are cooked in tightly covered containers. The steam pressure may get so high that the container could burst or explode.

If you use waxed paper or plastic wrap to cover foods, use a steam vent to let steam out. To make a steam vent, fold back a small section of paper or plastic used to cover the cooking container. See 6-12. Also, be sure to keep the waxed paper or plastic wrap from touching the food. The food can become so hot that it could melt the wax or plastic.

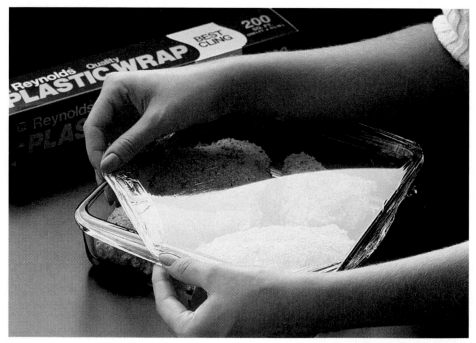

Sharp Electronics Corporation

6-12 Steam vents let steam escape. This will help prevent burns.

Microwave Oven Safety

Some people wonder about the safety of microwave ovens. Microwaves can harm you only if they escape from the oven and reach you. All microwave ovens have special features that protect you from exposure to microwaves. For example, the oven won't work if the door is open. When the closed door is totally sealed, no microwaves leak out. It is important to keep the door seal clean. If either the seal or door is bent or damaged, do not use the oven. Have a trained service person repair it before using it again.

Cooking with a microwave oven is a safe way of cooking. However, it's important to keep in mind that cooking with microwave ovens can be dangerous if certain safety guidelines aren't followed. There are some safety tips everyone should follow when using microwave ovens to prevent burns, fires, and explosions.

Avoiding Burns

Although the microwave oven does not get hot, burns can still result. These are ways to avoid burns when cooking foods in a microwave oven.

- Steam: When foods cook, steam builds up under the covers of cooking containers. Steam also builds up inside microwave popcorn bags. Be sure to remove covers and open bags by opening them away from you. This lets the steam escape and prevents steam burns.
- Jelly doughnut effect: Sugar heats very fast in a microwave oven. Foods, such as a jelly doughnut, may feel warm on the outside and be boiling hot on the inside. Sugary portions of foods get so hot they can burn your mouth and throat.
- Hot spots: Food in some areas of the oven get much hotter than others. Stir liquids after heating and carefully test the temperature.
- Oven location: Painful burns may occur if the oven is too high to be easily reached. For instance small children or short adults may reach up to pull out dishes and spill hot food on themselves.
- Cooking containers: Heat susceptors and hot food can make the cooking container fiery hot. Protect yourself with pot holders.

Preventing Fires

If a fire starts in your microwave oven, leave the door closed. Unplug or turn off the oven. The fire should go out when it uses up all the oxygen in the oven. If it doesn't, call the fire department.

To prevent fires in the microwave, you should be aware of what could cause them. The following should be avoided when cooking with a microwave oven:

- Cooking with large amounts of fat: This is dangerous in a microwave oven because fat heats quickly. Flash fires can occur.
- Arcing: Blue sparks, flames, or even a fire may occur when a metal container or aluminum foil touches the oven sides or door. Only use microwave safe cooking containers. If the use and care manual says aluminum foil is safe to use in your microwave oven, be sure to keep the foil from touching any part of the oven.

Avoiding Explosions

Some foods and containers can explode when using a microwave oven. This is because when water gets hot enough, it becomes steam. Steam takes up more space than water, so pressure is created inside the food or container, causing it to expand. If enough steam pressure forms, the food or container may expand so much that it explodes. To avoid explosions, follow these guidelines:

- Pierce the skins of foods such as potatoes, tomatoes, and hot dogs.
- Do not cook eggs in the shell. Crack eggs into a dish and pierce the egg yolk.
- Use loose-fitting covers, 6-13.
- Make a steam vent in waxed paper and plastic wrap covers.
- Slit plastic cooking bags.
- Never cook foods in an unopened can, jar, or bottle.
- Don't cook in bottles with narrow necks. If the opening is too small to let steam escape quickly, bottles may shatter, causing burns and cuts. Only use widemouthed containers.

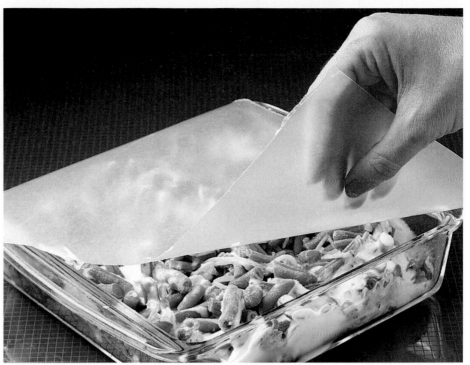

Whirlpool Corporation

6-13 Loose-fitting covers let steam escape.

Avoiding Possible Exposure to Microwave Energy

There are several tips to follow to avoid possible exposure to microwave energy. These include the following:

- Only use microwave ovens with doors that seal tightly. The tight seal prevents microwaves from escaping. Even with all the safety features, very tiny amounts of microwaves may escape. It's best to take two giant steps back from the microwave oven when you use it. That way, any escaped waves will dissipate before they reach you.
- Be sure not to run your microwave oven when it is empty. If an empty microwave oven gets turned on, there is nothing to absorb the microwaves. They may bounce back onto the magnetron and ruin it. Some families keep a cup of water in their microwave oven when they are not using it. If the oven gets turned on accidentally, the water will absorb the microwaves.

New Technology

Looking into the Future of Microwave Ovens

What will microwave ovens be able to do in the future? They will do more than just cook! There is a new microwave oven being developed that stirs, blends, mashes, and kneads food with a built-in blender bowl. It has a computer that automatically determines how long to cook a food and when to mix it. All you have to do is pick a food from the microwave oven's menu, and the appliance does the rest. It's almost like having a little cook inside the microwave oven! Another new microwave oven that's being developed reads the bar code on food packages. The oven uses the bar code information to determine how long to cook the food. It also decides which

power setting is best. Still another new microwave oven that you may see in the future fits on top of your plate. You will just position this small microwave oven over your plate, and it will start cooking!

Today, most microwave ovens are in homes. In the future, you'll also find them in cars! Dashboard dining is expected to take off in a few years when mini microwave ovens are expected to show up in the glove compartments of cars. Also, watch for more microwaveable foods that can be eaten with one hand. These foods will make it easier to drive and eat. That's really life in the fast-food lane!

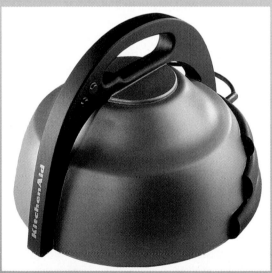

Kitchen Aid

In the future, microwave ovens may fit right over a plate.

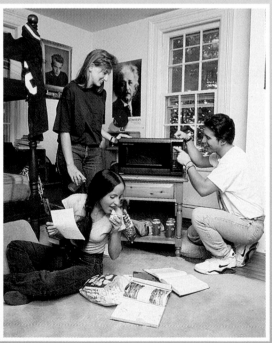

Sharp Electronics Corporation

Microwave ovens are often found in other places other than the kitchen.

Care and Cleaning

The use and care manual that comes with a microwave oven describes how to care for the appliance. Your microwave oven will last longer and the foods you prepare will be more tasty if you follow the manual's directions.

The oven is easy to clean. Food spatters don't bake onto microwave oven walls. That's because the appliance itself doesn't get hot. Cleaning the oven is as simple as washing it with a damp, soapy cloth. Always remember to wipe up spills. They will absorb microwaves the next time you use the oven. The microwaves they absorb can't be used to cook food. This can lengthen cooking time.

Microwave cooking clean-up is easy, too. Many foods can be cooked and served in the same dish. That means fewer dishes to wash. Microwaveable foods often can be cooked in their packages. These foods don't need a cooking dish at all.

Microwave ovens certainly can help you save time and energy. They make working in the kitchen easier. There are many other pieces of equipment that cooks can use, too. The next chapter explores the tools cooks use.

In a Nutshell

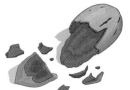

- Microwaves are a type of electromagnetic energy.
- Some foods, such as vegetables and leftovers, are more suited to microwave cooking than other foods.
- Baked foods do not get brown or crisp in a microwave oven.
- Microwaves pass through glass, paper, and plastic. Metal reflects microwaves.
- Microwave cooking time is affected by the type of food, amount of food, size of food pieces, and location where the food is placed inside the oven.
- Safety features help prevent microwaves from escaping from the oven.
- To use a microwave oven safely, use caution to prevent burns, fires, and explosions.

In the Know

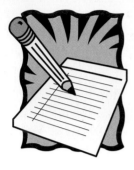

1. What part of a microwave oven converts electricity into microwaves?
2. True or false? Microwaves heat food by causing the food's molecules to vibrate.
3. Describe three differences between a microwave oven and a conventional oven.
4. True or false? Moist, solid foods cook faster than dry, spongy foods.
5. Foods cook faster in a microwave oven when _____.
    A. large amounts of food are cooked
    B. food is cut into square chunks
    C. food is placed near the sides of the oven
    D. food contains little fat
6. Which type of cookware is safe to use in a microwave oven?
    A. dishes with silver trim
    B. aluminum pans
    C. glass bowls
    D. None of the above.
7. Explain why you should wipe up spills and spatters from the microwave oven.
8. Explain why sealed containers may explode in a microwave oven.
9. Give three tips for avoiding explosions in the microwave oven.

What Would You Do?

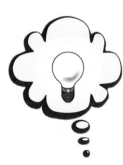

Suppose that your family has just bought a microwave oven. Everyone in the family knows that plastic, glass, and paper can be used to cook foods in the microwave oven. What advice would you give before they use any of these items to cook foods in the microwave oven?

Expanding Your Knowledge

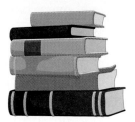

1. Compare muffins made in a conventional oven, microwave oven, and convection oven. Find a muffin recipe. Bake one-third of the muffins in a conventional oven. Bake one-third in a microwave oven. Bake the other third in a convection oven. Do a taste test. Compare their color, flavor, and texture.

2. Visit an appliance store. Examine four different microwave oven models. Make a list of the features of each. Write down the prices. Which model do you think would be best for a small apartment? Why? Report your findings to the class.

3. Take an inventory of the cooking equipment in a school foods lab or your kitchen at home. Make a list of all the items that could be used as cookware in a microwave oven. Test any cookware you aren't sure is safe to use. (Do not test metal items, since you already know they are not safe to use.)

4. Read the care booklet that comes with a microwave oven. Examine the appliance as you read the booklet. Make a small poster to tape to the microwave oven that describes how to care for it.

5. Design a bulletin board on microwave oven safety tips. Include as many safety tips as you can.

6. Compare the effect of cooking time on the quality of foods cooked in a microwave oven. Wash two stalks of broccoli. Place each stalk in a separate glass dish. Cover both dishes with plastic wrap that is vented. Microwave one dish on high for 1 minute. Allow to stand, covered, for 2 minutes. Microwave the second dish on high for 5 minutes. Allow to stand, covered, for 2 minutes. Conduct a taste test to compare the appearance, texture, and flavor of the broccoli. How does the broccoli cooked for one minute compare to the broccoli cooked for five minutes? Which looks most appealing? How can you use this information?

7. Observe how foods cooked in a microwave oven may not heat evenly. Place four cups of water in a glass measuring cup. Put the measuring cup in the center of a microwave oven and microwave it on high for 5 minutes. Do not move the measuring cup or stir the water. Use a thermometer to carefully measure the temperature of the water in the center of the measuring cup. Wait 10 seconds before reading the temperature. Don't let the thermometer touch the measuring cup. Record your findings. Now, place the thermometer at the edge of the measuring cup without letting it touch the cup. Wait 10 seconds before reading the temperature. Record the temperature. Stir the water for 15 seconds. Measure the temperature at the center and the edge of the cup again. Record the temperatures. How did the temperature of the water in the center of the cup compare to the temperature near the edge? What caused this temperature difference? After heating a liquid, what should you do before testing its temperature?

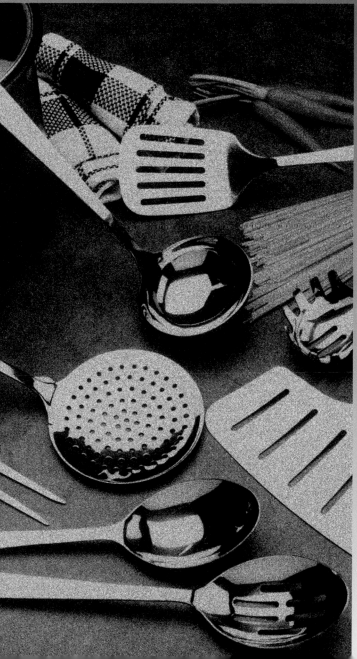

Chapter 7

The Cook's Tools

Objectives

After reading this chapter, you will be able to
- identify kitchen tools and small appliances.
- decide which kitchen tools and small appliances suit your needs.
- describe how to care for tools and small appliances.

New Terms

small appliances: electrical tools that can be moved easily from one place to another.
serrated: having a sawtooth edge.

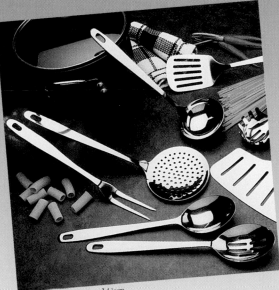

Progressive International Corp.

147

Almost every job requires some sort of tool. A *tool* helps you perform a certain task. For instance, artists use paintbrushes. Surgeons use scalpels. Writers use word processors. Cooks use rolling pins and blenders.

Tools make tasks easier and safer. For instance, it is easier to cut a pizza with a knife than to tear it with your hands. It is safer to reach a high shelf with a stepladder than a chair.

Cooks use many tools. That's because there are many types of jobs in the kitchen. To get ready to cook, you might measure, cut, or mix ingredients. During cooking, you may need to lift, turn, or drain foods. When you are finished cooking, you'll need to serve the foods. After the meal, it's time to clean up. Tools can help you do all of these jobs.

Small Appliances

Small appliances are electrical tools that make cooking easier. They can be moved easily from one place to another. Small appliances also save you time and energy. Small appliances can be used to perform many tasks. Mixers, blenders, food processors, and electric skillets are just a few examples of small appliances found in the kitchen.

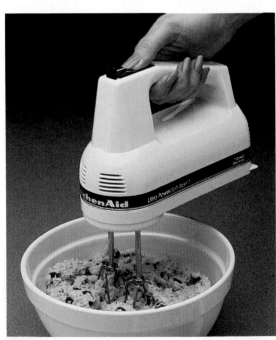

Mixer   KitchenAid Portable Appliances, St. Joseph, Michigan

Mixers are used to blend ingredients. They have a motor that turns the beaters. The most useful mixers have several speeds. Slow speeds are used to gently mix ingredients. High speeds are used to beat egg whites. Look for mixers with beaters that are easy to insert and remove.

⚠️ *Safety tip: Always unplug the mixer before inserting or removing the beaters.*

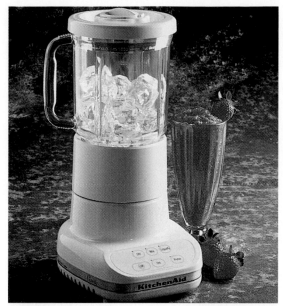

Blender KitchenAid Portable Appliances, St. Joseph, Michigan

Blenders have three basic parts. These include the base, container, and blades. The base contains the motor that turns the blades. The blades quickly cut, blend, and liquefy foods placed in the container. The best blenders have several speeds. Their containers have wide openings, sturdy handles, and pouring spouts. Blenders are easy to clean if the containers and blades are removable.

 Safety tip: Stop the motor before removing the cover. Wait until the motor stops before lifting the container off the base.

Food processors have the same three parts as a blender. However, they have more than one type of blade. Some blades are used to slice fruits and vegetables. Others grate cheese and grind nuts. Still others mix ingredients. The most useful food processors have blades and containers that can be washed in a dishwasher. The safest food processors only work when the cover is in place.

 Safety tip: Be certain the cover is locked in place before turning on the food processor. Wait until the blade stops turning before removing the cover.

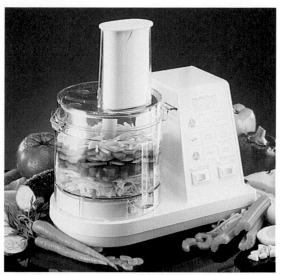

Food processor Hamilton Beach/Proctor-Silex

An *electric skillet* is a pan with its own heat source. It has a lid and a temperature control. You can cook foods in an electric skillet instead of using a cooktop or oven. Foods can be fried or roasted in an electric skillet. You can bake cakes in it, too.

 Safety tip: Unplug the electric skillet and let it cool before washing it.

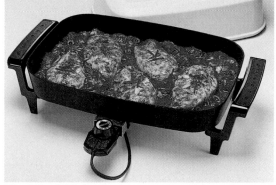

Electric skillet National Presto Industries, Inc.

Toasters brown both sides of bread at the same time. They have a control that lets you decide how brown the bread will become.

 Safety tip: Unplug the toaster before trying to remove foods that are stuck in it.

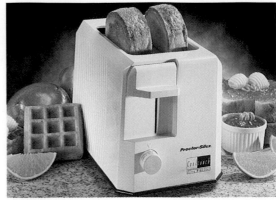

Toaster Hamilton Beach/Proctor-Silex

A *toaster oven* can do the same jobs as a toaster and full-size oven. It toasts bread and bakes small amounts of food. A toaster-oven uses less energy than a full-size oven. It doesn't heat up the kitchen as much as a full-size oven does.

 Safety tip: Unplug the toaster oven if a fire starts inside. Leave the oven closed until the fire goes out.

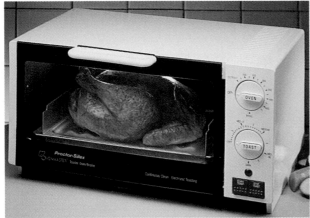

Toaster oven Hamilton Beach/Proctor-Silex

Coffeemakers brew coffee and keep it warm. The temperature is controlled by the coffeemaker. Some coffeemakers have a timer. The timer lets you set the coffeemaker to start at a certain time.

 Safety tip: Unplug the coffeemaker when the coffeepot is empty.
Set the coffeemaker in a place where the hot coffee won't get knocked over.

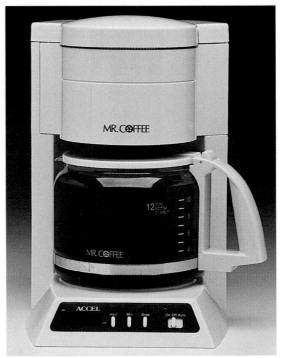

Coffeemaker Mr. Coffee

There are many other small appliances like these. Electric knives, can openers, woks, ice cream makers, waffle irons, and popcorn poppers perform special jobs. Before buying a special small appliance, check to see if you have another tool or appliance that will do the same job. For example, a large pan and cooktop can be used instead of an electric wok. Add a lid to the pan and you can pop popcorn.

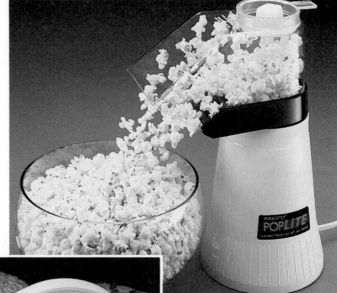

Popcorn popper   National Presto Industries, Inc.

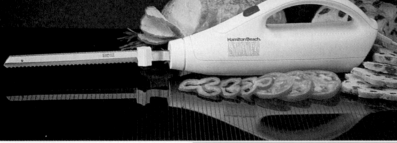

Electric knife   Hamilton Beach/Proctor-Silex

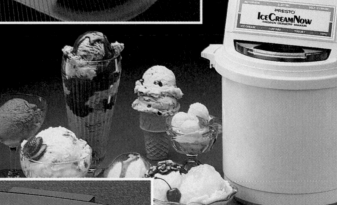

Ice cream maker   National Presto Industries, Inc.

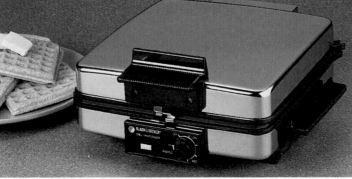

Waffle iron   Black and Decker

Measuring Tools

Many ingredients must be measured. This is because the directions for preparing a food usually call for a specific amount of each ingredient. If the specific amount called for isn't used, the food might not turn out right.

Ingredients are measured using liquid measuring cups, dry measuring cups, and measuring spoons. These measuring tools are available in both metric and standard measures. Measuring cups and spoons help you get the exact amount needed. It's a good idea to store them in the preparation and storage center.

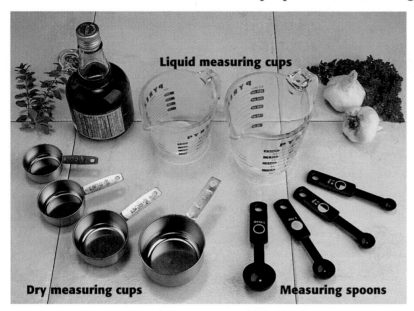

Liquid measuring cups

Dry measuring cups   Measuring spoons

Different tools are used to measure liquid and dry ingredients. *Liquid measuring cups* are used to measure liquids. Examples of liquid ingredients are water, milk, and syrup. *Dry measuring cups* are used to measure dry ingredients. Common dry ingredients are flour, sugar, and shortening.

Liquid measuring cups have handles and pouring spouts. Most are made of clear glass or plastic. Measurements are marked on the side of the cup. The top marking is below the edge of the cup to prevent spills. Liquid measuring cups come in many sizes. The most common sizes are 1-cup, 2-cup, 4-cup, 250-milliliter, and 500-milliliter. Some have both standard and metric measurements.

Most dry measuring cups are made of metal or plastic. They may not have pouring spouts. Dry measuring cups are often sold in sets. Common standard dry measuring cup sizes are ¼-cup, ⅓-cup, ½-cup, and 1-cup. The common metric dry measuring cup sizes are 50-milliliter, 125-milliliter, and 250-milliliter. To obtain accurate measurements, ingredients should be level with the top of the cup.

Kitchen Math

Going Metric!

There are two measuring systems often used in the kitchen. They are the *metric system* and the *standard system*. The United States mostly uses the standard system. The standard system includes teaspoons, tablespoons, cups, ounces, and pounds.

The United States is slowly changing to the metric system. Most of the world already uses the metric system. It is the system used by scientists.

The metric system is based on multiples of 10. It's easy to learn because it works like our money. For instance, the basic unit of money in the United States is the dollar. There are 10 dimes in a dollar. It takes 10 pennies to equal a dime. There are 100 pennies in a dollar.

The chart below shows common metric prefixes. It shows how they are added to the basic units of measure to show specific amounts.

Metric Prefixes

kilo = 1000 times the basic unit
A kilogram equals 1000 grams.

deci = $1/10$ of the basic unit
A decigram equals $1/10$ of a gram.

centi = $1/100$ of the basic unit
A centigram is $1/100$ of a gram.

milli = $1/1000$ of the basic unit
A milligram is $1/1000$ of a gram.

In the metric system, prefixes are added to the basic units to show specific amounts. These are the most common prefixes.

The liter is the basic unit of volume in the metric system. There are 10 deciliters in one liter. It takes 10 centiliters to equal one deciliter. There are 10 milliliters in a centiliter. It takes 1000 milliliters to equal one liter.

The gram is the basic unit of weight. There are 10 decigrams in a gram. It takes 10 centigrams to make one decigram. There are 10 milligrams in one centigram. A gram equals 1000 milligrams.

The following chart shows the metric amounts equivalent to common standard measurements. Today most recipes are written using standard measurements. Many new cookbooks are being written with metric measurements. Getting to know the metric system now will help you in the future.

Metric and Standard Measure Comparison

Metric	Standard
Volume	**Volume**
5 milliliters	1 teaspoon
15 milliliters	1 tablespoon
30 milliliters	1 fluid ounce
250 milliliters	1 cup
Weight	**Weight**
28 grams	1 ounce
454 grams	1 pound
1 kilogram	2.2 pounds

Metric measurements are similar to standard measurements.

Most measuring spoons are made of metal or plastic. They are often sold in sets. The common standard measuring spoon sizes are ¼-teaspoon, ½-teaspoon, 1-teaspoon, and 1-tablespoon. The common metric measuring spoon sizes are 1-milliliter, 2-milliliter, 5-milliliter, 15-milliliter, and 25-milliliter. Measuring spoons are used to measure both liquid and dry ingredients. Use them to measure amounts less than ¼ cup or 50 milliliters.

Cutting and Spreading Tools

There are many cutting, trimming, and chopping jobs in the kitchen. You will need several tools to do all these tasks. Like the measuring tools, cutting and spreading tools should be stored in the preparation and storage center of the kitchen.

Knives are used for many cutting tasks. Knife blades are made of metal. The blade may have a smooth or **serrated** (sawtooth) edge. Knife handles may be made of metal, wood, plastic, or bone.

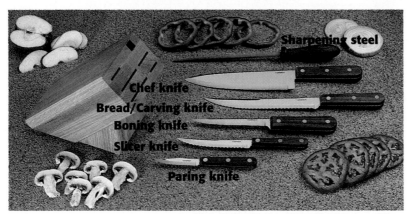

Tomer Cutlery–Division of Bemis Manufacturing and Nasco

The best knives have a hardwood handle that feels comfortable in your hand. The *tang* is the part of the blade that is attached to the handle. It should extend at least one-third of the way into the handle. At least two rivets should be used to attach the handle. A *sharpening steel* is often used to sharpen knives, but many people have them sharpened professionally.

There are many types of knives. *Chef's knives* have long, triangular blades. Use them to chop and cut vegetables and fruits. *Bread/carving knives* have serrated blades. They are used to slice bread, cake, and sandwiches without crushing them. They are also used to carve and slice large pieces of meat such as roast beef. *Boning knives* have long, narrow blades. They are for trimming fat from steaks and roasts, removing fins from fish, and deboning chicken. *Slicer knives* are used to slice cake, cut chunks of cheese, shred lettuce, and slice tomatoes. *Paring knives* have short blades. The skins of fruits and vegetables are removed with paring knives.

Other tools are used for cutting, too. A *vegetable peeler* is used to remove the skin from fruits and vegetables. You also can use it to thinly slice vegetables. Its blade floats over the food's surface and slices off very thin layers.

Cutting boards protect countertops from getting scratched when food is cut. Cutting boards may be made of wood or plastic. Plastic cutting boards are easier to clean than wooden ones. Bacteria and food odors can become trapped in the wood.

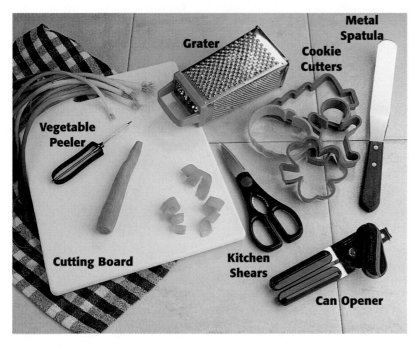

Graters are used to shred and grate vegetables and cheese. Most graters have at least two sizes of holes.

Kitchen shears can be used to snip fresh herbs. They also can be used to remove the skin from poultry and to trim vegetables.

Cookie cutters are used to cut cookie and biscuit dough into shapes. They come in many shapes and sizes. They may be made of plastic or metal.

Can openers cut through lids of metal cans to open them. Can openers may be handheld or mounted on a cabinet. Easy-to-use can openers have a sharp blade and handles long enough to be gripped easily. An electric can opener is a small appliance.

A *metal spatula* has a dull, long, flexible, metal blade. You can use it to spread frosting and smooth ingredients. Also, metal spatulas are used to loosen cakes, cookies, and bread from pans.

Mixing Tools

Mixing tools are used to make many foods. For instance, a sifter and pastry cutter are used to make biscuits and pie crusts. A wooden spoon is used to stir soups and sauces. A wire whisk can be used to whip cream. The most common mixing tools are shown here. These tools should also be stored in the preparation and storage center.

Spoons are used to mix and stir foods. They may be used to serve foods, too. Spoons come in many sizes and shapes. They may be made of wood or metal. Wooden spoons don't scratch pans and bowls. They also do not become hot when stirring hot foods. Metal spoons do get hot when stirring hot foods.

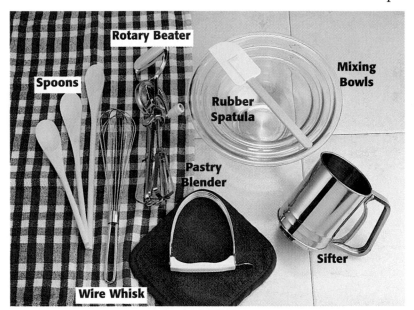

 Safety tip: Protect yourself from burns by using metal tools that have long, heat-resistant handles.

Wire whisks and *rotary beaters* are used to blend ingredients. Wire whisks come in many sizes. They often are used to whip cream or beat egg whites. Rotary beaters work like an electric mixer, except you provide the energy. The blending speed depends on how fast you turn the crank.

Pastry blenders are used to blend flour and shortening. They cut the shortening into tiny pieces that become coated with flour. You can do this task with two knives if you do not have a pastry blender.

Sifters add air to dry ingredients such as flour. They also blend and remove lumps from dry ingredients. *Wire mesh sieves* are used for the same tasks as sifters.

Ingredients are blended in *mixing bowls.* There are many mixing bowl sizes. Mixing bowls can be made of metal, plastic, or glass.

Rubber spatulas clean food from pans and bowls. You can use them to gently blend ingredients, too.

Lifting and Turning Tools

Lifting and turning tools move food from one place to another. For instance, a ladle is used to lift punch out of the bowl into a cup. A turner is used to flip a pancake over. Some common lifting and turning tools are shown here. Store them near the cooktop and oven.

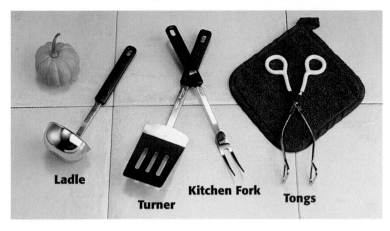

Ladle

Turner

Kitchen Fork

Tongs

Ladles are used to lift and serve sauces, soups, stews, and punches. Ladles look like a cup with a long handle.

A *turner* is used to turn hamburgers, pancakes, and eggs. You can use it to remove foods from a pan and serve pie or cake, too. A turner may be solid or slotted. It also is called a spatula.

A *kitchen fork* helps you to turn or lift large pieces of meat. You can use a kitchen fork to hold roasted meat or turkey in place while carving. Kitchen forks should have a long, heat-resistant handle.

Tongs can be used to lift and turn foods such as bacon and baked potatoes. They make it easy to remove food, such as corn-on-the-cob, from hot liquids.

Draining and Straining Tools

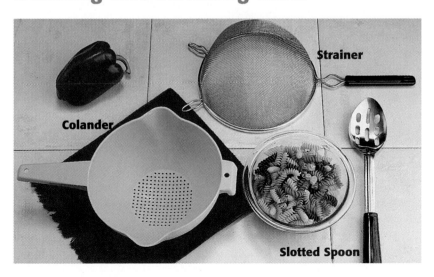

Strainer

Colander

Slotted Spoon

Draining and straining tools are used to separate liquid and solid foods. For instance, a colander separates noodles from the cooking water. These tools are shown here. They should be stored near the sink.

A *colander* looks like a bowl with many holes in it. It can be used to drain foods. You also can use it to wash fruits and vegetables. Colanders may be made of metal or plastic.

Strainers are used to remove solid pieces from liquid foods. For instance, you could pour brewed tea through a strainer to remove tea leaves. You could use a strainer to remove seeds from freshly squeezed lemon juice. Strainers come in many sizes.

Slotted spoons are used to remove solid foods from liquid. Slotted spoons should have long, heat-resistant handles.

Baking and Cooking Tools

Some cooking and baking tools, such as rolling pins and pastry brushes, are used to prepare foods. Store these tools in the preparation and storage center. Thermometers are used during cooking and baking. Cooling racks are used after cooking and baking. Store these items near the range.

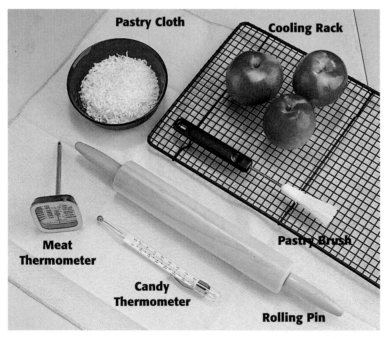

Cookie, piecrust, and biscuit dough are kneaded and rolled out on a *pastry cloth*. The pastry cloth keeps the dough from sticking to the counter. A *rolling pin* is used to flatten the dough. A *pastry brush* may be used to brush dough and other foods with butter or a sauce.

There are many types of *thermometers*. Oven-safe meat thermometers stay in roasts and whole turkeys. These thermometers measure the temperature of the food as it cooks. Instant-read thermometers are inserted in foods for a few seconds. You can use these thermometers to quickly check the temperature of almost any food. They can even be used for thin foods, such as hamburger patties. Deep fat thermometers measure the temperature of oil used to fry foods such as French fries. Candy thermometers measure the temperature of candy ingredients as they are cooking.

⚠️ *Safety tip: Always use a thermometer when heating oil. Oil that becomes too hot can suddenly burst into flames.*

Cooling racks let air circulate around the food. The foods are able to cool quickly. Cooling racks also keep hot pans off the counter. This prevents pans from scorching the countertop.

Special Tools

Many other cooking tools are available. Most special tools do only one or two jobs. For instance, a *nutcracker* only cracks nuts and lobster shells.

Often another tool can do the same job as a special tool. For example, a *pizza cutter* only slices pizza. A *garlic press* only crushes garlic. Both of these jobs could be done with a knife.

Many cooks only buy tools they will use often. For instance, if you serve tortillas only once a year, you can buy ready-made tortillas. If you serve tortillas often, a tortilla press may be an important tool in your kitchen.

Cookware and Bakeware

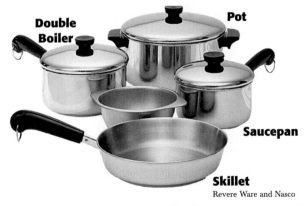

Double Boiler **Pot** **Saucepan** **Skillet**
Revere Ware and Nasco

Cookware and bakeware are used for cooktop, oven, and microwave oven cooking. Most cookware and bakeware is made of metal or heat-resistant glass. Some metal cookware has a special coating that keeps foods from sticking. Special plastic cookware is used in microwave ovens. Cookware and bakeware come in many sizes and shapes. It is best to store these tools in the cooking center.

Cookware is most often used for cooking on the cooktop. Some basic cookware is shown here.

Saucepans have one handle. *Pots* are the same as saucepans, except they have two handles. Some saucepans and pots have matching lids. Use saucepans and pots to cook foods in liquid on the cooktop.

A *double boiler* is a small pan that fits fairly tightly on top of a slightly larger pan. Food is placed in the top pan. Water is put in the bottom pan. As the water gets hot, steam rises and gently cooks the food. Double boilers are used to melt chocolate and cook sauces.

Skillets have a wide bottom and low sides. Some have lids. Skillets also are called frying pans. Foods fried in a small amount of fat are cooked in a skillet. A griddle is a skillet without sides. You can use it to grill sandwiches and cook pancakes.

Steamers are placed in saucepans or pots. They hold foods above boiling water. The steam rises and cooks the foods.

Woks often are used in Chinese cooking. They are shaped like large bowls. Woks are used to fry foods quickly in a very small amount of fat.

Bakeware is shown here. *Bakeware* is used in the oven.

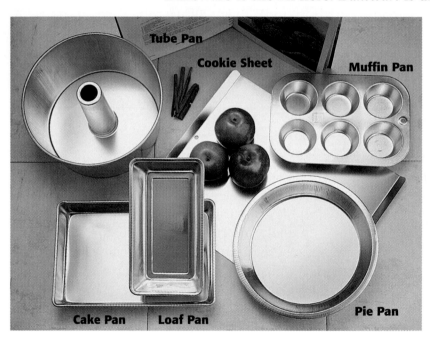

A *cookie sheet* is a flat sheet of metal with a low rim. You can bake cookies and pizzas and toast bread on it. Foods bake evenly on a cookie sheet. That's because there are no sides on the pan to block the flow of hot air.

Cake pans come in many sizes and shapes. Cakes and some cookies are baked in cake pans. One special type is called a *tube pan.* It is deep and round and has a tube in the center. A tube pan is wider at the top than at the bottom. The bottom may be removable. Angelfood and sponge cakes are baked in this type of pan.

A *muffin pan* is like many small, round cake pans connected together. You can bake muffins, cupcakes, and rolls in a muffin pan.

Loaf pans are deep, narrow, and long. They are used to bake bread, pound cake, and meat loaf.

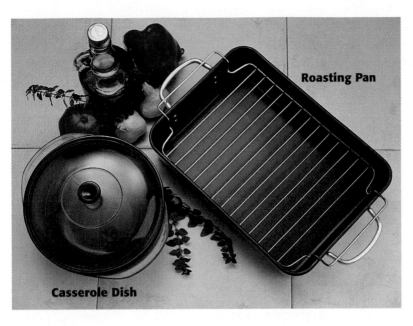

Pie pans are round and shallow. They have sloping sides. Pies and quiches are baked in pie pans.

Casserole dishes have high sides and often come with lids. Many entrees, side dishes, and desserts are baked in casserole dishes.

Roasting pans are large. They have low sides and a rack inside. Some have high, domed lids. You can use roasting pans to bake fish and roast meat or poultry.

Tableware

Tableware is all the items used to serve and eat a meal. Tableware may be fancy or simple. Your choice of tableware depends on your likes, budget, and type of meal. You might choose paper and plastic tableware for a picnic. You could use stemware, cloth napkins, and table decorations for a birthday dinner. Store tableware in the eating center.

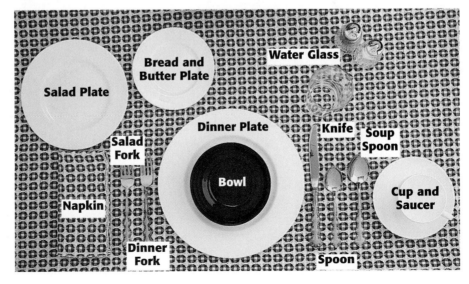

The tableware each person might need to eat a meal is shown on the previous page. Tumblers and stemware are called *glassware*. A *tumbler* is a glass without a stem. Juice is served in small tumblers. Iced tea, water, and other beverages are served in large tumblers. *Stemware* has a stem between the glass and its base. Any beverage can be served in stemware. Stemware is more fragile than tumblers. *Dinnerware* includes plates, saucers, bowls, and cups. Dinnerware may be made of paper, plastic, wood, or glass. It comes in many colors. *Flatware* includes forks, spoons, and knives used for eating. Flatware may be made of plastic or metal.

Serving utensils include large spoons and forks used to serve food. Most of these utensils are made of metal. They are placed on the table next to or in serving dishes. Beverages and foods are placed in hollowware. *Hollowware* includes pitchers, tureens, and serving bowls. Hollowware may be made of plastic, metal, or glass. It may match the dinnerware. *Serving trays* make it easy to carry many items to the table at once. You can also use a tray to carry used tableware back to the kitchen after a meal.

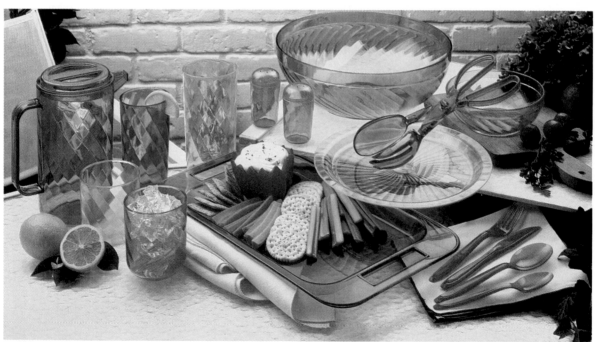

Serving Utensils

Hong Kong Trade Development Council

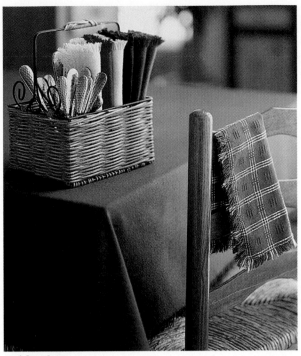

Table Linen   Spiegel

Table linen includes placemats, tablecloths, and napkins. Placemats and tablecloths cover the table and protect it. They also add color and interest to the table. A napkin is kept on your lap. You can use it to wipe your mouth and hands during a meal. Table linen may be made of paper, plastic, or cloth. It comes in many colors.

Table decorations add interest to a meal. The most attractive table decorations complement the other tableware. Many objects can be used to decorate a table. You could use candles, a flower arrangement, baskets, or fresh fruit. You can place the decorations anywhere on the table. The decorations should not get in the way of people as they eat and talk.

Cleanup Tools

Cleanup tools help you make the kitchen a clean, safe place. You will study more about the importance of keeping the kitchen clean in Chapter 9.

Most cleanup tools can be stored near the sink. These items include rubber gloves, scouring pads, sponges, a dish drainer, dish towels, and a scrub brush. You can store pails, mops, brooms, dust pan, and stepladders in a nearby closet.

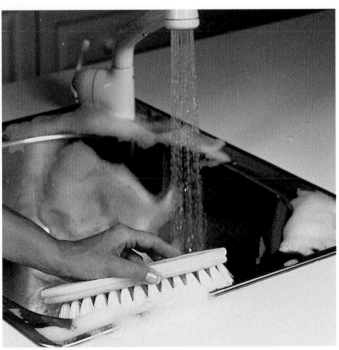

Scrub Brush   HMP Professional Cleaning Products

Buying Tools and Small Appliances

You have many choices to make when choosing kitchen tools and small appliances. Some special stores feature only these items. Department stores may devote a large area to selling these items. Discount stores often offer the best prices on kitchen tools and small appliances.

When you are deciding to buy a kitchen tool or appliance, think about your needs, the space you have to store it, and your budget. These and other factors can help you decide whether to buy a tool or appliance.

 Kitchen Basics

Buying Cookware and Bakeware

When shopping for cookware and bakeware, look for pots and pans with these features:

- Pots and pans should be sturdy. They should stand up to everyday use and last for many years.
- Pots and pans should conduct heat evenly. Copper, cast iron, aluminum, and stainless steel with copper or aluminum bottoms conduct heat evenly.
- Pots and pans should have a flat bottom, smooth finish, and no rough edges. The bottoms of pots and pans used on the cooktop should be the same size as a surface unit.
- Pots and pans should be well-balanced so they will not tip over.
- Pots and pans should be light enough to carry easily and safely. They should be heavy enough to last many years and not warp.
- Check the outside finish of bakeware. The outside finish of the pan affects how baked products will look. A shiny finish reflects part of the heat away from the food. A dull finish absorbs heat. Use a bright, shiny pan if you want a soft, light crust. Use a dark, dull pan if you want a darker, crisper crust.
- Pots and pans should be easy to clean. There should be no seams where food can build up.
- Handles on pots, pans, and lids should be heat-resistant. The handles should be securely attached. They should be large enough to grasp with pot holders.
- Lids should fit tightly. Loose-fitting lids let too much moisture and some nutrients escape.

Do I Need the Tool or Appliance?

Some tools and appliances are needed in almost every kitchen. These tools usually include measuring cups and spoons, knives, a cutting board, mixing bowls, pans, tableware, and dish towels. The other tools and appliances you need depend on the foods you prepare. For example, you can chop foods with a food processor or a knife. You can chop more food faster with a food processor than with a knife. If you seldom chop foods, a knife is all you need. If you chop large amounts of food often, you may need a food processor.

Many tools and appliances do the same job. For example, a strainer does the same job as a sifter. If you have a strainer, you can use it instead of buying a stifter. Also, two knives can do the same job as a pastry blender.

How Often Will I Use It?

Some tools and appliances are used often. For instance, mixing bowls, knives, and pans are needed to make many foods. You might use them every day. Others may get used only a few times each year. Tools and appliances that are seldom used can be borrowed or rented.

Do I Have a Convenient Place to Store It?

Many kitchens have limited storage space. You may have to store some tools and appliances in places that are hard to reach. It takes extra time to get out appliances and tools that are not handy. You may not use them much if they are not convenient.

Is It Easy to Use?

The most useful tools and appliances are easy to use. Tools and appliances are supposed to help you. If they are complex to use or set up, you may avoid using them. If you don't use them, they aren't helpful at all.

Is It the Right Size for Your Family?

Some appliances come in more than one size. For instance, some coffeemakers make only four cups. Others make 20 cups or more. Look for the size that is right for your family.

Is It Easy to Clean?

The easiest to clean tools can be washed in warm, soapy water or in the dishwasher. Cookware and bakeware that are easy to clean have nonstick surfaces. Appliances with smooth surfaces can be wiped clean easily. Cleanup time increases as the number of parts a tool or appliance has increases.

Is It of Good Quality?

Quality tools last a long time. They are sturdy and comfortable to use. For example, knives of good quality have hardwood handles that fit your hand. Quality kitchen shears open and close easily. Pots of good quality won't tip when they are empty.

Is It Safe to Use?

Check to see that a safety seal is on all electrical appliances. Such a seal indicates the appliance has met safety standards. Some appliances have important safety features. For instance, a mixer may shut off if the beaters get stuck. A food processor may not work if the cover is not locked in place. Look for smooth edges on tools and appliances. Rough or sharp edges can cause cuts.

Does the Appliance Have a Warranty?

A *warranty* is the seller's promise that a product will perform as specified and be free of defects. Check to see how long the warranty is in effect. Also check to see what the warranty covers.

Does It Fit into My Budget? _____

You can find most tools and appliances at a range of prices. The price depends on the brand, model, and the store. To find the best buy, compare the quality and features of different brands and models. Visit several stores and compare prices.

_____

Caring for Kitchen Tools

Kitchen tools last longer and perform better when they receive proper care. *Use and care manuals* often come with kitchen equipment. These manuals describe how to use, care for, and clean the equipment. Appliances and tools will last longer if you carefully follow the advice given in the manual. Clean electrical appliances with a damp cloth. Don't immerse them in water unless the manufacturer's directions say you can.

Glass, metal, and plastic tools can be washed in warm, soapy water. Most also can be washed in the dishwasher. Before washing plastics in the dishwasher, check the manufacturer's directions. Some plastics melt in the dishwasher.

Steel wool pads and scouring powder will scratch glass, metal, and plastic tools. They also damage nonstick finishes on pots and pans.

Wash and dry wooden tools as soon as you are finished with them. Soaking them or washing them in the dishwasher may cause them to crack or warp.

In the next chapter, you'll learn more about kitchen tools and how to use them safely.

In a Nutshell

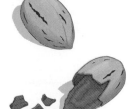

- Tools make tasks easier and safer.
- Small appliances are small machines that can be moved.
- Measuring cups and spoons help you get the exact amount of an ingredient needed for a recipe.
- Cutting and spreading tools are used to cut, trim, chop, and spread ingredients.
- Mixing tools are used to blend ingredients.
- Lifting and turning tools are used to move food.
- Foods are separated using draining and straining tools.
- Cookware and bakeware are used to cook foods.
- The best cookware and bakeware are sturdy, well balanced, and good conductors of heat.
- All the items used to serve and eat a meal are called tableware.
- Cleanup tools are used to make the kitchen a clean, safe place.
- Your appliance and tool needs depend on the foods you prepare often, your storage space, and your budget.
- Tools and appliances last longer when they are cared for properly.

In the Know

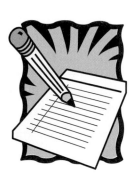

1. Explain how blenders and food processors are alike.
2. _____ _____ are used to measure small amounts of liquid and dry ingredients.
3. The _____ knife has a serrated blade.
   A. chef
   B. bread
   C. paring
   D. boning
4. Name four mixing tools.
5. Which lifting and turning tool would be best for removing food from hot liquids?
6. When buying cookware, which features should you look for?
   A. Pots and pans with loose-fitting lids.
   B. Pots with a rough finish.
   C. Pots and pans that distribute heat evenly.
   D. Very thin, lightweight pots and pans.
7. Explain how saucepans differ from pots.
8. A _____ _____ is a flat, metal pan with a low rim.
9. True or false? The best way to clean glass and plastic tools is to use steel wool pads.
10. List three factors to consider when buying a tool or appliance.

What Would You Do?

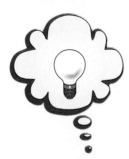

Your older brothers are moving into their first apartment. They have a tight budget. They know they need to buy some kitchen tools. They aren't sure what to buy. How can they decide what to buy? What would you suggest they buy?

Expanding Your Knowledge

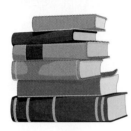

1. Visit the housewares section of a department store. Make a list of the types of kitchen tools you see. Do some research to find out how tools not covered in the chapter are used.

2. Select an appliance in your school or home kitchen. Read the care manual that came with it. Practice using the appliance. Prepare a demonstration showing how to use it. Include safety tips in your demonstration.

3. Arrange a tour of a restaurant's kitchen. Ask the chef to show you the tools used in the restaurant. Ask the chef to explain how the tools are used. How do the tools differ from the ones you use at home? Ask the chef to demonstrate how to use a sharpening steel.

4. Make an inventory of the tools in the school kitchen. Find out how to use any unfamiliar tools. Also note where the tools are stored. Are they stored in a convenient location? Are there any changes in storage location you would recommend?

5. Visit the dinnerware, flatware, and glassware section of a department store. Note the materials used to make the tableware. Also, note the prices. Write a report describing what you saw.

6. Select four recipes from a cookbook. Make a list of all the tools needed to prepare the foods.

7. Create an idea book of simple table decorations. For example, in the autumn you could use a basket of colored leaves and nuts. A Valentine's Day table decoration could be a heart-shaped cake.

8. Do some research to find out about all the materials that can be used to make cookware. Make a poster describing the advantages and disadvantages of each type of material.

9. Interview an elderly person. Ask him or her to describe kitchen tools used in the past that are not used today. Write an article for the school newspaper to share your findings.

Chapter **8**
Play It Safe!

Objectives

After reading this chapter, you will be able to
- ❑ identify safety hazards in the kitchen.
- ❑ prevent kitchen accidents.
- ❑ explain how to help an accident victim.

New Terms

carbon monoxide: a colorless, odorless deadly gas.

first aid: treatment given right after an accident that helps to relieve pain and prevent further injury.

cardiopulmonary resuscitation (CPR): a lifesaving technique that helps save a victim who isn't breathing and whose heart has stopped.

antidote: a substance that works against a poison.

abdominal thrust: a technique that can help save a choking victim.

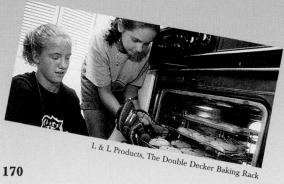

L & L Products, The Double Decker Baking Rack

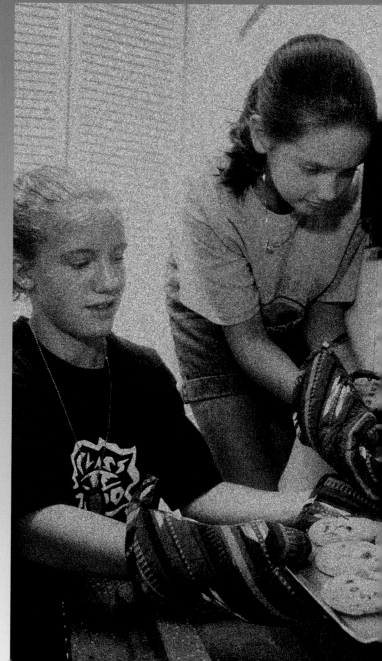

Kitchens are warm, inviting places where tasty foods are prepared. However, many dangers lurk there. In fact, more accidents occur in the kitchen than in any other room. Thousands of people are hurt in kitchen accidents every year.

Did you ever cut yourself while slicing an apple? Have you burned your finger on a hot pan? Did you ever slip on a wet floor and fall down? If so, you have been a victim of a kitchen accident. This chapter describes how to work safely in the kitchen. It also explains what to do if an accident happens.

Preventing Kitchen Accidents

Knives are sharp. Ovens and pans can be fiery hot. Wet floors are slippery. Everyone knows these facts! Why, then, are so many people injured in the kitchen every day?

Accidents are caused when people don't know the safe way to work. Being careless causes accidents, too. Some people think that accidents happen so fast you can't do anything to stop them. In most cases, that's not true. You can prevent many accidents. A little care and knowing how accidents occur helps you to stop most accidents before they happen.

To Prevent Cuts

Cuts can be caused by many things. Sharp kitchen tools, such as knives, graters, and the blades in blenders, are the most common cause. Broken glass and the edges of lids from opened cans can cause cuts, too.

Small cuts are painful and can become infected. Large, deep cuts are especially dangerous. A person can bleed to death in a few minutes. To protect yourself, keep these safety points in mind when using knives.

- Always pick up a knife by its handle. To give a knife or sharp tool to another person, lay it on the counter. Let the other person pick it up from the counter. This way, no one has to touch the blade.

Kitchen Basics

How Do Accidents Happen?

Many accidents are caused by a chain of events. The first three links in the chain lead up to the accident. The fourth link is the accident itself. The last link is the injuries or damage the accident causes. You can prevent accidents by breaking the first three links of the chain. Here is an example of how the chain of events might occur.

- **Link 1** - *The Setting:* Jack, who is in eighth grade, is making a special spaghetti dinner for his parents. His five-year-old sister, Marla, is helping him. Jack begins by putting a pan of water on the range to boil. Then, he and Marla set the table.
- **Link 2** - *Careless Habit:* As a cook, Jack is often in a hurry. He knows how to prepare many foods, but forgets to take the time to follow basic safety rules. For instance, he may leave a pan handle turned outward so that it extends over the edge of the range. Sometimes he stands on a chair to reach a high shelf.
- **Link 3** - *The Unsafe Action:* Tonight is like other nights. Jack left a pan handle turned outward.
- **Link 4** - *The Accident:* Dinnertime is near. While Jack is busy putting the salad on the table, Marla decides she wants to help cook the meal. She is small and can't see the cooktop. Last week she saw Jack stand on a chair to

reach a high shelf. So, she pulls a chair over to the range. As she steps onto the chair, her head bumps the pan handle. The pan falls off the cooktop. The chair tips over.

- **Link 5** - *The Outcome:* Marla fell on the floor and was soaked with the water from the pan. This time, Marla was very lucky. She could have been badly burned and broken some bones. Luckily, the water was only warm. It made her wet and upset, but she was not burned. Falling off the chair gave her a few small bruises.

Marla's accident could have been prevented. What would you do to break the first three links in the chain of events?

It's easy to prevent accidents when you keep safety in mind. Injuries are painful. Some are deadly. So, it pays to be careful.

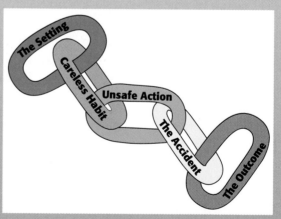

Gene R. DeFoliart

Accidents can be prevented by breaking links one, two, or three.

- Keep knives sharp. A sharp knife is safer than a dull knife. This may surprise you, but a sharp knife cuts through food easily. If a knife is dull, you will need to press harder to get it to cut the food. Hard pressure can cause the knife to slip and may cause you to cut yourself instead of the food.
- Cut away from your body and others. Also, keep your fingers out of the way. If the knife slips, no one will get hurt.
- Use kitchen knives only to cut food. The blade can break if it is used to pry open a can, saw cardboard boxes, or tighten a screw.
- Wash knives one by one. Keep them separate from other dishes so that they aren't hidden. Also, don't let knives soak in soapy water. You might not see them when you reach into the water.
- When loading a dishwasher, place the tips of knives and other sharp tools pointing down into the utensil basket.
- Store knives in racks or special containers. See 8-1. If they are stored loose in drawers, you could cut yourself badly when you reach into the drawer.

8-1 Special storage racks provide a safe way to store knives.

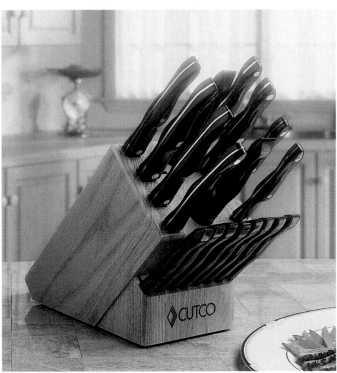

Cutco Cutlery, Olean, NY

Other items in the kitchen also can cause cuts. Follow these safety practices.

- Use a can opener that leaves a smooth edge. Ragged edges are very dangerous. Open the can completely and remove the lid. Leaving the lid attached to the can or bending it can cause painful cuts.
- Keep your fingers away from the blades in blenders and food processors. Unplug the appliance if food becomes stuck in the blades or if you need to remove the blades.
- Discard cracked or chipped glasses and cups.
- Sweep up broken glass right away. Don't pick it up with your fingers. Wipe up the tiny slivers with a damp paper towel. If a glass or dish breaks in the sink, wrap your hand in a towel. Slowly find the drain and open it. When the sink is empty, use the towel to remove the broken pieces.

To Prevent Falls

Falls are the most common cause of accidental death in the home. They also cause serious injuries such as broken bones. A wet floor, objects left laying on the floor, and chairs used as ladders can cause falls.

Here are some ways to avoid falls.

- Keep floors clean and dry. Just a little water or food makes floors slippery. Always wipe up spills right away. If the floor is wet, wait until it dries before walking on it.
- Be sure all rugs have a nonskid backing. These rugs do not slide easily. You will be less likely to slip on rugs with this backing.
- Keep the walkways in the kitchen clear. Open drawers, electrical cords, toys, shoes, and other objects may trip you.
- Use a sturdy stepladder to reach high shelves. See 8-2. A chair, box, or wobbly ladder may tip over.

To Prevent Burns

Burns can be caused by hot appliances, hot dishes, hot food, hot water, or steam. Minor burns make the skin red and sore. Blisters may form. Major burns can destroy skin and nerves.

8-2 A sturdy stepladder helps you reach high shelves safely.

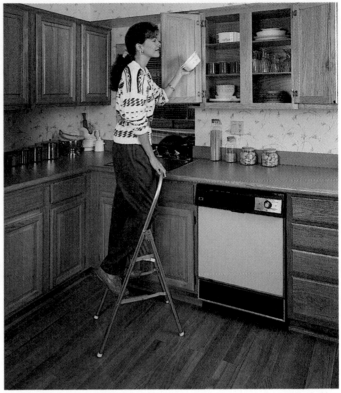

Kellar Ladders

Many people get burned in the kitchen every year. Some die from these burns. You can avoid burns by following these safety measures.

- Avoid wearing loose-fitting clothes or long sleeves when you cook. Clothes and hair can burn. Be sure to tie back long hair.
- Avoid reaching across a hot surface unit. The heat from the unit can scorch or burn your skin or clothes.
- Fill pots and pans no more than two-thirds full. A pot or pan that is filled too full may boil over. The hot liquid can cause severe burns.
- Turn the handles of pans toward the back of the range. See 8-3. If handles stick out over the edge of the range, pans might get knocked off. Also, be sure the handles don't project over a hot surface unit. The hot surface unit will heat the handle and make it fiery hot.
- Open a pan lid by tilting the lid up from the back of the pan. This method lets the steam escape away from you and prevents steam burns. Steam is hotter than boiling water and can cause serious burns.

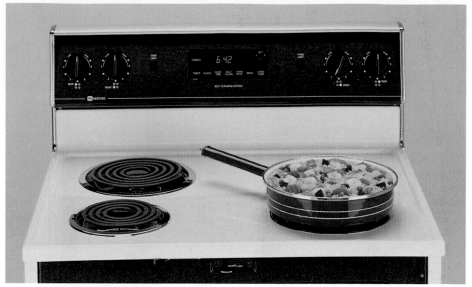

8-3 By turning the handles of pans inward, you can prevent them from being knocked off the range.

- Pick up hot pots and pans with thick, dry pot holders. If the pot holder is damp, the water in it heats up when it touches a hot pan. The heated water can burn you. Use pot holders that are thick and large enough to protect your hands. If the pot holder is too large, it may touch the surface unit and catch fire.
- Serve hot foods with care. A ladle, tongs, or serving fork can help you transfer hot food to plates or cups. Pot holders protect your hands when carrying containers of hot food to the table.
- Avoid reaching into a hot oven. Instead, use a pot holder to pull the oven shelf out. Then you can remove the pan.
- Close the door of a hot oven as soon as you put food in or remove it. People, especially young children, may touch the open door and get burned. Also, never use the oven to heat the kitchen.
- When you are finished cooking, be sure to turn off the surface units and oven. Keep in mind that some surface units can stay hot for a long time after they are turned off. Even though surface units don't look hot, they can still cause a burn.
- Water from the faucet can be very hot. Carefully test it before putting your entire hand in it. You may need to adjust the faucet to make the water cooler.

To Prevent Fires _____

Every year, fires and smoke kill many people. Fires leave a large number of families homeless.

For a fire to start, three ingredients are needed: fuel, heat, and air. Fuel can be paper, cloth, wood, gas, or food. Oil and fat are two foods that burn very easily. Fuel cannot burn without heat. A match, electrical wire, oven, surface unit, or cigarette can provide heat. Fires need oxygen from the air to burn.

If any one of these three factors is missing, a fire cannot burn. You can prevent or stop a fire by removing the fuel, heat, or air. The following points can help you prevent fires.

- Don't overload outlets. Most circuits are designed for two plugs. Overloaded outlets can become hot enough to burn. They are a major cause of electrical fires.
- Store matches and lighters in a secure place. Keep them out of the reach of children.
- Store towels, paper, pot holders, cookbooks, and plastic items away from the range. Also keep curtains and cloth-covered furniture away from the range. Cloth and paper items burn easily. Plastic may melt and produce toxic fumes.
- Keep appliances clean so that grease doesn't build up. Grease catches fire easily.
- Don't use aerosol sprays near a hot cooktop or oven. The heat may cause the spray to flame.
- When cooking with oil, watch it closely. Hot oil can easily catch fire.
- If the flame of a gas oven goes out, turn off the gas. Then, open the oven door and air out the room. When relighting it, always light the match first then turn on the gas.
- If you smell gas, turn off the range controls. Open a window to let the gas escape. Do not try to light the range. It could cause an explosion. Alert others in the house to leave. Call the gas company from a neighbor's house and ask them to inspect the range and gas lines.
- Install smoke alarms, 8-4. These appliances warn you when smoke is in a room. Smoke alarms save thousands of lives and homes every year.
- Keep a fire extinguisher handy. Be sure to learn how to use the fire extinguisher before a fire starts.

8-4 Smoke alarms check the air in a room. If smoke passes through it, the smoke alarm warns you.

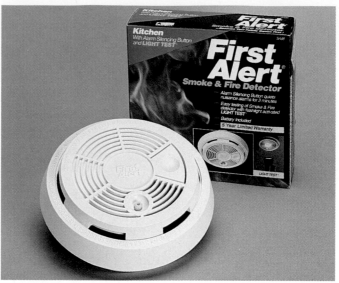

First Alert

Extinguishing Fires

Fires may start even when you carefully follow safety rules. This makes it important to know what to do if a fire does occur. Acting quickly and calmly can save your life, 8-5.

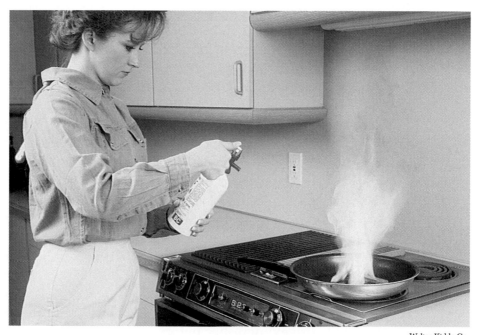

Walter Kidde Co.

8-5 Knowing how to use a fire extinguisher can help you stop a fire quickly.

If food cooked on the cooktop catches fire, here's how to put it out.

1. Turn off the heat if you can safely reach the controls.
2. Put the fire out with a fire extinguisher. You also can throw salt, baking soda, or flour on the fire to put it out. Placing a lid on the pan will put the fire out, too. Only put the lid on the pan if you won't get burned.

Do not do the following:

- Never try to put the fire out with water. If the food contains fat, the water will make the fat spatter. The spattered fat may spread the fire.
- Don't carry the flaming pan to the sink. You may spill the burning food. This can spread the fire and cause you to get burned, too.

This is how to extinguish oven fires.

1. Turn off the oven.
2. Leave the oven door closed. The fire will go out as soon as it uses all the oxygen in the oven. If you open the door, more oxygen goes to the fire. The fire may spread. Microwave oven fires are extinguished in the same way. If you can, unplug the microwave oven if a fire occurs.

If your clothing is on fire, this is how to put it out.

1. Do not run around because this will cause the fire to spread. Instead, stop and drop to the floor.
2. Roll on the floor until the fire is out. If a blanket is nearby, wrap yourself in it. It will reduce the fire's oxygen supply which helps to put out the fire.

Make a fire action plan before a fire starts. A fire action plan can help families be ready for any fire emergency. Here's how to make a fire action plan.

1. Plan an escape route from every room in your home. The whole family needs to know the fastest way to get out in case of fire.
2. Practice fire drills often. Everyone in the family needs to know what to do if a fire starts.

If you can't bring a fire under control quickly, put your fire action plan into motion. Alert others to get out quickly. If you need to escape from a burning building, keep your head below the smoke. You may need to crawl on the floor. If it's smoky, put a towel or pillow over your mouth and nose. If the door out of the room feels hot, don't open it. Instead, go to a window and let firefighters know you are inside. Once you escape, do not return to the burning building. Go to a neighbor's and call the fire department. If you live in an apartment, pull the fire alarm.

To Prevent Electric Shock

Electricity powers many kitchen appliances. These appliances save you time and energy and make your work easier. Electricity is helpful, but it can shock, burn, or kill you.

When electricity passes through your body, it creates heat that causes burns inside your body. The electricity may paralyze nerves and muscles and cause you to stop breathing. It may cause your heart to stop, too.

You can prevent accidents with electricity if you keep these points in mind.

- Worn or damaged plugs and cords can cause shocks. Plugs and cords can be damaged if you pull on the cord instead of the plug, 8-6. Also, placing cords under rugs can cause the cord's covering to wear through.
- Arrange the cord so others won't trip over it. Also, place it so that you won't get caught in the cord and pull the appliance off the counter.
- If an appliance has a cord that can be removed, plug the cord into the appliance first. Then, plug the cord into the electrical circuit. Unplug small appliances when you are not using them. Parts of the appliance may have electricity flowing through them even when the switch is off.
- If something seems to be wrong with an appliance, don't use it. Unplug it and have a trained service person examine it.
- Avoid using extension cords. If you must use one, select a heavy-duty one. Be sure the extension cord matches the appliance's plug. Some appliances have a plug with two prongs, others have three prongs.

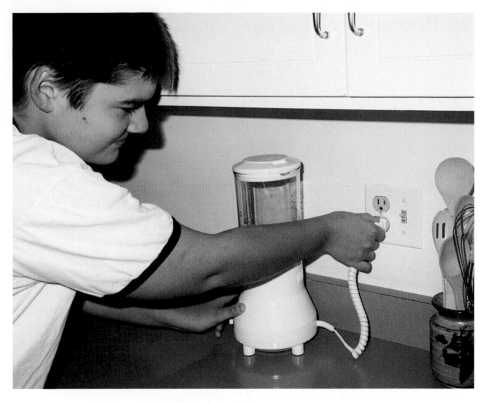

8-6 Always unplug an appliance by pulling on the plug instead of the cord.

- Don't overload circuits. Overloading them could cause a shock or fire.
- Food may get stuck in an appliance, such as bread in a toaster. If this happens, unplug the appliance and carefully remove the food. Never put a metal utensil in an appliance that is plugged in. You could get shocked.

Water and electricity don't mix. Here's how to prevent painful injuries and death caused by electrical shocks.

- Do not place appliances near water such as sinks and water pipes. If an appliance falls into water, unplug it right away. Do not reach into the water until the appliance is unplugged.
- Dry your hands before using an electrical appliance.
- Don't stand on a wet floor when using an electrical appliance.
- Unplug small appliances before washing or cleaning them.

To Prevent Poisonings

You may not realize that some of the products you use every day are deadly poisons. Household cleaning products such as dish washing detergent, ammonia, window cleaner, and bleach are poisons. Insect spray, gasoline, paints, lotions, and alcohol are poisons, too. Vitamin supplements and medicines can be harmful if they are not taken correctly.

Poisons can enter your body through three routes. They can enter through your nose and lungs if you inhale them. Poisons can enter through your mouth if you eat or drink them. Some can pass through your skin when you touch them. When you work with substances that can be poisonous, be sure to prevent them from entering your body.

Many people, especially children, are poisoned every day. To prevent poisonings, keep these safety points in mind.

- Before using a household cleaner, insect spray, or medicine, read the directions and warnings on the package. Use these products only as directed.
- Use spray products only in well-ventilated areas. Point the spray nozzle away from you. Never spray toward other people or inhale the spray yourself.
- Wear rubber gloves to prevent harmful substances from touching your skin. Cover your mouth and nose with a face mask to keep from inhaling dangerous fumes. You can buy gloves and masks at hardware stores.
- Never mix household cleaning products. Some produce deadly fumes when mixed together.
- Avoid using insect killers in the kitchen. If you must use them, cover all food and dishes. Insect killers can make you sick or even kill you.
- Don't trust childproof caps to keep children away from poisons. It is safest to put all poisons and medicines in a locked cabinet. Children can climb onto counters and reach cabinets near the ceiling. Also, do not tell children that medicine tastes good or that it is candy. They may want to take more when you aren't looking.
- Store household cleaning products in the containers in which they came. The container often tells what to do if someone swallows the product, gets it on his or her skin, or in his or her eyes. If the product is put in an empty food jar or bottle, someone might mistake it for food.

- Some household plants are poisonous. Examples are elephant ear, poinsettia, philodendron, dieffenbachia, and oleander. Keep plants away from food and out of children's reach.
- Put *Mr. Yuk symbols* on all poisons in your house. See 8-7. This symbol lets you know that a product is poison. Teach younger brothers and sisters about Mr. Yuk.

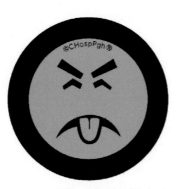

Children's Hospital of Pittsburgh

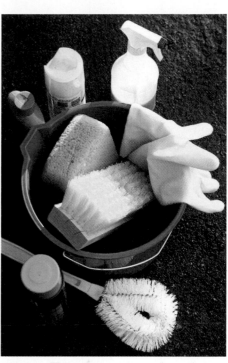

8-7 Mr. Yuk stickers help young children recognize poisons. You may want to place them on household cleaners and other poisonous products in your home.

Plan Ahead for Poison Emergencies

If a poisoning does occur, you'll need to get help for the victim fast. Here's what you can do to be ready to help victims who swallow, inhale, or touch a poison.

- Post a poison chart in your kitchen. This chart tells you what to do if someone swallows, inhales, or touches a poison. You can get a poison chart from a poison control center.
- Post the phone number of a poison control center near your phone. These centers have trained staff who know how to deal with poison emergencies. If you can't find the poison control center's number in the phone book, check with your local hospital.

- Get medical help right away if someone is poisoned. Have the poison's container nearby when you call the poison control center. Take the container with you to the hospital. The medical staff will need information from its label.

To Prevent Choking

A person chokes when an object becomes trapped in his or her throat. This blocks off the flow of air into the lungs. When air cannot reach the lungs, a person suffocates. Slippery, round foods, such as hot dogs, grapes, and hard candy, are the most common cause of choking. Hard foods, such as nuts, and thick foods, such as peanut butter, also are common causes of choking.

If choking does occur, fast action is needed. A person can die of suffocation in four minutes. A person is choking when he or she looks alarmed and can't talk, cough, or breathe. Some choking victims give the distress signal for choking. This signal is clutching the neck.

Here's what you can do to prevent choking.

- Take small bites. The larger the bite, the greater the chance you will choke. Chew each bite well. Tiny bits of food are easy to swallow. They aren't likely to get stuck in your throat.
- Sit down to eat. Running or talking while eating may cause you to swallow before food is well chewed.
- Avoid eating in the car. If you start to choke, it is difficult for others to give you aid in the car. Also, it takes time for the driver to pull off the road to assist you.
- Small children often don't chew food as well as they should. Avoid giving them foods that can choke them. These foods include grapes, carrots, popcorn, nuts, hot dogs, and hard candies. Peanut butter should be spread thinly on crackers or toast. (Toast is preferable to fresh bread because the combination of fresh bread and peanut butter can cause choking.) See 8-8.

To Prevent Other Hazards

There are many other safety hazards in the kitchen. Here are ways to prevent them.

- Store plastic bags out of children's reach. Children can suffocate if they cover their faces with plastic. A small child may bite off pieces that can get caught in his or her throat.

8-8 Making children sit while they are eating and encouraging them to chew their food well can help prevent choking.

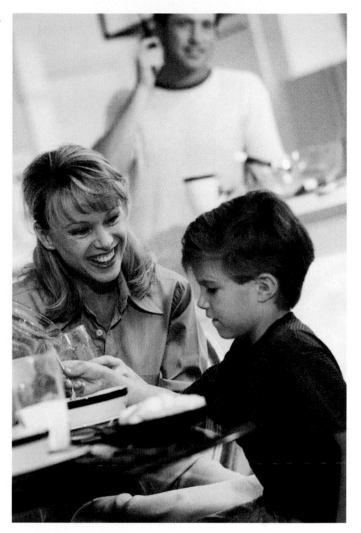

- Keep cabinets and drawers closed. Injuries occur when people bump into open cabinets and drawers.
- Store aerosol sprays in a cool place. These products are under pressure. Heat can cause their containers to explode. Dispose of aerosol cans in nonburnable trash. Burning the empty can may cause it to explode.
- Avoid shaking soft drinks. This could cause them to explode. Tilt them away from yourself and others when opening them.
- Only use a charcoal grill outside, 8-9. It produces a deadly gas called ***carbon monoxide***. Outside, this colorless and odorless gas can disperse. Inside, it is trapped by the walls and can build up and kill you in minutes. Charcoal grills also can cause fires when used inside.

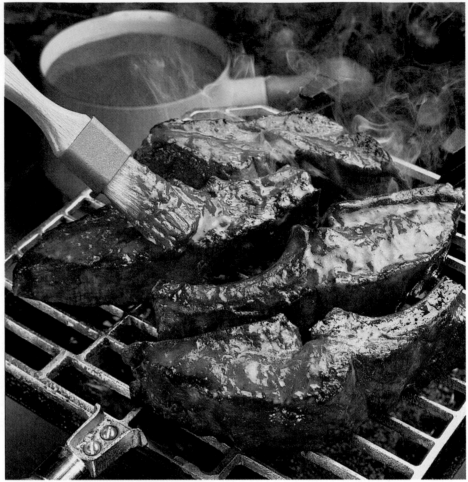

8-9 To prevent fires and buildup of carbon monoxide gas, always use charcoal grills outside.

Basic First Aid

Even when you are very careful, accidents sometimes happen. Injuries can result. A child bumps into an open drawer. You mistakenly pick up a hot pan without a pot holder and burn yourself. A glass shatters as you wash dishes in the sink. You get a bad cut. When an accident happens, you need to know what to do.

Treatment given to people right after an accident is called *first aid*. It helps to relieve pain and prevent further injury. Giving first aid takes knowledge and skill. If you lack these, you could cause more harm to yourself or others.

You can give first aid yourself if you or someone else has only a small injury. You may need to aid a victim with serious injuries before calling for help. For instance, severe bleeding must be stopped right away.

The information below describes basic first aid techniques.

Small Cuts

1. Wash area with soap and water.
2. Apply a mild antiseptic and bandage.

Deep Cut or Puncture

1. Place a clean cloth or bandage over the wound.
2. Press on the cloth with the palm of your hand. The pressure should stop the bleeding.
3. Get medical help right away.

Falls

1. Stop any bleeding (see cuts above).
2. Loosen the victim's collar and belt.
3. If you think the victim has a broken bone, don't move the victim. Get medical help.
4. Don't let the victim eat or drink anything.

Minor Burns

1. Place the burned area in cool water. You also can wrap ice in a clean cloth and place it on the burned area. Keep the area cold until pain subsides.
2. If a blister forms, do not break it. This could cause an infection. Don't apply grease or ointment.

Severe Burns

1. Keep the victim warm and lying down. Don't put anything on the burn or try to remove any material stuck to the skin.
2. Get medical help right away.

Electric Shock

1. Disconnect the appliance that caused the shock. Use a wooden broom handle or dry cloth to do this. Do not use metal. Never touch the victim or appliance with your bare hands. If you use metal or your bare hands, the electrical current will shock you. You will become a victim, too.
2. If the person isn't breathing, give *cardiopulmonary resuscitation (CPR)* if you are certified to do this. CPR is a lifesaving method. It includes rescue breathing and forcing the victim's heart to pump blood.
3. Get medical help right away.

Poisoning

1. Read the poison's label. If it lists an antidote, give it to the victim. An *antidote* reverses the effect of the poison.
   - If the poison is on the skin, rinse it right away. Remove any clothing that has the poison on it.
   - If the poison is in the eyes, flush the eyes with water. Do this for at least 15 minutes.
   - If the poison was inhaled, move the victim into fresh air.
   - If the poison was eaten or drunk, the victim may vomit. If this happens, be sure the victim can breathe. The vomit can block the throat and cause the victim to suffocate.
2. Call a poison control center. Take the poison's container with you to the phone.
3. Carefully follow the directions given by the poison control center's staff.

Choking

If the victim can't speak or breathe, perform the *abdominal thrust.* It can save the life of a person who is choking. The abdominal thrust is shown in 8-10. If you are choking and no one is around to help, you can perform the maneuver on yourself. This maneuver should not be used with infants and small children. It can harm them. There is a special method used to stop choking in infants and small children.

You can learn more about the abdominal thrust and other first aid measures by taking a course. Local Red Cross chapters, fire departments, and hospitals offer first aid courses. They will teach you how to handle emergencies. You can learn how to stop bleeding and do rescue breathing. They also can certify you to do CPR.

FIRST AID FOR CHOKING

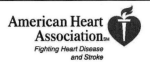

American Heart Association℠
Fighting Heart Disease and Stroke

CONSCIOUS VICTIM

1 Ask the victim, "Are you choking?"
If the victim can speak, cough, or breathe, do not interfere.

2 If the victim cannot speak, cough, or breathe, perform the abdominal thrust until the foreign body is expelled or the victim becomes unconscious.

IF VICTIM BECOMES UNCONSCIOUS

1  Activate Emergency Medical Services as soon as possible. Open mouth and perform finger sweep.

2 Open airway (head tilt–chin lift) and attempt to rescue breathing.

3 If unsuccessful, perform the abdominal thrust up to 5 times.

BE PERSISTENT

CALL-FOR-HELP NUMBER:

Repeat sequence of finger sweep, rescue breathing, and the abdominal thrust.

Continue uninterrupted until successful or advanced life support is available.

American Heart Association

8-10 The abdominal thrust is used when a person is choking.

Serious Injuries Require Medical Help

Get help at once if a person has a serious injury. A person who is bleeding badly, isn't breathing, or has taken a poison has a serious injury. Every second counts.

You can call the fire department, police department, paramedics, hospital, or a doctor for help. Some towns have a special phone number that directly connects you to rescuers. This number often is 911. When you call for help, you will need to provide some information. You'll need to give your phone number and location. You'll also need to describe the victim and the accident. The information you provide lets rescuers know how to prepare to aid the victim. Don't hang up until you are told to do so. The people you contact for help may give you instructions. Follow them carefully.

While you are waiting for help to arrive, you should closely follow any directions given to you. Be sure to stay calm and tell the victim that help is on the way. Also, keep the victim lying down. Only move the victim if he or she is in a dangerous place. Make the victim comfortable by loosening the victim's clothing and keeping the victim warm. Never give the victim anything to eat or drink. Do not leave the victim alone, unless you need to go for help.

Cuts, burns, falls, fires, electrical shocks, poisonings, and choking incidents are some of the dangers lurking in the kitchen. However, they aren't the only hazards in the kitchen. In the next chapter, you will learn about dangers in foods and how to protect yourself.

In a Nutshell

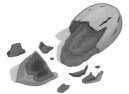

- Many accidents can be prevented.
- By learning safe methods for working in the kitchen, you can avoid most cuts, falls, burns, fires, electrical shocks, poisonings, choking incidents, and other hazards.
- A fire action plan can help you to respond quickly and calmly when a fire starts.
- Knowing basic first aid procedures can help you relieve an accident victim's pain and prevent further injury.
- When serious injuries occur, know how to call for medical help and provide the information rescuers need to find and care for the victim.

In the Know

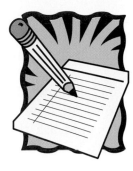

1. Review the chain of events that led up to Jack and Marla's accident in the boxed feature. Describe how the accident could have been prevented and how the first three links in the chain of events could have been broken.
2. Which is NOT a safety hazard?
    A. An electrical appliance set beside a sink.
    B. Damp, padded pot holders.
    C. Knives stored in a rack.
    D. Dull knives.
3. Explain how to prevent a steam burn when lifting a lid from a pot.
4. List the steps for removing a pan from the oven.
5. Name the three factors a fire requires to start and burn.
6. Describe how to put out a fire that occurs on the cooktop.
7. True or false? You should run cords under rugs so people won't trip over the cords.
8. List three ways poisons can enter your body.
9. How can you tell if someone is choking?
10. When calling for help after an accident, what information do you need to provide?
11. Explain why you should not touch a victim of electrical shock with metal or your bare hands.

What Would You Do?

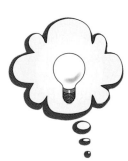

You notice that your friend has two small bandages on her fingers. She also has a bruised knee. "Every time I go in the kitchen, I hurt myself," she says. "This morning I cut myself with a knife and hit my knee on an open drawer. Accidents just seem to happen to me!" How can you help your friend? What could she do to avoid accidents? What advice would you give her?

Expanding Your Knowledge

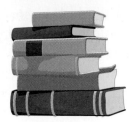

1. Invite a CPR instructor to visit your class. Ask the instructor to demonstrate how to perform rescue breathing, CPR, and the abdominal thrust. Have the instructor explain how you can become certified in CPR.

2. Interview the school nurse. You could ask the nurse to show you the first aid supplies. Also, ask the nurse to demonstrate how to give first aid to someone with a small cut. You could ask the nurse to describe the training needed to become a nurse, too.

3. Write a skit that shows what to do if someone is badly hurt. Perform the skit for your class.

4. Sign up for a first aid course. To find a course in your area, call the American Red Cross or fire department.

5. Post emergency numbers near every phone in your house. Write down the phone numbers for the police department, fire department, ambulance squad, and poison control centers. Many towns have one emergency number. This number often is 911. Find out if your community has this service.

6. Teach younger brothers and sisters how to call for help in an emergency.

7. Do a safety hazard search of your kitchen at home or the school food lab. Predict what might happen if a hazard remains in the kitchen. Ask your parents or teacher to help you remove any hazards that you find.

8. Write a safety rule for working in the kitchen. Make a poster about the rule. Display the poster in your school cafeteria or library.

9. Visit your school library and research home accidents. Find out what types of accidents are most common. Write an article for the school newspaper about home accidents. Describe how to prevent these accidents.

10. Read the labels on three household cleaning products. Review the warnings on the labels. Are any first aid instructions given? Report your findings to the class.

11. Give a presentation to your class entitled, "Safety Is No Accident."

12. Arrange a visit to the fire department. Ask a fire fighter to demonstrate how to use a fire extinguisher. Find out how to plan escape routes for your house. Also find out how to hold fire drills at home.

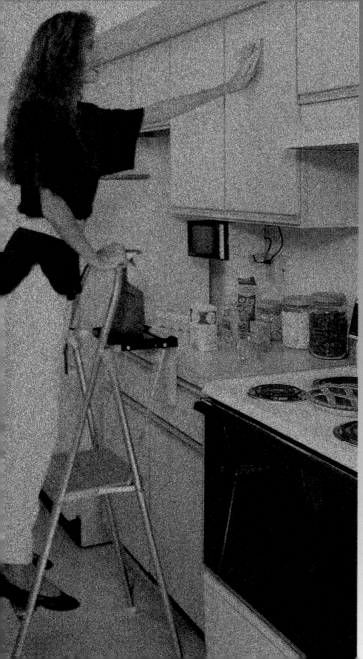

Chapter 9

Keep It Clean!

Objectives

After reading this chapter, you will be able to
- [ ] explain how food becomes contaminated with pathogens.
- [ ] describe common types of foodborne illness.
- [ ] list the symptoms of foodborne illness.
- [ ] prevent foodborne illness.

New Terms

foodborne illness: disease caused by a pathogen in food.

pathogen: an organism or substance that invades the body and damages its cells.

bacteria: tiny organisms that are found everywhere. A few types can cause foodborne illness.

danger zone: temperatures at which bacteria grow fastest (40°F to 140°F or 5°C to 60°C).

toxin: poison.

cross-contamination: spreading bacteria to a clean food from contaminated work surfaces, utensils, hands, or food.

sanitation: the study and use of methods that create a clean, healthy environment.

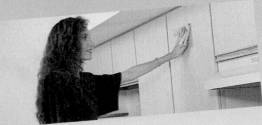

Keller Ladders

193

A community egg hunt was planned. Three days before the event, Ivan and his friends began hard-cooking and dyeing 3,000 eggs, 9-1. Soon the refrigerator was full, so Ivan started stacking the cooked eggs in boxes on the counter. A few hours after the hunt, many children who had eaten some eggs started vomiting. Some had diarrhea. What happened?

9-1 What mistake did Ivan make after cooking the eggs for the community egg hunt?

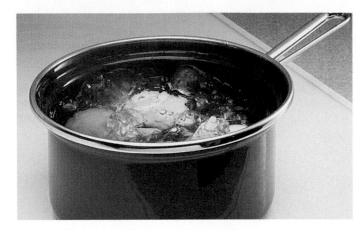

GE Appliances

Maria sliced some raw chicken into strips and put them in a bowl. "Jason," she called, "please come and help me make a tossed salad." Maria handed the cutting board she had used for the chicken to Jason. "Here, slice the salad ingredients on this." Later, Maria's family thought they had the flu. What happened?

The food for the party was ready, 9-2. "Wow! I'm way ahead of schedule," said Sonja. "My friends won't arrive for at least four hours. I'll take the lasagna out of the oven and cover it with foil. That should keep it hot. I'll pop it in the oven for a few minutes just before everyone arrives." Early the next morning, many of Sonja's friends felt ill. What happened?

What did happen to the children from the egg hunt, Maria's family, and Sonja's friends? The food they ate made them sick! They were victims of foodborne illness.

What Causes Foodborne Illness?

Foodborne illness is caused by foods that are not stored or prepared in a clean or safe manner. Foods prepared in a dirty kitchen can cause foodborne illness, too. Most foodborne illnesses just

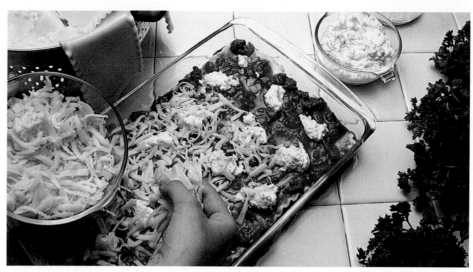

© American Heart Association

9-2 What should Sonja have done to have kept the lasagna safe to eat?

make you sick. Some can kill you. Foodborne illness is also called *food poisoning.*

Foodborne illness is very common. Health experts believe it affects more than one out of every 20 people in the United States each year. In fact, they think half of all diarrhea cases are caused by foodborne illness.

Many people who get foodborne illness don't even know it. They think they have the stomach flu. That's because the symptoms of many foodborne illnesses are the same as flu symptoms. Both often cause cramps, headache, diarrhea, vomiting, fever, and weakness. The next time you think you have the flu, you may really have a foodborne illness.

Foodborne illness can start any time, any place, in any food. It occurs when you eat a food that contains a pathogen. A ***pathogen*** (PATH-uh-jen) is an organism or substance that invades the body and damages its cells. Harmful bacteria, viruses, parasites, molds, and poisons are pathogens.

Bacteria

Bacteria are tiny animals. They have only one cell and are found everywhere! They are found in food, on your hands, and on tabletops. They are in the air you breathe and water you drink. Each day, you are exposed to billions of bacteria! See 9-3.

Bacteria are the most common cause of foodborne illness. Many bacteria are helpful. For instance, helpful bacteria are used to make yogurt and cheese. Some help fight disease. Others can make certain vitamins. Luckily, only a few types of bacteria pose a threat.

Almost all foods contain small amounts of harmful bacteria. Small amounts won't make you sick, but large numbers will. Bacteria increase in number quickly when they get a chance. All they need are nutrients, moisture, and warmth. Foods, especially protein-rich foods, are an ideal place for bacteria to grow. Protein-rich foods include meats, fish, poultry, eggs, and milk products.

Bacteria like warm temperatures. They grow fastest at temperatures of 40°F to 140°F (5°C to 60°C). This temperature range is called the ***danger zone,*** 9-4. Bacteria grow by dividing. In just two hours, foods left in the danger zone can contain thousands of bacteria. The danger zone includes room temperature and low cooking temperatures. Most bacteria die at higher temperatures.

9-3 Thousands of tiny bacteria can fit on the tip of a pin.

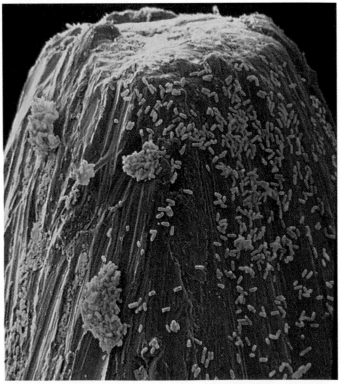

Dr. Tony Brian & David Parker/Science Photo Library

New Technology

Electronic Pasteurization

Pathogens in foods are a major health problem in the United States. To help fight pathogens, more and more food processors are using a powerful weapon called *electronic pasteurization*. This process uses electricity to make waves of energy that are like microwaves. These energy waves kill harmful bacteria on meat, poultry, eggs, seafood, and spices. The energy waves also kill insects and mold that may be on fresh fruits and vegetables. Electronic pasteurization keeps onions, garlic, and potatoes from sprouting, too.

Unlike microwaves, the energy waves from this process do not cook foods.

Fresh and processed foods that are electronically pasteurized stay fresh and safe to eat much longer than other similar foods. However, even foods that have been treated with this process need to be stored safely. Keep in mind, milk is pasteurized, but it still must be kept refrigerated. In the same way, treated meat, poultry, eggs, and seafood still need to be kept refrigerated or frozen. The next time you shop for food, look for electronically pasteurized foods. These foods can help you avoid foodborne illness.

9-4 Bacteria grow best in the danger zone.

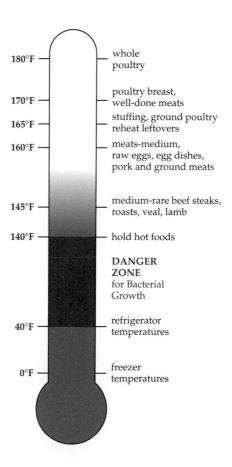

That means cooking helps make your food safe, 9-5. Bacteria grow very slowly at lower temperatures. You can protect yourself by storing foods in a cold refrigerator or freezer.

Bacteria can cause two types of foodborne illness. They can cause either an infection or poisoning. Bacteria that cause infections are *Campylobacter, Salmonella,* and *Listeria.* Bacteria that produce a ***toxin*** (poison) as they grow cause poisoning. *Staphylococci, Clostridium perfringens, Clostridium botulinum,* and *E. coli* are bacteria that produce toxins.

 ## Science in the Kitchen

Growing Bacterial Colonies

Bacteria reproduce by dividing. When they have nutrients, moisture, and warmth, they reproduce quickly. In fact, they can double in number every 20 minutes. That means in 20 minutes, 100 bacterial cells become 200. After 20 more minutes, these 200 become 400 bacterial cells. In a little more than three hours, there could be over a million bacteria!

One bacterial cell is so small you cannot see it, but you can see colonies of bacteria. This experiment will let you observe how bacteria grow. You will need cellophane tape, a packet of plain gelatin, sugar, a heavy-duty paper plate, and plastic wrap.

To begin, draw lines on the paper plate to divide it into eight sections (see drawing). Number each section. Now, bring ¼ cup of water to a boil. Add 2 teaspoons of sugar, and 1 packet of gelatin

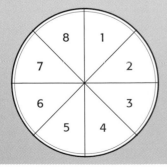

and stir until the gelatin dissolves. Remove the pan from the heat and cool for 2 minutes. Pour the mixture onto the paper plate and chill until firm.

Now, transfer bacteria to the gelatin from these seven items: sink drain, cutting board, tabletop, floor, unwashed hand, washed hand, and your hair. Use the following process to transfer bacteria. First, tear off a 2-inch strip of tape. Next, put the sticky side of the tape on the first item. Pull off the tape and then lay it, sticky side down, on the gelatin in the section marked with the number 1. Now, gently lift off the tape. Tear off a clean piece of tape and repeat this process for the other items. Don't transfer bacteria to the section marked with the number 8.

Cover the plate with plastic wrap. Place the covered plate in a warm (not hot) location for three days. Without removing the plastic wrap, describe what you see in each of the sections. Were any sections free of bacterial colonies? Which ones? Which sections had the largest colonies? Why do you think this occurred? How can you use your observations to keep food safe to eat? Dispose of the covered paper plate.

To determine the effect of refrigeration upon bacterial growth, you could prepare two plates as described above and store one of the plates in the refrigerator. Then compare the differences.

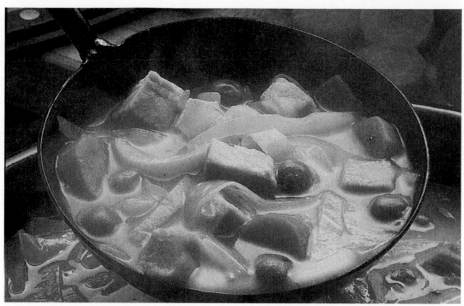

9-5 One way to prevent food-borne illness is to serve foods piping hot.

Campylobacter

Campylobacter (KAM-pee-loh-BAK-ter) bacteria are the most common cause of foodborne illness. Food scientists call these bacteria "Campy." These bacteria can be killed by cooking food. Raw or partly cooked poultry is the main source of the foodborne illness caused by these bacteria. Campy also can spread from one food to others. For instance, suppose you sliced raw chicken contaminated with Campy. Then, you sliced lettuce that was not contaminated. After slicing the chicken, the cutting board, knife, and your hands were contaminated with bacteria. You can spread bacteria to the lettuce just by touching it with an unwashed hand, cutting board, or knife. Spreading bacteria to a clean food from contaminated work surfaces, utensils, hands, or food is called ***cross-contamination.***

Salmonella

There are over 2,000 types of *Salmonella (sal-muh-NEHL-ah)* bacteria. All types can be killed by cooking. However, *Salmonella* is one of the most common causes of foodborne illnesses. Raw poultry and eggs are the main food sources of *Salmonella* bacteria. *Salmonella* can enter food through cross-contamination, too.

Listeria

Listeria (lih-STEER-ee-ah) bacteria are found mostly in raw milk. All milk sold in the United States must be heated before it is sold. The heat kills these bacteria. A few soft cheeses are made with milk that is not heated. Examples of these cheeses are Brie and Camembert. These are the main source of foodborne illness caused by *Listeria.* Unwashed fruits and vegetables may be a source of *Listeria,* too, 9-6. These foods become infected with *Listeria* when polluted water is used to water crops.

Staphylococci

Staphylococci (staff-low-COCK-eye), or Staph, are the most common type of bacteria that produce a toxin in foods. Protein-rich foods and cream filled pastries are the most common sources of these bacteria. Moist salads made with chopped foods (such as potato salad, macaroni salad, and ham salad) are common sources, too. These bacteria live in your nose, throat, and skin sores and enter food when you sneeze or cough. They also enter if your hands are dirty or have an open sore.

9-6 Thoroughly wash fruits and vegetables to reduce the risk of food-borne illness.

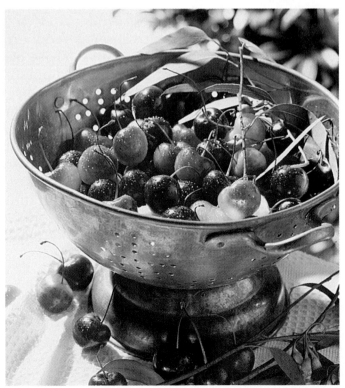

Harry & David

Neither the Staph bacteria nor their toxin are destroyed by heat. The only way to avoid this type of foodborne illness is to prevent the growth of the bacteria. Keeping foods out of danger zone temperatures stops the growth of Staph. It also prevents these bacteria from producing the toxin.

Clostridium Perfringens

Clostridium perfringens (clahs-TRIH-dee-um per-FRIHN-jens) bacteria are sometimes called "banquet germs." That's because most outbreaks occur at restaurants or events such as picnics and banquets. Foods served at picnics, banquets, cafeterias, and restaurants often are made ahead of time. Many times, foods are kept warm, but not hot. If foods are kept at danger zone temperatures, these bacteria grow fast and make their toxin. Gravy, protein-rich foods, stews, soups, and creamy foods are the most common sources of these illness-causing bacteria. See 9-7.

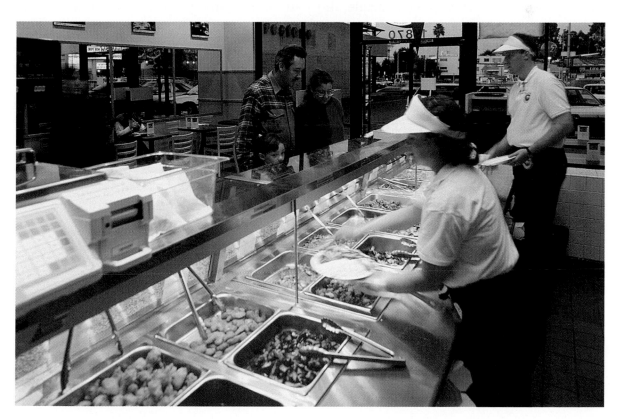

9-7 *Clostridium perfringens* growth is prevented by keeping buffet food steaming hot.

Clostridium perfringens bacteria are found in soil, water, milk, dust, and sewage. They enter food through polluted water and may be on unwashed fruits and vegetables. These bacteria also enter the food supply through dust that settles on food. They can enter food through cross-contamination, too.

Clostridium Botulinum

The toxin made by the *Clostridium botulinum (botch-you-lye-nuhm)* bacterium causes the disease called *botulism (BOTCH-you-lih-zum)*. These bacteria cause a deadly type of foodborne illness. Scientists believe the botulism toxin is the strongest poison known. An amount as small as a grain of salt can kill many people in less than an hour.

The bacteria that cause botulism live in soil and water. They can grow only if no air is present. This is why they thrive in foods sealed in airtight jars and cans. During the canning process, foods are sealed in cans or jars and heated. The heat kills these bacteria. If the food inside the can or jar isn't heated to a high enough temperature for a long enough time, these bacteria don't die. This rarely happens in canned foods sold in supermarkets. It happens mostly in foods canned at home. If you plan to can food, be certain to use safe techniques. The Cooperative Extension program in your state can teach you these techniques.

To avoid this foodborne illness, check food cans and jars closely. If a can or jar is leaking, rusting, bulging, or has holes, the food inside may contain the botulism toxin. If you suspect a food contains the botulism toxin, don't take any chances. Discard the food so no person or animal can eat it. Tasting one bean contaminated with botulism toxin can kill you.

E. coli

Most types of *E. coli (EE coal-EYE)* bacteria are harmless, but at least six types can cause serious illness. One of the most dangerous types is *E. coli 0157:H7*. Undercooked meat, especially hamburger, is often blamed for outbreaks of the foodborne illness caused by these bacteria. The illness can cause death, especially in children and the elderly.

To safeguard against these harmful bacteria, thoroughly cook all raw meats. If eating in a restaurant, always order meat cooked well done. Never eat undercooked meats. Before you eat meat, first cut into it. If it is red or pink, do not eat it.

Viruses

The most common foodborne illness caused by a virus is *hepatitis (heh-pah-TYE-tuhs)*. This virus is found in water contaminated with sewage. Raw fish, oysters, and clams caught in polluted water are common causes of hepatitis. This virus may be on skins of unwashed fresh fruits and vegetables, too. Cross-contamination is also a cause of hepatitis.

Hepatitis is a very serious disease. It can be deadly. It causes nausea, vomiting, weakness, and liver damage. Heat destroys the hepatitis virus. You can avoid this virus by cooking seafood thoroughly. Washing all fresh fruits and vegetables well also helps prevent hepatitis.

Parasites

A *parasite* is an organism that lives inside or on a host. The host can be any living plant or animal. The parasite takes its food from the host. Some worms are common parasites found in food. When they enter your body, you become the host. The most common source of parasites is raw or partly cooked meat and fish.

One of the most well-known parasitic worms found in food is *trichina (trick-EYE-nah)*. These roundworms cause a disease called *trichinosis (trick-ih-NOE-sis)*. You can become infected with this worm by eating raw or partly cooked pork or wild game meat.

Trichinosis causes vomiting, diarrhea, nausea, fever, thirst, and chills. This disease makes it hard to talk, swallow, and breathe. It causes puffy eyelids and swollen, sore muscles. The symptoms appear within a few days to a few weeks.

Heat kills parasites. You can protect yourself from them by thoroughly cooking meat and fish. Avoid eating raw or partly cooked meat. If you become a host to parasites, see your doctor right away.

Molds

Molds are fuzzy growths on the surface of foods. Molds can be any color. They spread to foods through the air. Some molds produce poisons. Their poisons are found below the mold you can see. Molds and their poisons can cause foodborne illness. To avoid mold growth, eat foods within a few days of buying them.

Poisons

Foodborne illness may be caused by poisons, too. Some poisons are a natural part of plants or animals. Others get into food through accidental contamination from the environment.

Natural Poisons

Certain plants and animals contain natural toxins. For instance, many mushrooms are tasty, while others contain a deadly poison. Poisonous mushrooms often look just like nonpoisonous ones. Poisonous and nonpoisonous mushrooms may grow side by side. Avoid picking wild mushrooms, fruits, and berries unless you are an expert, 9-8.

9-8 Dangerous or delicious? Only experts should pick wild mushrooms.

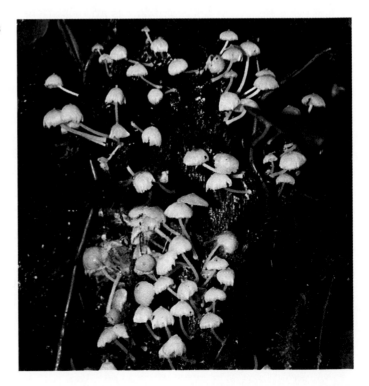

A natural poison is also found in potato peels. The amount is small, but it increases as the potato sprouts. It also increases if potatoes are stored in a brightly lit place. You can avoid this poison by removing the peel, green spots, and sprouts.

Poisons from the Environment

Toxic substances in the environment may get into foods through food containers, polluted water, and farming practices. Common toxic substances include lead and pesticides.

Lead is found in lead-glazed dishes, lead crystal glasses, lead solder, and old paint. The glazes on some handmade and old dishes often contain lead. Lead can leach out of lead glazes and crystal containers into food and beverages. Lead from solder can leach into food and beverages, too. In the past, lead solder was used to seal the seams of cans and copper water pipes. Lead solder is no longer permitted in cans manufactured for packaging food in the United States. However, lead seams can still be found on some imported canned food products. Many older homes may still have lead-soldered water pipes. Food can also be contaminated if lead paint chips fall into it.

The symptoms of lead poisoning are headaches, vomiting, and diarrhea. Lead poisoning can cause muscles to waste. It can also lead to mental retardation.

You can reduce the amount of lead that enters your body by using lead-glazed dishes only for decorative purposes. Such dishes are often handmade, old, or have a dusty or chalky look. New dishes made by large companies in the United States no longer contain lead. Save lead crystal containers for special events. Never store food or beverages in lead crystal containers.

It is also a good idea to remove food from cans soon after opening them. Lead from the solder on some imported food cans can leach into the food if you store leftovers in the can. Lead also leaches into water when the water sits in pipes. If you have lead or copper pipes, let water run a minute or two before using it. The lead that leached into the water will go down the drain with the water. You should always choose lead-free paint for your home, too.

Pesticides used in farming are another type of poison that can enter food. These poisons are used to keep insects, mice, rats, weeds, and diseases from attacking crops, 9-9. The United States Government has strict controls on pesticides, but sometimes a small amount of some pesticides remains on crops. You can reduce the amount of pesticides in your food by washing raw fruits and vegetables well.

Symptoms of poisoning can occur within a few minutes. Sometimes symptoms take weeks to appear. If you think you have eaten a poison, see a doctor right away. Try to take along some of the food you ate. (Review the steps in Chapter 8 for dealing with poisoning.)

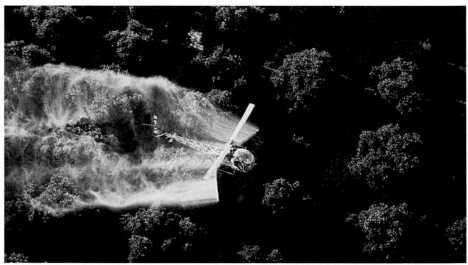

USDA

9-9 Pesticides protect crops, but they may contaminate the food supply.

What Should You Do If You Think You Have a Foodborne Illness?

Most foodborne illnesses last a few days. The usual treatment is to rest in bed and drink plenty of fluids. Foodborne illnesses may keep a person home from work or school, but they are not a threat to the health of most people.

Foodborne illnesses can be very dangerous for some people. The following victims of foodborne illness should see a doctor without delay:

- babies, children, and elderly people
- those who are sick with other diseases
- those with severe symptoms, such as a high fever, blood in the feces, constant vomiting and diarrhea, and dizziness
- those who don't recover within a few days
- those who think they have botulism

You or your doctor should report instances of foodborne illness to the health department. Health department workers will try to find out which food caused the illness, 9-10. Once they know the source of the illness, the workers can take steps to protect other people. For

9-10 Health department workers can often track down the cause of food-borne illnesses.

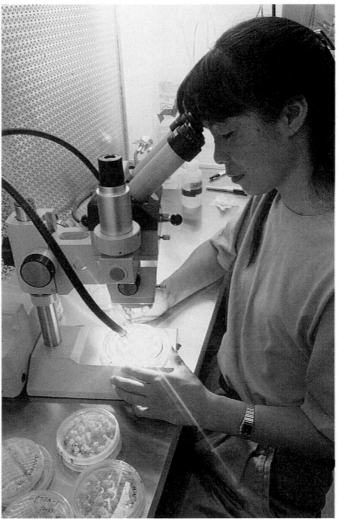

instance, if restaurant food caused the illness, the health department can order the restaurant to clean up. If a food in the supermarket is the problem, the health department can keep others from buying it and can tell others who already bought the food to return it.

Keeping Food Safe to Eat

Keeping food clean and safe to eat is the responsibility of every person who handles food. That includes food producers, processors, shippers, food store workers, and you.

Some government agencies also work to keep the food supply safe and clean. These agencies include the U.S. Department of Agriculture, the Food and Drug Administration, and health departments. These agencies write and enforce strict rules. They inspect food-processing plants, food stores, and restaurants to be sure the rules are followed. One place they don't inspect is your kitchen. That's your responsibility.

Many cases of foodborne illness begin in home kitchens. It's up to you to prevent them. It's easy to protect yourself if you follow good sanitation rules. ***Sanitation*** means to study and use methods that create a clean, healthy environment. You can practice good sanitation if you follow the four rules shown in 9-11.

Keep Yourself Clean

Bacteria are found on your body and clothes. These bacteria can get into food and cause foodborne illness. Chefs and other food workers must follow strict rules for keeping themselves clean. You can use the rules they follow to prevent foodborne illness.

Keep your hands clean. Your hands come in close contact with food. Even hands that look clean may be contaminated with harmful bacteria. It's easy to control the spread of bacteria from your hands. All you need to do is wash them before cooking. Scrub them for at least 20 seconds with plenty of hot, soapy water. Don't forget to wash between your fingers and scrub under your fingernails.

After washing your hands, try not to contaminate them again with bacteria. Your hands become contaminated every time you cough, sneeze, or use the bathroom. Touching raw meat or

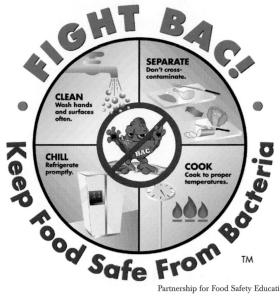

Partnership for Food Safety Education

9-11 Follow the four basic rood safety guidelines—clean, separate, chill, and cook—to keep foods safe to eat.

unwashed fruits and vegetables transfers bacteria to your hands, too. Bacteria also spread to your hands when you touch your face, hair, or pets. If you think your hands may be contaminated with bacteria, wash them right away.

Handle foods as little as possible. Even clean hands have small amounts of harmful bacteria on them. Try not to touch food you are preparing. Use utensils to mix or turn foods. If you must touch foods with your hands, you might want to wear disposable plastic gloves.

Only touch the parts of dishes and utensils that don't come in contact with food. You can reduce the spread of bacteria by picking up forks, knives, and spoons by their handles. Try to pick up plates and bowls by their bottoms and edges. Avoid touching the rims and inside areas of cups and glasses.

Wear clean clothes. Bacteria on dirty clothes can get into food. Roll up loose sleeves to keep them from dipping into food.

Tie back your hair if it is long. If it is tied back, hair won't fall into food. Also, you will be less likely to touch your hair and contaminate your hands with bacteria.

If you sneeze or cough, turn away from food and cover your mouth and nose. The air you exhale carries bacteria that can get into food. Always wash your hands after sneezing or coughing.

Avoid working with food when you are sick. The germs causing your illness could get into food. You could infect the food and pass the germs on to others.

Cover open cuts and sores with a clean bandage. Open cuts and sores contain harmful bacteria that can cause foodborne illness. Never touch a wound while you are cooking. The liquid oozing from wounds contains harmful bacteria that will contaminate your hands. If you have a cut or sore on your hands or arms, protect the wound and food by wearing disposable plastic gloves.

Keep Your Kitchen Clean

Bacteria thrive in damp, dirty areas of the kitchen. They love cracks and corners where food, moisture, and dirt collect. Pests, such as insects, mice, and rats, like dirty kitchens, too. They move in when crumbs, food spills, and garbage are left in the kitchen. These pests spread bacteria every place they go. They climb over counters, dishes, and food. Bacteria and pests don't like kitchens that are clean and dry. See 9-12.

Here's how you can keep bacteria under control and pests out of your kitchen.

- Wash work surfaces. Work surfaces include countertops, tables, and cutting boards. Wash them with soap and water and rinse well before using them. Clean them again after using them. Wooden cutting boards need special care. Bacteria like to nestle into the small, damp spaces of the scratches in wooden cutting boards. Damp plastic cutting boards provide an ideal breeding ground for bacteria. To kill the bacteria, wash cutting boards with a mixture of one cup of water and one tablespoon of bleach. Then wash them in the dishwasher or with hot, soapy water and dry them thoroughly.
- Consider using paper towels. If you use dishtowels and sponges, be sure they are clean. Bacteria thrive in damp or dirty dishtowels, so be sure to wash them often. After using a sponge, wash it in very hot, soapy water. This will kill many bacteria. Then rinse it with cold water, squeeze out the clean sponge, and let it dry. Wash dishtowels on the hot cycle of your washing machine.

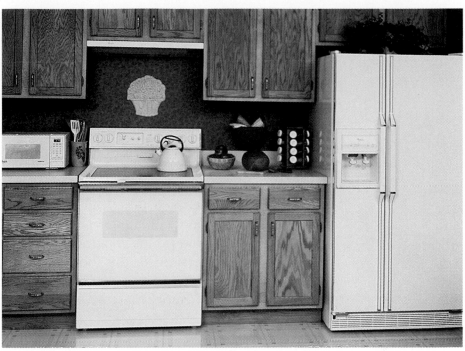

9-12 A clean kitchen helps prevent food-borne illness.

- Wipe up spills as soon as they happen. Bacteria grow quickly in spills. Pests like to feast on spills.
- Keep pets out of the kitchen. Pet fur can carry harmful bacteria. Hairs may float in the air and get into food.
- Each time you taste a food during cooking, use a clean spoon. Bacteria can spread to food if the spoon is dirty. Always wash the spoon before using it again.
- Throw away foods in torn or damaged containers. Bacteria and pests can enter damaged or open food containers. The food inside the package may be spoiled or unsafe to eat. When you shop, reject open packages and leaking, dented, or bulging cans. Choose jars that are tightly closed. Some jars have a safety button on their lids. You know the jar has been opened if the safety button has popped up. Soft, soggy, or stained frozen food packages are signs that food has thawed. When frozen foods thaw, bacteria begin growing right away. If you find foods in torn or damaged containers at the store, bring them to the attention of the manager.

- Clean out your refrigerator and freezer often. Discard spoiled foods. If you don't know how old the food is, don't take chances. Discard it. Often you cannot tell a food will cause food-borne illness just by looking at it or smelling it. The food may look, smell, and taste fine and still make you sick. See 9-13.
- If you aren't sure a food is clean or safe to eat, discard it. Foods that look or smell strange may not be safe to eat. Food from a can that spouts and sprays when you open it is not safe to eat. Dispose of these foods so no person or animal can eat them.
- Cover your garbage can with a tight lid. Empty it at least once a day. Garbage attracts pests and bacteria.
- Rinse empty food containers before recycling or discarding them. Bacteria and molds can grow on the tiny bits of food left in food containers. Also, the food and odors from dirty food containers attract pests.
- Sweep the floor. Crumbs make tasty morsels for pests and bacteria.

9-13 Keep your refrigerator clean and be aware of how long foods have been stored. To prevent foodborne illness, throw away foods if you are in doubt about how fresh or safe they are.

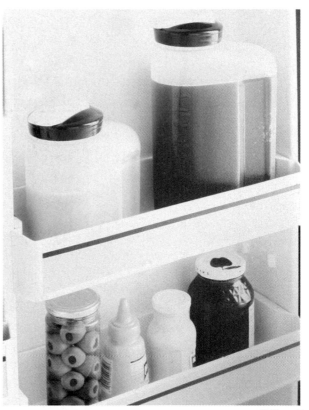

Rubbermaid

Separate: Don't Cross-Contaminate

Cross-contamination spreads bacteria from contaminated areas and items to clean food. Raw food and dirty hands, clothing, dishtowels, sponges, utensils, and dishes all carry bacteria that can contaminate your clean food. You can take several steps to prevent cross-contamination.

- Never dry dishes with the same towel used to dry your hands. Bacteria from your hands are spread to the towel. These bacteria can end up on clean dishes if you dry dishes with the same towel. Some families have two colors of dishtowels. They use one color to dry dishes and the other color to dry their hands. This makes it easy to keep towels for dishes and towels for hands apart.
- Keep dirty items away from clean dishes and food. Bacteria can spread from dirty utensils and dishes to clean dishes and food. Put dirty dishes and utensils in the sink or dishwasher. If you wash them in the sink, use plenty of hot, soapy water. Then, rinse them in hot water. If you can, let dishes and utensils air-dry. If you need to dry them quickly, use a clean dishtowel.
- Be sure to wash every item raw foods touch before using the item again. This rule will help you avoid cross-contamination. Keep in mind that raw foods carry bacteria that contaminate everything they touch. You can spread bacteria just by touching a clean food with an unwashed knife. A common cause of cross-contamination is placing cooked meat on the same unwashed plate used for raw meat.
- Raw meat, poultry, fish, and their juices often contain harmful bacteria. Therefore, separate raw meat, poultry, and fish from other foods in your grocery cart to prevent cross-contamination. Also, put raw meat, poultry, and fish on plates before refrigerating them. This will keep their juices from dripping on other foods.

Chill and Cook: Keep Food out of Danger Zone Temperatures

Bacteria grow fastest at temperatures between 40°F and 140°F (5°C and 60°C). For safety, keep foods out of the danger zone. You can do this by serving cooked food while it's hot. Also, keep cold foods cold until you are ready to use them. The following tips can help you to keep foods out of danger zone temperatures.

- Store foods safely. Take groceries home right after shopping. Put frozen and refrigerated foods away as soon as you get home. It's a good idea to put a date on frozen foods so you know how old they are. Keep canned and dry foods in a cool, dry place. Bacteria prefer moist, warm places, such as those under a sink or above an oven. You'll learn more about storing food in Chapter 12.
- Keep cold foods in the refrigerator or freezer until you need them. Return them to the refrigerator or freezer as soon as you can. Refrigerator temperatures should be between 32°F and 40°F (0°C and 4°C). Keep freezer temperatures at 0°F (-18°C). You can check the temperature by keeping special thermometers in your refrigerator and freezer.
- Sometimes cold foods will need to be out of the refrigerator for a few hours. Picnic foods and packed lunches are examples. These foods need to be kept cold, too. An insulated carrier with a cold pack inside keeps food cool for a few hours. Be sure to keep the carrier closed and out of the hot sun, 9-14.

9-14 An insulated carrier helps keep packed lunches cool and safe to eat.

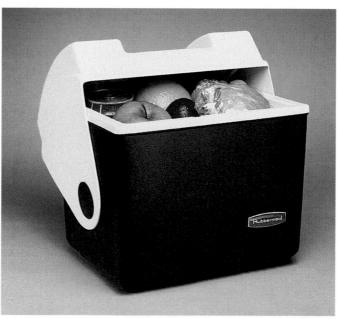

Rubbermaid

- Thaw frozen food in a microwave oven or refrigerator. Letting food thaw on the countertop gives bacteria a chance to grow. Bacteria start growing on the outer parts of the food even before the inside thaws.
- Keep hot food hot until it is served. Hot means 140°F (60°C) or higher. Bacteria cannot grow above this temperature. Hot temperatures kill many bacteria and their toxins. If food cools slightly, it enters danger zone temperatures.
- Thoroughly cook meat, fish, poultry, and eggs. Cooking kills harmful bacteria. You're taking chances when you eat meat, poultry, fish, or eggs that are raw or only partly cooked.
- A food thermometer is the only way you can tell for sure that meat and poultry are safe to eat. The color of cooked meat can fool you. For instance, hamburgers may be brown and still be undercooked. Use a clean food thermometer to measure the internal temperature of cooked foods. The internal temperatures in 9-15 will help you know when food is safe to eat. Fish is done when it is opaque and you can flake it with a fork.

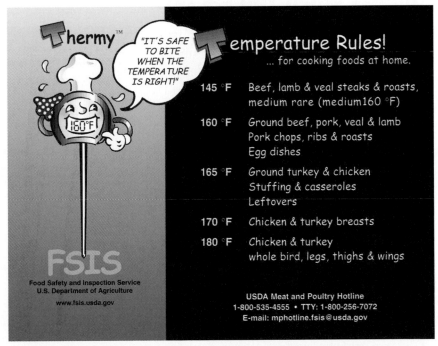

9-15 Keep cooked foods safe to eat by using a food thermometer to make sure they have reached these recommended temperatures.

- Many eggs are contaminated with salmonella. These bacteria can grow inside fresh, unbroken eggs. You should cook eggs until the yolk and white are firm. Some older recipes, such as eggnog, may call for raw eggs. Don't use recipes in which eggs remain raw or only partly cooked. You'll learn more about preparing eggs safely in Chapter 22.
- Cool leftovers right away. Bacteria grow fast as hot foods start to cool. Leaving them at danger zone temperatures for more than two hours makes them unsafe to eat. Place leftovers in the refrigerator immediately. Don't leave them out to cool. You can speed the cooling of large amounts of leftovers by dividing them into small containers. Small amounts of leftovers cool faster than large amounts. Bacteria have less time to grow when foods cool quickly.

 Focus on Food

Avoiding Foodborne Illness When You Eat Out

Restaurants must follow strict sanitation rules. Experts from the health department inspect restaurants to be sure the rules are followed. Sometimes problems occur and customers get a foodborne illness. You can avoid foodborne illness by asking yourself these questions before eating at a restaurant.

- Does the restaurant look clean? The tabletops should be clean. Look for clean walls and floors and tidy rest rooms.
- Are the workers healthy and neatly groomed? The workers should not appear sick. They should be wearing clean clothes. If they have long hair, it should be tied back. Make sure the workers do not touch the parts of utensils or dishes that will touch your food.
- Does the food look clean and smell fresh? Check to see that hot foods are hot and cold foods are cold. Take a close look at salad bars and hot buffets. Salad bar foods should be kept chilled. Hot buffet foods should be hot, not warm. Make sure custard and cream pies are refrigerated. Be extra careful if you are buying milk or sandwiches from a vending machine. Check the dates on the foods. If the date has passed or the food is not cold, don't eat it.
- If you have any leftovers, take them home right away. They need to be put in the refrigerator within two hours of the time the food was served. Be sure to reheat leftovers well before eating them.

If you have a problem with foodborne illness, call your local health department. They can look into the problem and warn others.

- Thoroughly reheat leftovers. Bacteria have a chance to grow while hot foods cool. Bacteria also can grow slowly in the refrigerator. Leftovers are safest to eat when they are heated to at least 165°F (74°C). You should boil leftover sauces, soups, and gravy.
- If a firm-textured food has molded, remove a large area around the mold. The mold you see is only part of the problem. The poisons molds can form are found under the surface of the food. Sometimes you can save parts of molded bread, cheese, fruits, and vegetables by cutting off the mold. Discard the food if the mold covers a large part of the food. Also, discard any soft or liquid foods that become moldy.

Now that you know how to keep food clean and safe, you're ready to begin preparing it. The next chapters will help you do just that.

In a Nutshell

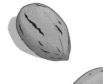

- Many people become victims of foodborne illnesses every year.
- Foodborne illness is caused by pathogens that get into food you eat.
- Bacteria, parasites, molds, and poisons are pathogens.
- Bacteria grow quickly when foods are stored in danger zone temperatures.
- *Campylobacter, Salmonella,* and *Listeria* are bacteria that cause infections.
- *Staphylococci, Clostridium perfringens, Clostridium botulinum,* and *E. coli* are bacteria that produce toxins that cause poisonings.
- The virus that causes hepatitis is found in contaminated water.
- Worms are the most common parasites found in foods.
- Certain plants and animals contain natural poisons. Other foods may be contaminated by poisons from the environment.
- The treatment for most people with foodborne illnesses is to rest in bed and drink plenty of fluids.
- Most foodborne illnesses can be avoided if you keep yourself clean, keep your kitchen clean, and keep foods out of danger zone temperatures.

In the Know

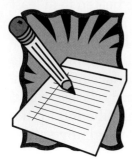

1. Describe how cross-contamination occurs.
2. Which food is most likely to cause foodborne illness if left at room temperature for more than two hours?
   A. A raw carrot.
   B. A loaf of bread.
   C. A bowl of pudding.
   D. An open can of cola.
3. True or false? Almost all bacteria cause foodborne illness.
4. Danger zone temperatures range from ___ to ___.
5. _____ is a common source of *Salmonella* and *Campylobacter*.
   A. Milk
   B. Apples
   C. Chicken
   D. Honey
6. Name the foodborne illness you are likely to get by eating raw or partly cooked eggs.
7. The most deadly type of foodborne illness is caused by _____.
   A. *Clostridium botulinum*
   B. *Clostridium perfringens*
   C. *Staphylococci*
   D. *Listeria*
8. Which type of foodborne illness is caused by a parasite?
   A. *Clostridium perfringens.*
   B. *Trichinosis.*
   C. *Staphylococci.*
   D. *Campylobacter.*
9. Describe the symptoms of most types of foodborne illnesses.
10. List three rules for preventing foodborne illness.
11. True or false? You can usually tell if a food will cause foodborne illness by smelling or tasting it.
12. Which is NOT a way to prevent foodborne illness?
    A. Allow food to cool to room temperature before refrigerating it.
    B. Cook pork until it is no longer pink.
    C. Scrub wooden cutting boards with a mixture of bleach and water.
    D. Keep pets out of the kitchen.

What Would You Do?

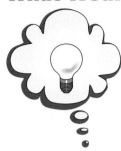

Nick stared at the bowl of ham salad on the counter. "I can't believe I forgot to put this in the refrigerator! I guess I was in a big hurry to get to bed last night. Let's see, the salad smells good and tastes all right. I wonder if it is safe to eat? I really wanted to use it to make sandwiches!" Should Nick use the ham salad? Why or why not? What advice would you give Nick?

Expanding Your Knowledge

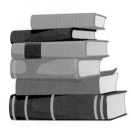

1. Write a booklet to teach children how to prevent foodborne illness. Cut out magazine pictures to illustrate the booklet.
2. Create a card game on the pathogens that cause foodborne illness. Play the game with friends.
3. Research home canning. Start your research by contacting your local Cooperative Extension office. Find out how canning preserves food. Compare the steps for canning peaches and cherries with the steps for canning beans and corn. Why do the steps differ? Report your findings to the class.
4. Interview a local health inspector. Ask the inspector to describe the sanitation rules restaurants must follow. You could ask questions such as these: How is a restaurant inspected? What happens if a rule is broken? Have there been any outbreaks of foodborne illness in your town? What does the health department do if there is an outbreak?
5. Create a video on how to avoid foodborne illness. Show the video to younger children.
6. Observe the sanitation rules followed in your school cafeteria. Ask the cafeteria manager to explain how the workers prevent foodborne illness. Adapt the sanitation rules the cafeteria workers use to your school or home kitchen. Make a poster of the rules.
7. Write a skit about how to handle a food that has an odd color, odor, texture, or flavor. Perform the skit. Ask your classmates to describe what might happen if you ate the food.
8. Do a sanitation check of your school or home kitchen. Be sure to inspect the refrigerator and freezer and check their temperatures. What changes could be made to make the kitchen more sanitary?

9. Find out how hot the danger zone is. Bring a cup of water to a boil. Remove it from the heat and pour it into a cup. Record its temperature with a thermometer. Let it cool to 140°F (60°C). Carefully take a sip of the water. Let it cool to 120°F (49°C) and taste it again. Each time it cools 20°F (7°C), taste it again. Repeat until the water reaches 40°F (5°C). (Once the water reaches room temperature, put it in the refrigerator to continue cooling it.) Describe your reactions to danger zone temperatures. How do they compare to the temperatures of foods you eat?

10. Write an article for your school newspaper on how to keep a picnic lunch safe.

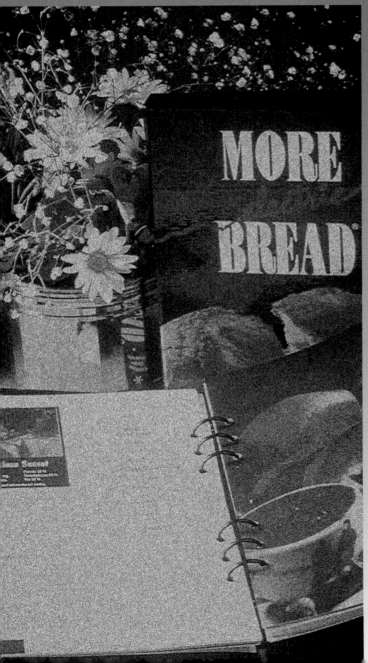

Chapter 10
Recipes – Blueprints for Food

Objectives

After reading this chapter, you will be able to
- describe the parts of a recipe.
- define recipe terms.
- measure ingredients accurately.

New Terms

recipe: a list of ingredients and directions for preparing a food.
yield: the number and size of portions a recipe will make.

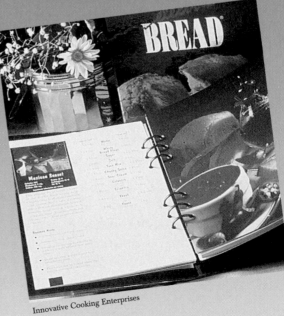

Innovative Cooking Enterprises

A recipe is a blueprint for preparing food. A blueprint is a plan that tells a builder how to construct a house. A recipe is a plan that tells a cook how to "build" a food.

A builder looks at the blueprint to see what building supplies are needed. A cook looks at a recipe to see what ingredients are needed. If the builder follows the blueprint exactly, he or she will get the same house every time. If you follow the recipe exactly, you'll get the same food every time.

Where can you find recipes? There are many sources. Cookbooks are the first source that might come to mind. There are thousands of cookbooks. You can find recipes in many newspapers and magazines, too. Some people like to collect recipes and trade them with friends. Many family recipes are passed down from one generation to the next.

The Parts of a Recipe

A *recipe* tells you exactly what you must do to make the food. It also tells you what ingredients you will need. A recipe can be divided into five parts. The parts are an ingredient list, cooking equipment needed, cooking time and temperature, steps to follow, and yield. See 10-1.

Ingredient List

The ingredient list tells you which ingredients are needed to make the recipe. It also lists the amount of each ingredient you will need. Recipes that are the easiest to use list the ingredients in the order they are needed.

The ingredient list also states the exact form of each ingredient. For example, you might need canned corn, low-fat cheese, or fresh orange halves.

The list of ingredients helps you make your shopping list. Compare the ingredient list to the foods you have on hand. If you don't have a needed ingredient, add it to your shopping list. Sometimes you can substitute one ingredient for another. Cookbooks often suggest ingredients that can be used in place of items you don't have on hand.

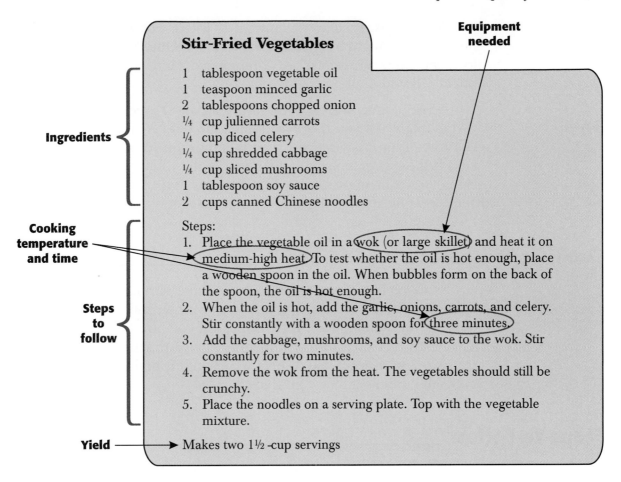

Equipment needed

Stir-Fried Vegetables

Ingredients {

1 tablespoon vegetable oil
1 teaspoon minced garlic
2 tablespoons chopped onion
¼ cup julienned carrots
¼ cup diced celery
¼ cup shredded cabbage
¼ cup sliced mushrooms
1 tablespoon soy sauce
2 cups canned Chinese noodles

Cooking temperature and time

Steps to follow {

Steps:
1. Place the vegetable oil in a wok (or large skillet) and heat it on medium-high heat. To test whether the oil is hot enough, place a wooden spoon in the oil. When bubbles form on the back of the spoon, the oil is hot enough.
2. When the oil is hot, add the garlic, onions, carrots, and celery. Stir constantly with a wooden spoon for three minutes.
3. Add the cabbage, mushrooms, and soy sauce to the wok. Stir constantly for two minutes.
4. Remove the wok from the heat. The vegetables should still be crunchy.
5. Place the noodles on a serving plate. Top with the vegetable mixture.

Yield → Makes two 1½-cup servings

10-1 A well-written recipe has these five parts.

The ingredient list can save you time, too. Before making a recipe, use it to get out all the needed ingredients. Arrange them in the order they are needed. You'll be able to make the recipe without stopping to search for ingredients.

Cooking Equipment Needed

Most recipes tell you how to prepare a food, but don't state what equipment you will need. For instance, a recipe may tell you to boil noodles or slice carrots. Everyone knows that a saucepan and a cooktop are needed to boil noodles. A knife and cutting board are needed to slice carrots. Take a look at the recipe in 10-1. Is there any equipment you will need that's not named in the recipe?

Sometimes, specific equipment is listed. For instance, a large mixing bowl might be specified for a cake recipe. You might be told to "beat with a wire whisk" or "drain in a colander." A biscuit recipe might tell you to use a rolling pin.

A recipe may instruct you to use a pan of a certain size. A pie recipe might tell you to use a 10-inch pie pan. A stew recipe might call for a four-quart saucepan. It is important to use the right size pan. If the pan is too small, the ingredients will overflow. If the pan is too large, the ingredients will spread out. This may cause them to cook too quickly and dry out.

Cooking Temperature and Time

Some recipes give you an exact cooking temperature and time. For example, a recipe might tell you to cook the food at 350° F (175° C) for 30 minutes. Other recipes tell you how to cook the food. They may not give exact temperatures and times. For instance, a recipe might instruct you to heat water until it boils. A sauce recipe may tell you to simmer it until it's thick.

Steps to Follow

The steps describe what you must do to prepare the recipe. The steps are listed in the order they should be done. Sometimes, the steps are numbered. Other times, the steps are written in paragraph form.

Some recipe steps tell you how to get ingredients and equipment ready. For example, an omelet recipe might tell you to beat the eggs. A muffin recipe might tell you to grease the pan and preheat the oven. Other steps state how and when to combine ingredients. For instance, a hot cocoa recipe might direct you to combine the cocoa and milk before heating them.

The recipe steps also will explain what to do with the blended ingredients. A pizza recipe might instruct you to bake the blended ingredients. A salad recipe may tell you to chill the ingredients.

Yield

The *yield* is the number and size of portions a recipe will make. A pudding recipe may yield four half-cup servings. An iced tea mix may make 12 eight-ounce servings.

The yield tells you how many people you can serve. It also tells you how much each person will get. The yield helps you decide if you need more or less food than the recipe will make. If you are serving more people than the yield, you can increase the recipe or serve smaller portions. If you need fewer servings than the yield, you could decrease the recipe. You also could choose to make a whole recipe and serve the leftovers later.

Recipe Language

Recipes have a language all their own. This language is made of terms that describe exactly how to prepare, combine, or cook ingredients.

This language is easy to learn. You already know some of the terms. For example, you know what stir and slice mean. You can learn more terms each time you make a new recipe. Soon you will become a skilled cook who knows all the terms in the recipe language.

The meanings of some terms are very much alike. Grate, grind, and mince are examples. They all mean to cut food into very small pieces. Their meanings do differ, though. When you know the recipe language, you will know how they differ. Your recipes are more likely to be a success if you know the recipe language.

Getting Ready to Cook

Some cooking equipment needs to be prepared before you use it. These terms tell you how to get cooking equipment ready.

Grease: To rub or spray lightly with fat or oil.

Preheat: To heat a conventional oven to the cooking temperature before putting food in the oven.

The success of your recipe depends on the way you handle ingredients. These terms tell you how to handle ingredients.

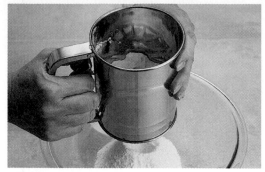

Sifting

◄ *Sift:* To put dry ingredients through a flour sifter or fine sieve.

Baste: To moisten foods during baking or roasting with fat, juice, or sauce. Basting adds flavor and keeps the food moist. ➤

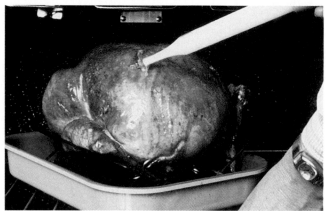

Basting   National Turkey Federation

Drain: To remove liquid from a food by pouring off the liquid or drying the food with paper towels.

Getting Under the Skin

Some fruits and vegetables need to have their skin removed. Recipes will tell you when to do this.

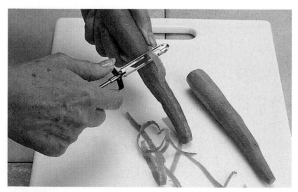

Scraping

◄ *Scrape:* To remove a very thin layer of outer skin by rubbing it with a knife or vegetable peeler.

Pare: To cut off outer skin with a knife ➡ or vegetable peeler.

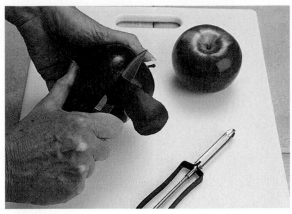
Paring

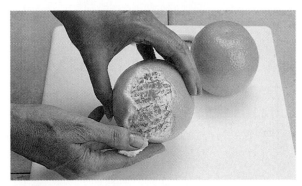
Peeling

⬅ *Peel:* To strip or pull off the outer skin using your fingers or a knife.

Anyway You Slice It

There are many ways to cut foods. Some foods are cut into large pieces. Others are cut into very small pieces. The terms used in your recipe tell you how to cut the ingredients.

The most common ways foods are cut are listed here. The terms are arranged from the largest pieces to the smallest pieces.

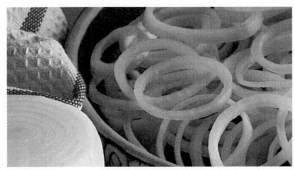
Slicing   National Onion Association

⬅ *Slice:* To cut into flat pieces. The pieces may be thick or thin.

Julienne: To cut into long, thin strips ➡ the size of matchsticks.

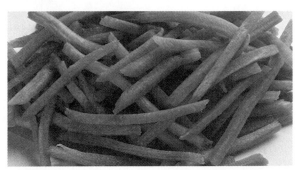
Julienne   Mann Packing Company, Inc., Salinas, CA

Shred: To cut into long, very thin strips using a knife or the large holes of a grater. ➡

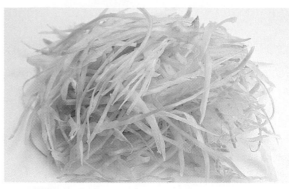

Shredding

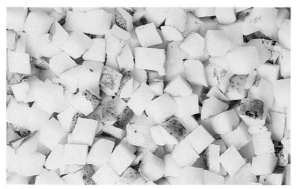

Cubing   Hobart Corporation

⬅ *Cube:* To cut into cubes about ½-inch in size. Dice means the same thing as cube.

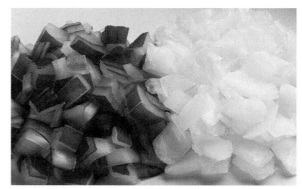

Chopping   Mann Packing Company, Inc., Salinas, CA

Chop: To cut into small, uneven ➡ pieces.

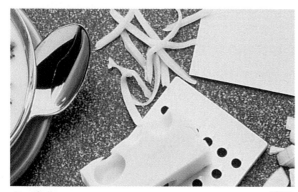

Grating   USDA

⬅ *Grate:* To cut into small pieces using the small holes of a grater.

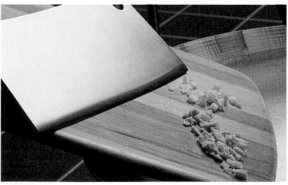

Mincing   American Heart Association

Mince: To cut into very small pieces. ➡

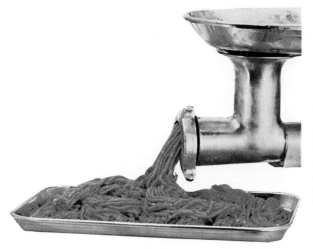

Grinding

National Turkey Federation

Grind: To crush into very tiny bits by putting food through a food grinder.

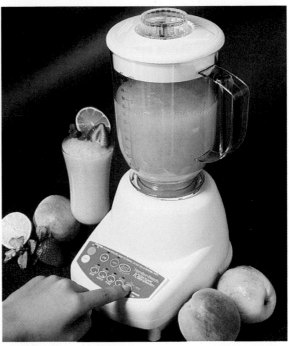

Puréeing

Hamilton Beach/ Proctor-Silex, Inc.

Purée: To grind or mash food until it becomes smooth and liquid.

Mixing Ingredients

There are many ways to combine ingredients. Some ingredients are combined using slow, gentle motions. Other ingredients are combined using fast, forceful motions. Stir, mix, blend, beat, cream, and whip have similar meanings. They all mean to combine ingredients with a spoon, wire whisk, beater, or electric mixer. The main differences in these terms are the speed and force of the motion used.

The terms that describe how to combine ingredients are listed here. These terms are arranged in order from the most gentle motion to the most forceful.

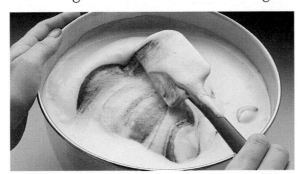

Folding

General Mills, Inc.

Fold: To gently combine ingredients. To fold ingredients, slide a spatula down through the center of a mixture. Then, slide the spatula across the bottom of the bowl and up the side, gently lifting and turning the ingredients. Repeat these steps until the mixture is blended.

Knead: To press and fold a ball of ➡ dough with the heels of your hands until the dough is smooth and elastic.

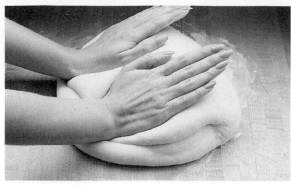

Kneading   General Mills, Inc.

⬅ *Cut in:* To combine solid fat, such as shortening, with a flour mixture by cutting the fat into tiny pieces with knives or a pastry blender.

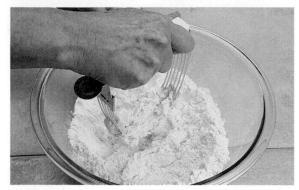

Cutting-in

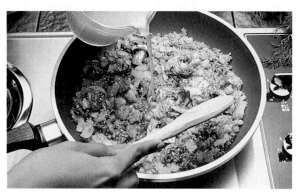

Stir: To slowly move a spoon in a cir- ➡ cle to combine ingredients.

Stirring   American Heart Association

Mix: To combine ingredients by stirring or beating them.

Blend: To mix ingredients until they are very smooth.

Beat: To stir quickly with a spoon, wire whisk, beater, or mixer until ingredients are smooth.

Cream: To beat sugar and a solid fat, such as butter, together until they are smooth, light, and fluffy.

Whip: To beat rapidly with a wire whisk, beater, or mixer in order to make a mixture smooth and fluffy.

Cooking with Fat

Foods cooked in hot fat are called fried foods. These foods are cooked in an uncovered pan. Fat is added to the pan in all types of frying except pan-broiling. The amount of fat added to the pan varies. Deep frying uses the most fat. Stir-frying requires the least fat. The fat used in pan-broiling comes from the meat being cooked.

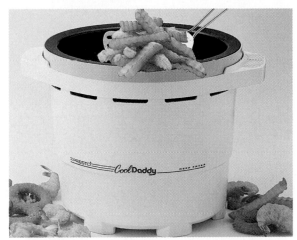

Deep frying   National Presto Industries, Inc.

Deep-fry: To cook food by completely immersing it in hot fat. This is also called French frying.

Sauté: To brown or cook lightly and quickly in a small amount of hot fat. This also is called panfrying.

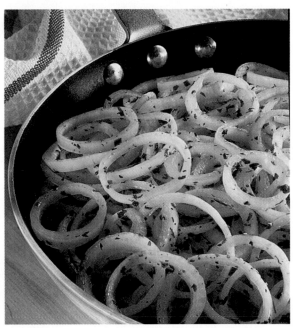

Sautéing   National Onion Association

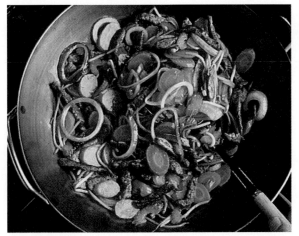

Stir-frying   USDA

Stir-fry: To cook small pieces of food quickly in a very small amount of hot fat. The food is stirred throughout cooking.

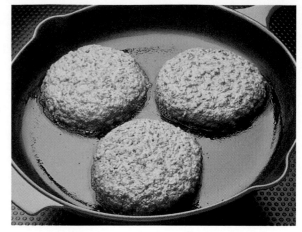

Pan-broil: To cook meat in its own fat. The fat melts as the meat cooks. The fat is poured off as it collects. ➡

Pan-broiling

National Cattlemen's Beef Association

 ## Cultures of the World

Chinese Stir-Fry

China is one of the largest countries on earth. The cuisine of China varies as you move from region to region. For example, in the western region of Szechwan (SESH-wan), many foods are very spicy. In the eastern region of Shanghai (SHANG-hi), foods often have a sweet taste.

The taste of the food may differ as you travel from one region to the next. However, you'll see the same kitchen equipment and cooking methods used all around the nation. In fact, the most common Chinese kitchen equipment and cooking methods have changed hardly at all in over 2,000 years.

The most important equipment in Chinese kitchens includes a wide blade knife and a wok. The knife is used to cut

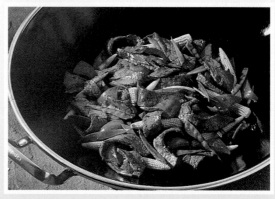

National Cattlemen's Beef Association

Chinese cooking involves several techniques studied in this chapter.

foods into small pieces. Cabbage is shredded. Eggplant is thinly sliced. Other foods may be diced or minced. Foods are cut into small pieces so they will cook quickly and be easy to eat with chopsticks. Once foods are cut, they are combined and cooked in the wok.

1

1—*Enrich:* Have students research China and stir-frying. Have them prepare the stir-fry recipe in 10-1. If desired, serve it with hot tea.

Stir-frying is a widely used cooking method. This is because stir-frying cooks food quickly and uses little fuel. Cooking fuel is scarce in China, so fast cooking is important. Woks also are sometimes used for boiling, steaming, and deep-frying.

People in China eat mostly vegetables and either rice or wheat. Rice grows well in the hot, rainy, southern areas of China. Rice is eaten at every meal. It is considered impolite to not eat every grain of rice served.

In the northern part of China, wheat grows well. It is used to make steamed buns, pancakes, and dumplings. Wheat is also used to make noodles. Chinese diners prefer long noodles because they stand for "long life." It is a tradition to give noodles as a birthday gift in some areas of China.

Tea is a popular beverage in China. Hundreds of types of tea grow there. Two teas many people drink are Dragon's Whiskers tea and Silver Needles tea. There is a legend that hundreds of years ago, tea farmers taught monkeys to gather tea leaves for them!

Chinese foods are delicious. The next time you plan to eat out, consider going to a Chinese restaurant.

You may want to be adventurous and try some recipes for Chinese foods at home.

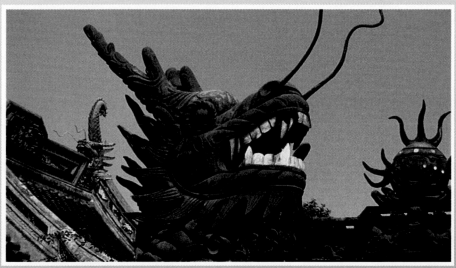

Abercrombie & Kent International

Exploring the cuisine of China can be an exciting adventure.

Cooking with Liquids

Foods can be cooked in any hot liquid. The liquid is often water or milk. Other liquids may be used, too. For instance, yogurt is often used as a cooking liquid in Northern Africa.

Some foods are cooked in a large amount of liquid. Others are cooked in a small amount. Boiling and poaching use large amounts of liquid. Small amounts are used to steam or braise foods.

Most foods cooked in liquid are prepared on the cooktop. Some are cooked in the oven. The foods may be cooked in a covered or uncovered pan. Your recipe will tell you the type and amount of liquid to use and how to heat it. It also will tell you if the pan needs to be covered.

Blanch: To put a food in boiling water for a very short time to pre-cook it.

Boil: To cook in hot liquid that has bubbles that rise and break on the surface of the liquid.

Braise: To cook large pieces of meat or poultry slowly in a small amount of hot liquid.

Parboil: To boil until partly cooked. Cooking is finished using another method.

Poach: To cook gently in enough hot liquid so that the food can float.

Scald: To heat milk just until tiny bubbles form at the edge of the pan.

Simmer: To cook in liquid that is almost boiling, but is not hot enough to bubble.

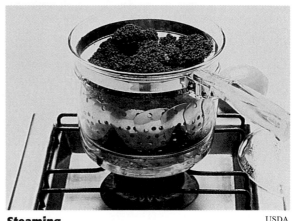

Steaming USDA

Steam: To cook in a pan using steam ➡ that rises from boiling liquid.

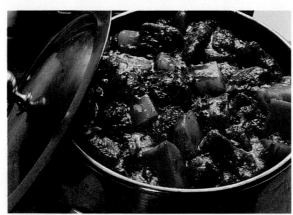

Stewing Del Monte Corporation

⬅ *Stew:* To slowly cook small pieces of food in moderate amounts of liquid.

Cooking with Dry Heat

What do cake, toast, and barbecued chicken have in common? All are cooked with dry heat. No fat or liquid is added. Foods cooked with dry heat are mostly cooked in an oven or toaster or on a grill.

Bake: To cook in hot air in an oven.

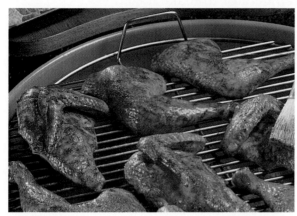

Barbecuing

National Broiler Council

Barbecue: To roast slowly over hot coals or in an oven and baste with a spicy sauce.

Broil: To cook directly under a very hot heating unit in an oven.

Brown: To make the surface of a food brown by baking, broiling, or toasting it.

Roast: To bake meat, fish, or poultry uncovered in hot air in an oven or over hot coals.

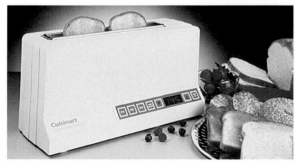

Toasting

Cuisinart

Toast: To brown foods using dry heat, usually in an oven or toaster.

Cooling Foods

Some foods are served cold. Recipes for these foods may instruct you to cool, chill, or freeze ingredients. For instance, a lemonade recipe may tell you to chill the drink for four hours. A cake recipe may tell you to cool the cake before frosting it.

Chill: To put food in the refrigerator to make it cold.

Cool: To let heated food come to room temperature.

Freeze: To lower a food's temperature to its freezing point or below.

Measuring Matters

Success with recipes depends on accurate measurements. If the measurements are off, even the best recipe won't look and taste good. Many recipes use abbreviations. An *abbreviation* is a shortened form of a word. Abbreviations save space. Common recipe abbreviations are listed in 10-2.

10-2 These common abbreviations, often used in recipes, are the cook's shorthand.

Recipe Shorthand	
Abbreviation	**Word**
c.	cup
°C degrees	Celsius
°F degrees	Fahrenheit
g or gm	gram
kg	kilogram
l	liter
lb. or #	pound
ml	milliliter
oz.	ounce
pt.	pint
qt.	quart
t. or tsp.	teaspoon
T. or Tbsp.	tablespoon

Ingredient Amounts

The amount of each ingredient you need may be given as units, weights, or volumes. Units tell you how many of an ingredient you should use. For instance, a recipe might call for one egg or two slices of bread.

Weights tell you how heavy an ingredient should be. An ounce of sugar and a kilogram of cherries are examples. Weighed ingredients are measured on a scale. Recipes used in restaurants and bakeries list ingredient weights. That's because it is easier for chefs to weigh 20 pounds of flour than to measure 80 cups.

Volume is the space an ingredient occupies. A cup of flour and a liter of milk are volume measurements. These measurements are made with measuring cups and spoons. Recipes written for use at home list ingredient volumes.

The ingredients you'll need to measure by volume are either dry or liquid. *Dry ingredients* include sugar, flour, and shortening. *Liquid ingredients* include milk, water, and oil.

Math in the Kitchen

Measurements Count

Skilled cooks know that accurate measurements are the key to success. Too little or too much of an ingredient can cause a recipe to fail. You can perform this experiment to see how important accurate measurements really are.

Gently fill a one-cup dry measuring cup with spoonfuls of flour. When it's heaping full, weigh it and record its weight. Now, level off the flour-filled cup, weigh it, and record its weight. Next, shake the flour-filled cup, add flour, shake, and add flour until no more can be added. Level off the cup, weigh it, and record its weight.

Place an 18-inch-long piece of waxed paper on the counter. Empty the flour in the measuring cup into a sifter. Place the measuring cup in the center of the waxed paper. Sift the flour until the cup is heaping full. Weigh the flour and record its weight. Next, level off the flour-filled cup, weigh it, and record its weight.

Which cup of flour weighed the most? Which cup of flour weighed the least? What was the difference in the weight of the cup of flour that weighed the most and the cup of flour that weighed the least? Why do the weights vary? What conclusions can you draw from this experiment?

The method used to measure dry ingredients differs from the method used to measure liquid ingredients. Knowing how to measure each type of ingredient helps you to get the exact amount needed. Success depends on accurate measurements.

Measuring Dry Ingredients

Dry ingredients are measured using measuring spoons or dry measuring cups. These ingredients are measured the same way whether you use standard or metric measuring spoons and cups. Here's how to measure dry ingredients, 10-3.

1. Fill the measuring cup or spoon with the ingredient.
2. Drag the straight edge of a metal spatula or knife over the cup or spoon to level off the ingredient.

Some dry ingredients need special treatment. Flour, brown sugar, and solid fats are examples.

10-3 Fill dry measuring cups until they are overflowing and then level off ingredients with a spatula. This helps you make sure you get the exact amount of dry ingredients you need.

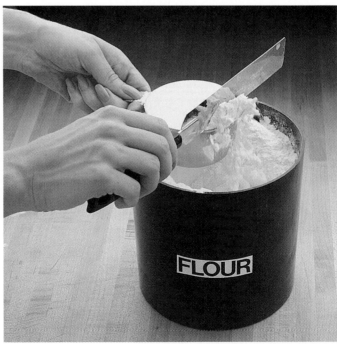

General Mills, Inc.

Flour

Before measuring flour, stir the flour with a spoon or fluff it with a fork to loosen it. Then gently place spoonfuls of flour into the measuring cup. If the flour is lumpy, or if your recipe calls for sifted flour, you can sift the flour into the measuring cup. Powdered sugar is measured in the same way.

Dipping the measuring cup into flour causes the flour to pack down. Shaking the filled measuring cup also causes the flour to pack down. If you pack flour down, you will end up with more flour than called for in the recipe. The food will be too dry or tough.

Brown Sugar

Press the brown sugar into the measuring cup. Pack it down until the measuring cup is full and level it off. When you empty the brown sugar out of the cup, it should hold the shape of the cup.

Solid Fats

Shortening, butter, and margarine are solid fats. Measure solid fat by pressing it into the measuring cup and leveling it off. Use a rubber spatula to remove the fat from the measuring cup. Another way to measure sticks of butter and margarine is to use the markings on their wrappers. One stick usually equals one-half cup. The wrapper markings often show tablespoons.

Measuring Liquid Ingredients

Liquid ingredients are measured using liquid measuring cups. Small amounts are measured with measuring spoons. Liquid ingredients are measured the same way whether you use standard or metric measuring spoons and cups. Here's how to measure liquid ingredients in a measuring cup:

1. Place the liquid measuring cup on a level surface.
2. Bend down and look at the measurements written on the side of the measuring cup. Pour the liquid into the measuring cup until you have the amount you need.

Be sure to bend down to read the measurements. See 10-4. If you lift the cup to check the amount of liquid, the cup will tilt. You will end up with more or less liquid than you need.

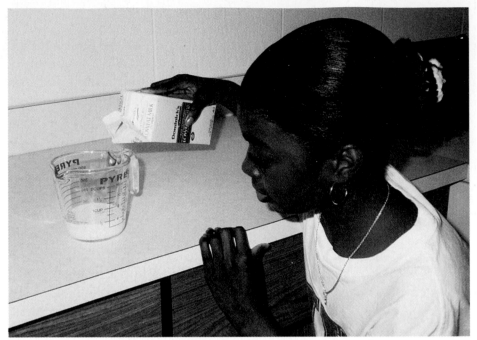

10-4 Measuring liquid ingredients at eye-level will help you make sure you get just the right amount for your recipe.

Adjusting Recipe Yields

There are times when you may want to adjust a recipe to yield more or fewer servings. For instance, if you are having friends over for a party, you may need more servings than one recipe would yield. If you are making a meal for only two people, you may need to adjust the recipe to yield a smaller amount.

To adjust the yield of a recipe, you need to decide how many servings you need. Then, divide the servings you need by the servings one recipe yields. The answer you get is the number you will use to adjust your recipe. This is the formula to use.

$$\frac{Servings}{You\ Need} \div \frac{Servings\ One}{Recipe\ Yields} = \frac{Recipe\ Adjustment}{Number}$$

You will need to multiply the amount of each ingredient by the recipe adjustment number.

For example, you may want to serve one cup of fruit punch to each of 16 people. Your recipe yields 8 cups. You would need to multiply the amount of each ingredient by 2. To obtain the recipe adjustment number, follow this equation:

$$\frac{\text{Servings You Need}}{} \div \frac{\text{Servings One Recipe Yields}}{} = \frac{\text{Recipe Adjustment Number}}{}$$
$$16 \div 8 = 2$$

If you only need 14 servings, your recipe adjustment number would be $1\frac{3}{4}$ ($14 \div 8 = 1\frac{3}{4}$). It is easier to increase a recipe when you don't have to work with fractions. It would be easier to make 16 servings even when you only need 14 servings. You could save the extra two servings to have as a snack later.

If you wanted to serve fruit punch to only four people, you would use the same formula. You would need to multiply the amount of each ingredient by $\frac{1}{2}$. To obtain the recipe adjustment number, follow this equation:

$$\frac{\text{Servings You Need}}{} \div \frac{\text{Servings One Recipe Yields}}{} = \frac{\text{Recipe Adjustment Number}}{}$$
$$4 \div 8 = \frac{1}{2}$$

Sometimes you may want to make a whole recipe even when you only need part of it. You could save the leftovers for another meal.

Using Equivalents

Increasing or decreasing recipes is easier when you know equivalent amounts of ingredients. Equivalents are two ways of saying the same thing. For example, seven days equal one week. A dozen eggs equal 12 eggs. One cup equals 16 tablespoons. The chart in 10-5 lists the most common standard measures and equivalents. Equivalents help you adjust recipes.

10-5 Knowing equivalent amounts makes it easy to adjust recipe yields.

Standard Measurement Equivalents		
3 teaspoons	= 1	tablespoon
16 tablespoons	= 1	cup
2 cups	= 1	pint
2 pints	= 1	quart
4 quarts	= 1	gallon

Let's say your recipe adjustment number is ½. Your recipe calls for 1 tablespoon of sugar. That means you will need ½ tablespoon of sugar (1 tablespoon × ½ = ½ tablespoon). Most measuring spoon sets don't include a ½ tablespoon measure. How can you accurately measure ½ tablespoon? You know from 10-5 that 1 tablespoon is equivalent to 3 teaspoons. So, ½ tablespoon is equivalent to 1½ teaspoons (3 teaspoons × ½ = 1½ teaspoons). You can accurately measure this amount with 1-teaspoon and ½-teaspoon measuring spoons.

Some recipes are easier to adjust than others. See 10-6. Exact amounts are not as critical when you make soups, stews, and salads. Exact measures are very important when making cookies, cakes, bread, and other baked goods. These foods won't turn out right if the measurements are not accurate.

Recipe Adjustments

Fruit Punch:

4 cups pineapple juice
2 cups orange juice
2 cups ginger ale

1. Blend all the ingredients together.
2. Serve over ice.

Yield: 8 one-cup servings

Original Recipe
(This recipe makes 8 one-cup servings.)

Fruit Punch:

4 cups pineapple juice × 2 = 8 cups
2 cups orange juice × 2 = 4 cups
2 cups ginger ale × 2 = 4 cups

1. Blend all the ingredients together.
2. Serve over ice.

Yield: 8 one-cup servings × 2 = 16 one-cup servings

Doubled Recipe
(To make twice as much, you need to double each ingredient.)

Fruit Punch:

4 cups pineapple juice × ½ = 2 cups
2 cups orange juice × ½ = 1 cup
2 cups ginger ale × ½ = 1 cup

1. Blend all the ingredients together.
2. Serve over ice.

Yield: 8 one-cup servings × ½ = 4 one-cup servings

Halved Recipe
(To make half as much, you need to divide the amount of each ingredient by two.)

10-6 Write down recipe adjustments so you won't forget to adjust the measurement of any ingredient.

If you need to adjust ingredient amounts, write down the exact amount of each ingredient you will need. This will help you to remember to use the right amount of each ingredient.

Knowing how to read recipes and adjust yields is the first step in planning menus. In the next chapter, you will learn how to select recipes and use them to create nutritious, delicious meals.

In a Nutshell

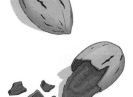

- A recipe is a list of ingredients and directions for preparing a food.
- The five parts of a recipe are the ingredient list, cooking equipment needed, cooking time and temperature, steps to follow, and yield.
- Recipe terms tell you exactly how to prepare, combine, or cook ingredients.
- Foods can be cooked in hot fat, hot liquid, or hot, dry air.
- Recipe success depends on accurate measurements.
- Ingredient amounts may be given as units, volumes, or weights.
- To adjust a recipe's yield, divide the servings you need by the servings one recipe yields. Multiply the amount of each ingredient in the recipe by this number.

In the Know

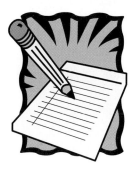

1. The ingredient list tells you _____.
   A. the method for measuring ingredients
   B. how to combine ingredients
   C. the amount of ingredients needed
   D. the yield
2. _____ is the number and size of portions a recipe will make.
3. Write the word that each of the following abbreviations represents.
   A. # _____
   B. tsp. _____
   C. oz. _____
   D. kg _____
   E. ml _____
   F. c. _____

4. Which term below would result in the smallest pieces of food?
   A. Julienne.
   B. Mince.
   C. Cube.
   D. Shred.

5. _____ means to moisten food during roasting to keep the food from drying out.

6. Which term below is the most gentle way to combine ingredients?
   A. Whip.
   B. Cream.
   C. Fold.
   D. Beat.

7. Which cooking method uses the most fat?

8. What do blanch, braise, and poach have in common?

9. True or false? Liquid and dry ingredients should be measured with liquid measuring cups.

10. It is best to use _____ to level ingredients in a dry measuring cup.
    A. the straight edge of a knife
    B. your finger
    C. a spoon
    D. any of the above

11. Explain how to measure one cup of water.

What Would You Do?

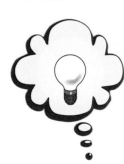

Your friend wants you to help him make brownies. He has the recipe and all the ingredients sitting on the counter. He gets out a coffee cup and iced tea spoon to measure the ingredients. You suggest that he should use measuring cups and spoons. He tells you that being a little off in the amounts won't matter. What advice would you give him?

Expanding Your Knowledge

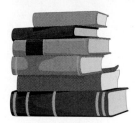

1. Find a recipe in a magazine or newspaper. Circle and label each part of the recipe.
2. Make a vegetable salad. Cut each vegetable in a different way. For instance, you could shred cabbage, julienne carrots, slice tomatoes, and mince onions.
3. Invite a chef to speak to your class. Ask the chef to demonstrate creative ways to cut foods. Prepare a list of questions to ask the chef ahead of time. You might ask how a person prepares to become a chef. Ask the chef to describe his or her job.
4. Locate two recipes. Choose a salad, beverage, cookie, soup, or pizza recipe. List all the cooking terms you find in the recipes and define them. Also write down any abbreviations you find in the recipes.
5. Make a set of cooking term flash cards. Write the cooking term on one side of the flash card. On the back of each card, write the meaning of the cooking term. Create a game using the flash cards.
6. Select four cooking terms. Demonstrate to the class what you should do to a food when you see these terms in a recipe.
7. Teach a friend how to measure ingredients. Explain why accurate measurements are important.
8. Measure the amount of water a coffee cup holds. Find some different shaped coffee cups and measure the amount of water they hold. What would happen if you used these cups instead of a measuring cup to measure a cup of water? Repeat this experiment with a soup spoon, iced tea spoon, and measuring spoons.

Chapter 11
What's on the Menu?

Objectives

After reading this chapter, you will be able to
- ❏ plan meals that are nutritious, tasty, and appealing.
- ❏ create menus that use the resources you have.
- ❏ identify types of convenience foods.
- ❏ decide when to use convenience foods.

New Terms

garnish: a decoration you can eat that adds color to meals.
resources: ways and means, such as time and money, that are used to complete a task.
convenience food: food that has been partially or totally prepared when you buy it.

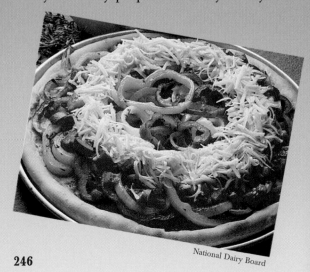

National Dairy Board

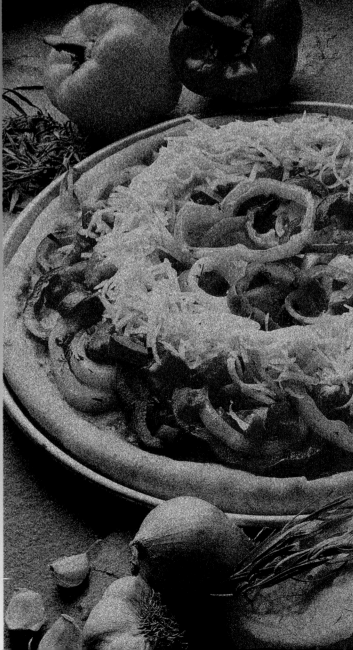

Planning menus can be fun. It gives you a chance to be a detective, scientist, and artist, all at once. As a detective, you gather clues about who will be eating the meal. You also track down why, when, and where they will be eating. You'll need to find out what they like, too.

As a scientist, you invent menus that are good for you. The kitchen becomes the lab where you put your nutrition knowledge to work.

As an artist, you get to use your creativity. You can try new color, flavor, and texture combinations in the foods you select. A blend of these helps you create a meal that is a work of art you can eat.

Taking the time to plan your meals pays off in many ways. It helps you be sure the meals are good for you. It also helps you create meals that look as good as they taste. Planning meals can help you in other ways, too. You know before you begin what you will need to prepare the entire menu. You can choose foods that can be made with the time, money, skills, and equipment you have. The best meals are planned meals.

Who? Why? When? Where? What?

Before planning a meal, think about who will be eating it. Will your menu be for a family lunch? Will it be an after school snack with friends? Maybe you are planning a birthday party menu. Knowing who will be eating helps you plan a nutritious menu that everyone will like, 11-1.

As you plan the meal, keep in mind why you will be making it. Try to match your menu with the occasion. Will it be a lunch to take to school? Perhaps it will be a meal for a special event. Meals served to celebrate events often differ from everyday meals. For instance, a holiday dinner might include a special dessert and table decorations.

Now you must decide when the menu will be served. This will help you plan a menu that fits your schedule. For example, if time is limited when you are serving an early morning breakfast, you need to plan a menu that is quick to prepare. You might select foods that could be made ahead of time. Your menu choices may differ if you have plenty of time.

11-1 Who do you suppose will eat this meal? Why, when, and where will the person eat it?

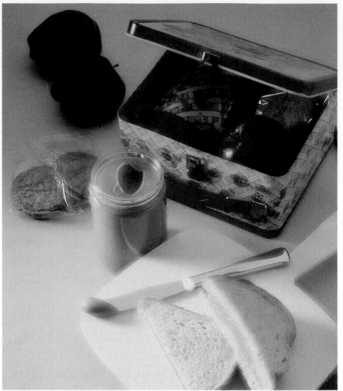

Knowing where the meal will be prepared and served helps you plan the menu, too. You can check to see how much space there is to prepare and serve foods. If the meal is to be served at home, you already know how much space you have. Preparing meals is easy when the space needed to make the menu matches the space you have.

What will you serve? You can answer this question best when you know who, why, when, and where. What you choose to serve depends on all of these. It depends on nutrient needs and food likes, too. Choices also depend on the time, money, cooking skills, and kitchen equipment you have.

Planning Nutritious Meals

You learned about the Food Guide Pyramid in Chapter 3. The major food groups are a quick and easy way to keep track of nutrients. They can help you plan meals that meet the nutrient needs of the people you are serving.

Cultures of the World

Sunny Mexico...Just South of the Border

Mexico is a southern neighbor of the United States. Mexican cuisine is a blend of foods from old Mexico and Spain. Spanish explorers arrived in Mexico in the 1500s. They brought rice, wheat, olives, spices, peaches, apricots, cattle, and cheese. Today, these foods from Spain are raised along side native Mexican foods. Foods native to Mexico include corn, beans, avocados, chilies, tomatoes, squash, potatoes, and vanilla.

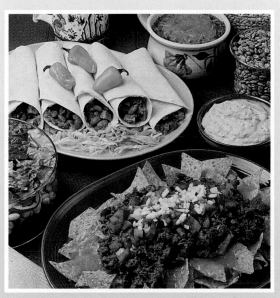

Idaho Bean Commission

You can use the Food Guide Pyramid to plan nutritious meals in any cuisine.

Corn and beans are Mexico's major crops. They are served at almost every meal. Beans are called frijoles (free-HOH-layz). They range in color from dark red to pink to black. Some are spotted! Beans are usually boiled, mashed, and fried to make frijoles refritos (reh-FREE-tohs).

A famous bean from Mexico is the cacao (kuh-KOW) bean. Cacao beans are the source of chocolate. In the 1500s, a group of Native Americans, the Aztec Indians, made a bitter drink from cacao beans. Only the priests and rulers were allowed to drink it. Now, chocolate is sweetened and eaten all over the world.

Tortillas (tor-TEE-yuhs) are the most important use for corn. This bread is made by flattening a mixture of cornmeal and water until it is paper-thin. The cornmeal dough is toasted, fried, or baked. Many people make this flat bread every day. Some buy fresh tortillas from a factory called a tortilleria (tor-tee-yuh-REE-uh).

Dozens of foods are made with tortillas. Enchiladas (ehn-chee-LAH-dahs) are tortillas wrapped around meat or cheese. They are baked and topped with a chunky tomato sauce called salsa (SAHL-sah). Tortillas are folded, fried, and filled with beans or meat and cheese to make tacos (TAH-cohs).

Quesadillas (keh-sah-DEE-yahs) are tortilla turnovers that are filled with cheese or vegetables. Nachos (NAH-choz) are crisp, fried tortillas served with a bean dip.

Chili (CHEE-leh) peppers add flavor to many Mexican dishes. Chilies come in many sizes, shapes, and flavors. Some are as small as a bean. Other are more than a foot long. Chili peppers can be any shade of green, yellow, orange, or red. Many have a sweet, mild flavor. Others, such as jalapeño (hah-lah-PAYN-yoh) peppers are fiery hot. You can give almost any dish a Mexican flair by adding a few chili peppers.

In the past, meal planners chose foods from the meat group first. Then they chose the other foods to go with it. The meat group was given the central role in meals. It was almost always served as the main dish.

Today, nutritionists feel that the central role belongs to the bread, cereal, rice, and pasta group; vegetable group; and fruit group. Meal planners should select these foods first. The meat group should be given a small role in meals. Breads, cereals, rice, pasta, fruits, and vegetables should be the main dish, and meat should be a side dish. That's because many foods in the meat group are high in fat. Too much fat in your diet can increase your chances of having heart disease and certain types of cancer. High-fiber foods, such as grains, cereals, fruits, and vegetables, can help prevent these diseases.

The most nutritious meals are planned in this order:

1. Bread, cereal, rice, and pasta group (Plan two or three servings.)
2. Vegetable group (Choose one or two.)
3. Fruit group (Choose one or two.)
4. Milk, yogurt, and cheese group (Choose one serving of a low-fat food from this group.)
5. Meat, poultry, fish, dry beans, eggs, and nuts group (Choose one serving of a low-fat food from this group. Foods from this group only need to be served twice daily.)
6. Fats, oils, and sweets group (Limit servings to one or two).

The meal shown in 11-2 was planned in the manner described above.

There are many foods to choose from in each of the major food groups. You can serve any food. The best choices are foods that are low in fat, sugar, and salt and high in fiber.

Try to serve a variety of foods from each food group every week. The more variety you get, the better your diet will be. The foods you serve depend on your likes and needs.

Some family members may have special needs. For instance, some may want to eat fewer calories or less fat. To lower calories, you could plan fresh fruit for dessert instead of pie or cake. You could serve plain broccoli instead of broccoli in butter sauce. To reduce fat, you could plan to bake fish instead of frying it. All family members will be able to enjoy the meal if you plan for special needs.

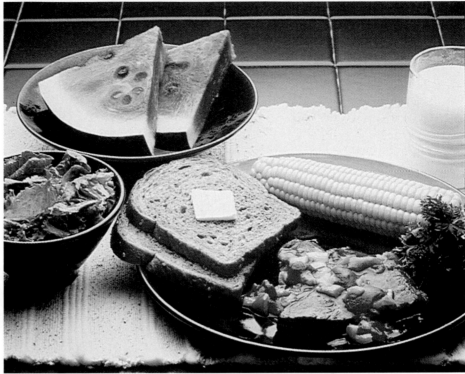

USDA

11-2 Check out this meal. How do the number of servings from each food group compare to the recommended number of servings?

Planning Meals with Appeal

What's the first thing you notice about a meal? Most people say how it looks. You want to begin eating right away. The most appealing meals include a variety of colors, shapes, textures, temperatures, and flavors.

Colors

Planning a meal with eye appeal is like painting a picture. Meal planners use foods the way artists use paint colors. The colors of the foods complement each other and create a picture on a plate. The colors in the most appealing meals look good together.

Garnishes add color to meals, too. A ***garnish*** is a decoration you can eat. It makes the food look more appealing. For instance, paprika sprinkled on fish is a garnish. Parsley sprigs, lemon slices, and carrot curls are other garnishes. Can you think of others you have seen?

Choose foods that are different colors. Color adds zest to a meal. See 11-3. All the foods in Meal A are white. The meal looks dull. With some simple changes, Meal A becomes Meal B. The colors in Meal B complement each other to create a meal with eye appeal. Choose food colors that do not clash with each other. For instance, red beets and spaghetti sauce would not be a pleasing combination.

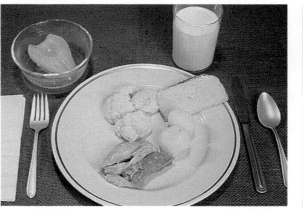 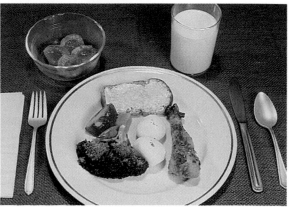

Meal A   **Meal B**   USDA

11-3 Why is Meal B more appealing than Meal A? How could you change Meal A to make it more appealing?

Shapes and Sizes

A variety of shapes and sizes gives meals eye appeal, too. The vegetable plate in 11-4 looks interesting. This is partly because of the variety of shapes and sizes of the foods being served.

You can change the shape and size of foods by cutting them. For example, you could serve fruits whole, halved, sliced, cubed, or puréed. Meat can be sliced, ground, or cut into strips.

11-4 The different shapes and sizes add interest to this vegetable plate.

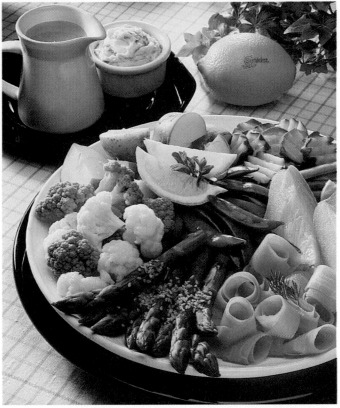

Sunkist Growers, Inc.

Textures

Texture is the way foods feel in your mouth. Foods may be soft, crispy, smooth, chewy, sticky, dry, or moist. The most appealing meals include a variety of textures.

In 11-3, Meal A has too many soft foods. Meal B has more variety. It includes soft, firm, and crisp foods.

Temperatures

Serving both hot and cold foods makes meals appealing, too. The cold foods contrast with the hot foods. Hot cocoa tastes good with a cold sandwich. The cold watermelon and milk in 11-2 contrast with the hot meat and corn.

Hot foods should be served hot. Cold foods should be served cold. Imagine eating lukewarm soup and drinking lukewarm milk. They aren't as pleasing as piping hot soup and icy cold milk.

Cooking Methods

You also can add appeal by using a variety of cooking methods. Imagine a meal of fried chicken, fried squash, fried cornbread, and fried cherry pie. This meal lacks variety. It would be more appealing if it included steamed squash, baked cornbread, and fresh cherries.

Flavors

The way a meal looks is only part of its appeal. Appealing meals include a variety of flavors that complement each other. It's a good idea to limit the number of foods with strong flavors at each meal. Too many strong flavors would overpower your taste buds. It's also smart not to repeat the same flavor. For instance, tomato soup and tomato salad are very much alike. You could serve clam chowder or fruit salad instead.

In 11-3, Meal A has too many mild flavors. The flavors of the apricots and broccoli in Meal B contrast with the mild flavors of the other foods. They add variety to the meal.

Planning Meals with Your Resources in Mind

The foods you are able to serve depend on the resources you have. ***Resources*** are the ways and means you have to complete a task. Four resources are needed to complete the task of preparing and serving a meal. These are time, money, food preparation skills, and kitchen equipment.

Time

It takes time to shop, store, prepare, and serve food. You need to decide how much time you can spend on each of these tasks. If you have plenty of time (and have the food preparation skills), you can prepare complex recipes. Easy-to-prepare foods will help if you need to whip up a meal in minutes.

If your resource of time is limited, you may need to buy the time of others. You buy time when you buy partially prepared or ready-to-eat foods. You also buy time when you eat out. You save your time when someone else does part or all of the work for you. You use your money to pay for their time. Busy families may choose to buy prepared foods or eat out when their food budgets will allow.

The time needed to make the meal in 11-5 can range from a few minutes to two hours or more. The meal is ready in minutes if you buy chicken at a fast-food restaurant. You could buy rice salad and instant ice tea mix at the supermarket. If you made some or all of these foods from scratch, this meal would take longer to prepare.

The cooking method you choose also depends on your time. If you are in a hurry, you can heat foods in a microwave oven or on a cooktop. You will need to give these foods more attention than foods cooked in a conventional oven. That's because they cook quickly. Many foods need to be watched closely or stirred often.

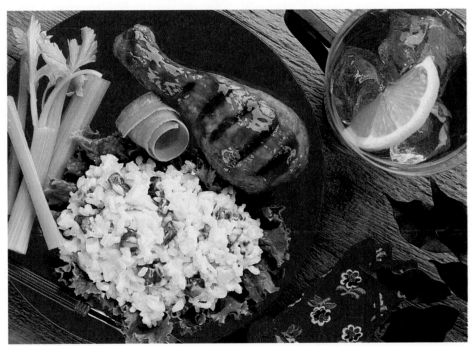

USA Rice Council

11-5 The resources needed to prepare this meal depend on the food forms you choose.

Money

A second resource is money. Most families set aside a certain amount of money for food each week. The money can be used to buy foods at the supermarket or in restaurants. Money also can be used to buy the time of others. For instance, when you eat out or buy ready-to-eat foods, you pay for the time of others to prepare the food.

Planning meals can help you stay within your food budget. You will need to decide the amount you will spend on ingredients for making foods from scratch. You will also need to decide how much you will spend on ready-to-eat foods and restaurant foods.

You can save money by buying ingredients to make foods from scratch. Foods made from scratch often cost less than partially prepared, ready-to-eat, and restaurant foods.

Food Preparation Skills

Your food preparation skills are also a resource that affects your menu choices. The skills needed to make the meal in 11-5 can range from few to many. A beginning cook could make the iced tea and prepare the fresh vegetables. A cook with more skill might prepare the chicken, too. A highly skilled cook may make all the foods from scratch.

You can improve your food preparation skills with practice. Start with simple recipes, such as one for baked potatoes. Then move on to more complex recipes, such as a recipe for scalloped potatoes. As you gain experience, complex recipes will seem easier.

Kitchen Equipment

Your kitchen equipment can affect your food choices, 11-6. Most recipes don't require any special equipment. If special equipment is needed, you often can use something else. For example, if you don't have a wok, you can stir-fry vegetables in a large skillet.

The equipment you have can affect your whole menu. For instance, you can't heat three pots at the same time if you have only two surface units on your range.

The kitchen equipment needed to prepare the menu in 11-5 depends on your choices. You only need tableware if you buy instant ice tea mix and ready-to-eat chicken, rice salad, and vegetables. To prepare this meal from scratch, you would need a range or hot plate to cook the chicken and rice. You would need a vegetable peeler, knife, and cutting board to prepare the fresh vegetables.

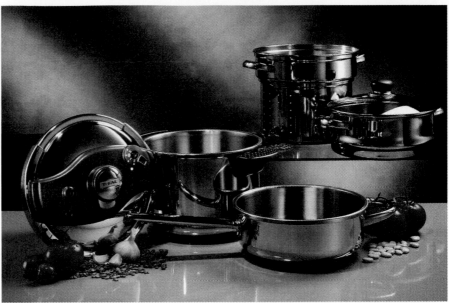

T-Fal

11-6 A variety of cookware is a resource that would allow you to prepare a range of foods.

Using Your Resources

The amount of each resource you have affects menu choices. People with a great deal of each resource can plan to serve almost any food. However, most people have a limited amount of one or more resources. Having limited resources doesn't mean you have to give up favorite foods or good nutrition. You will simply have to decide how to use your resources to prepare the foods you want to serve.

You can compare the amount of each resource you need with the resources you have for each recipe in a menu. If you need more resources than you have, you can alter your menu. For instance, you could serve a less costly food if your money is limited. You could buy ready-to-eat foods if your time, skills, or equipment are limited.

Using Convenience Foods

Forms of food that need little or no preparation are called *convenience foods*. These foods have been partially or totally prepared for you. They can help you serve tasty, nutritious meals in minutes.

With the help of convenience foods, you could serve the meal in 11-7 in less than 30 minutes. You could use bottled salad dressing, spaghetti sauce from a jar, dried spaghetti noodles, and ready-made bread. You could use canned peaches, instant pudding mix, and frozen lemonade concentrate, too. All you would have to do is heat the sauce and prepare the pudding and lemonade mixes. Then wash and cut the lettuce and boil the spaghetti noodles, and you'd be ready to eat.

This same meal made from scratch might take two hours or more to prepare. You would need to measure and mix ingredients to make the salad dressing, noodles, spaghetti sauce, bread, pudding, and lemonade. Then you would have to cook the noodles, sauce, bread, and pudding. After that, you would need to wash and slice the lettuce and peaches.

There are two main types of convenience foods. They are ready-to-eat and partially prepared foods.

11-7 Convenience foods can be used for many of the items featured in this menu. With the help of convenience foods, this meal can be prepared in minutes.

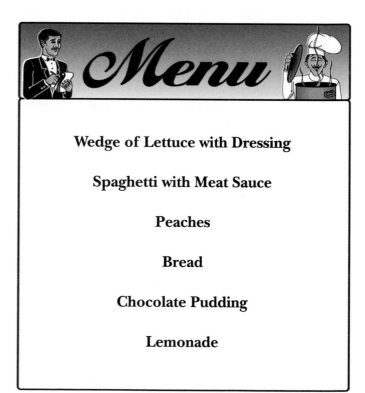

Menu

Wedge of Lettuce with Dressing

Spaghetti with Meat Sauce

Peaches

Bread

Chocolate Pudding

Lemonade

Ready-to-Eat Foods

Ready-to-eat foods don't need any preparation. There is no need to wash, peel, slice, mix, or cook. Just open the package and serve. Foods from every food group are sold in ready-to-eat form.

- Bread, cereal, rice, and pasta group: breakfast cereals, packaged breads, and bakery products.
- Vegetable group: canned vegetables. Fresh vegetables are almost ready to eat. Most only need to be washed before serving.
- Fruit group: canned fruits. Fresh fruits are almost ready to eat. Most only need to be washed before serving.
- Milk, yogurt, and cheese group: milk, cheese, yogurt, and ice cream. Almost all milk products are ready to eat.
- Meat, poultry, fish, dry beans, eggs, and nuts group: luncheon meats, canned tuna, and canned beans.
- Fats, oils, and sweets group: butter, margarine, mayonnaise, salad dressing, jelly, honey, and candy.

Restaurants and delicatessens sell a form of ready-to-eat food called take-out food. See 11-8. This food is bought and taken out of the store to be eaten. Take-out foods range from fancy meals to simple sandwiches.

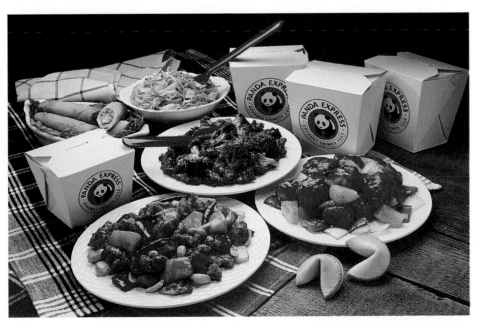

Panda Management Company, Inc.

11-8 Take-out foods are bought at restaurants, supermarkets, or delicatessens. These are ready-to-eat foods.

Some ready-to-eat foods may be canned or frozen. Canned foods may be packed in a can, bottle, or jar. They are cooked during the canning process. There is no need to wash, peel, or cook these foods. They can be served right from the package or heated. For example, you can buy canned plums, corn, tuna, chicken, pudding, and milk. Fats and sweets also are canned. Examples are vegetable oils, salad dressing, soft drinks, and syrup. You can buy canned mixtures of foods such as stew and chow mein, too.

Some frozen foods, such as ice cream and juice bars, are ready to eat. They don't need any preparation at all. Some, such as frozen fruits, only need to be thawed. Others, such as fish sticks, carrots, and waffles, taste best if they are warmed.

Many frozen foods can go straight from the freezer to the oven or cooktop. Some need to be thawed before cooking. The directions on the package will tell you if you should thaw the food before cooking.

Foods from every food group are sold in a frozen form, 11-9. Frozen pancake mix, whole turkeys, peas, orange juice, and milk shakes are examples. Frozen foods may be plain, in sauce, or mixed with other foods to make a main dish. For example, you can buy frozen plain peas, peas in a sauce, and pot pies that contain peas. You also can buy frozen meals.

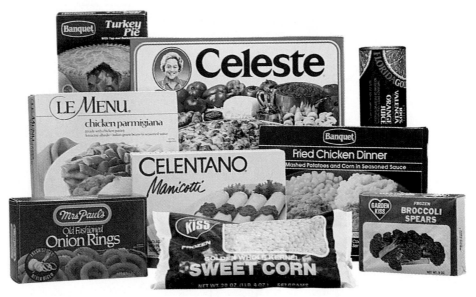

USDA

11-9 There are many frozen food choices.

Partially Prepared Foods _____

Partially prepared foods need some preparation. Most need to be blended with other ingredients. Cake mixes are an example. Most need to be mixed with eggs and water before being baked. Stuffing mixes, dried soups, and macaroni and cheese are other examples.

Buying Convenience Foods _____

Before deciding to buy a convenience food, consider the following:

- *The amount of time you have to prepare meals.* Many convenience foods can be prepared quickly. For example, a can of soup is ready to eat in a few minutes. Making soup from scratch takes more time.
- *Your cooking skills and kitchen equipment.* Special skills or equipment aren't needed to prepare most convenience foods. For example, you only need to open a can of soup and heat it before serving. Many recipes made from scratch require special skills or equipment. A beginning cook may not have all of the skills or equipment needed to prepare some recipes. Convenience foods might be a good alternative.
- *The money you have to spend on food.* Most convenience foods cost more than the same food made from scratch. Remember, too, that the total cost of a convenience food includes the food itself and any other ingredients you must add. For example, you will need to add eggs to a cake mix. Milk is added to pudding mixes. The less work you have to do to prepare a convenience food, the higher the price will be. The higher price reflects the time and energy spent by the food processor to prepare the food. To decide whether a convenience food fits into your budget, you must consider the value of your time. See 11-10.
- *The availability of foods.* Your food choices are determined by the foods available in food stores. Convenience foods are sold year-round. You can buy them anytime. Some fresh foods are available only at certain times of the year. Availability affects price, too. When fresh foods are in-season, they often cost less than convenience forms. If fresh foods are out of season, convenience foods may be a less costly choice. For instance, peas are out of season in the fall and winter. Your supermarket may not have fresh peas to sell at these times. Any fresh peas they do have are likely to be very costly.

11-10 To decide whether a convenience food is the best choice, you must consider your budget and time.

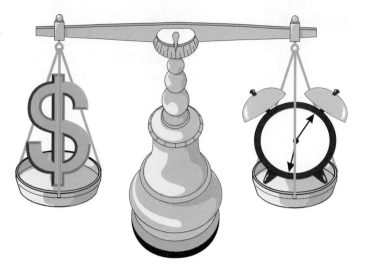

- *The nutrient content of the food.* Many convenience foods contain more fat, sugar, and salt than foods made from scratch. They may have fewer vitamins and minerals than foods made from scratch. Convenience foods may skimp on costly ingredients such as meat and vegetables. Information on food packages can help you make wise food choices.
- *Your taste preferences.* Your food choices depend on the flavors you prefer. Many people prefer the taste of fresh foods, but use convenience foods to save time. Food scientists work to make convenience foods taste like fresh foods. Some brands of convenience foods are more tasty than others. Comparing brands will help you find those that you like best.
- *How you plan to use the food.* Almost any form of food can be used in most recipes. For example, fresh, canned, or frozen carrots are fine in soup. Fresh foods work better than convenience forms in some recipes. For instance, fresh carrots are best for carrot raisin salad.
- *How long it will stay fresh.* Carefully stored canned, frozen, and dried foods will stay fresh for weeks or months. You can buy them long before you will need them. Most fresh foods are best when used within a week or two. Some can be kept for only a few days.

Science in the Kitchen

Is the Earth Becoming a Giant Garbage Heap?

Why are millions of Americans stacking newspapers and separating bottles and cans? These people are recycling their trash. They are trying to make a small dent in the world's garbage heap.

Why is recycling so important? After all, the average person in the United States creates only four pounds of trash each day. What's the big deal? Here's the big deal. There are 260 million people living in the United States. Just multiply the four pounds of trash each person makes by 260 million. Then multiply that by 365 days each year. That's one big pile of trash!

If you add the trash that businesses and industries throw away, the pile gets 22 times bigger. Oh, by the way, don't forget about the other 6 billion people living in other countries. They create trash, too, but Americans create much more trash per person than people in any other country.

Day after day, year after year, the trash heap grows. Where does all that trash go? Most of it goes into large holes in the ground called *landfills*. Some trash is dumped in the ocean. Some of the trash is burned.

These sound like good ways to dispose of garbage until you realize that the landfills are filling up. There isn't much space left in them. Trash dumped in the ocean is washing up on the beaches. It makes the beaches ugly and unsafe to use. The animals living in the ocean are getting sick and dying. How would you feel if

someone dumped tons of garbage on your home? The smoke from burning garbage is filtered, but many people are worried that poisons will be released into the air they breathe.

More and more of the trash Americans produce is being recycled. That means it can be processed and used again. Metal, glass, paper, and cardboard can be recycled. Some plastic can be recycled, too.

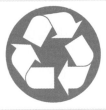

Look for this symbol. It tells you the container can be recycled.

Recycled trash is collected and sent to processing plants. At the plants, raw materials are separated and reused to make new products. For example, used aluminum soft drink cans are washed and melted down to make new cans. Recycled paper is used to make more paper. This saves a lot of space in landfills. Paper makes up 36 percent of all landfill waste!

Not all products are as easy to recycle as aluminum and paper. Plastic containers are an example. Recycling plants are working to invent new uses for them. One company has found a way to make them into park benches! It's important to find more ways to recycle plastic because it makes up seven percent of the waste in landfills.

Some progress has been made toward saving the earth. There's much, much more to be done. Everyone has a stake in the future. Here are some steps you can take to help.

- Buy foods and other products in containers that can be recycled. Then, be sure to recycle the container when it's empty!
- Buy products made from recycled materials.
- Buy foods in one large container instead of several smaller ones. Individually packaged foods, such as one-serving cereal boxes, create much more trash than larger packages of foods. You can divide the larger packages into smaller, reusable containers at home.
- Cut down on the amount of paper you use. Use cloth napkins instead of paper napkins at mealtime. Clean the kitchen with a sponge instead of paper towels.
- Make a compost heap. You can dispose of your food scraps, leaves, and grass clippings there. In the compost heap, these items will break down, then you can use the compost to fertilize soil.
- Reuse paper and plastic shopping bags. Take your own bags to the supermarket.
- Clean your house with chemicals that won't harm the earth. For example, baking soda is great for cleaning kitchen counters and sinks. White vinegar makes windows and mirrors gleam.
- Set up your own recycling center at home! Show your family how to sort products that can be recycled.
- Learn more about recycling and teach others how they can get involved. Take an active role in community recycling efforts. If your community doesn't have a recycling program, help get one started. Volunteer to help pick up items for recycling.
- Celebrate Earth Day on April 22. Keep celebrating every day. Make every day Earth Day.

You may wonder what difference one person can make. It's important to remember that every person has the power to change the environment. If everyone makes the effort, the changes will be enormous. The garbage heap will get smaller. The earth will be saved.

- *The packaging used.* Many fresh foods have simple packages. Some, such as fresh fruit, don't have packages at all. Most convenience foods have colorful packages that tell you about the food. The packages try to persuade you to buy the food. The packages add to the cost of the food. Some convenience foods can be cooked in their packages. Boil-in-bag vegetables and microwaveable pizza are examples. Some convenience foods, such as frozen dinners, can be cooked and served in their packages. These types of packages are costly and increase the price you pay for the food. When you eat the food, the package is thrown away. Choosing foods with packages that can be recycled helps to reduce your garbage and America's growing trash heap.

Once you've created your menu and decided which forms of food to use, you're ready to buy your ingredients. The next chapter will help you become a smart shopper.

In a Nutshell

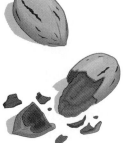

- The Food Guide Pyramid can help you plan nutritious meals.
- The most appealing meals include a variety of colors, shapes, textures, temperatures, and flavors.
- The time, money, cooking skills, and kitchen equipment you have affect your menu choices.
- Convenience foods have been partially or totally prepared before you buy them.
- Ready-to-eat and partially prepared foods are the main types of convenience foods.
- Convenience foods take less time, skills, and equipment to prepare than fresh foods.

In the Know

1. What changes would make this meal more appealing?
   Meatballs
   Cherry Tomatoes with Salad Dressing
   Small Boiled Potatoes
   Blueberries and Melon Balls
2. Menu choices depend on your _____.
   A. nutrient needs and food likes
   B. food budget
   C. time
   D. All of the above.
3. _____ are the ways and means you have that are used to complete a task.
4. Explain how you can use money to save time in the kitchen.
5. Which food group should be given the central role in meals?
   A. Meat, poultry, fish, dry beans, eggs, and nuts group.
   B. Bread, cereal, rice, and pasta group.
   C. Milk, yogurt, and cheese group.
   D. Fats, oils, and sweets group.

6. Which food is a ready-to-eat food?
   A. Lemonade mix.
   B. Refrigerator biscuits.
   C. Canned pears.
   D. Instant mashed potatoes.
7. Plan a meal that uses mostly convenience foods. The meal should include at least one food from each of the major food groups.
8. Explain why most milk products can be thought of as convenience foods.
9. Which is true about convenience foods?
   A. Most cost less than the same foods made from scratch.
   B. Most are available in the supermarket year-round.
   C. Special equipment is needed to prepare most of them.
   D. Most have less fat, sugar, and salt than foods made from scratch.

What Would You Do?

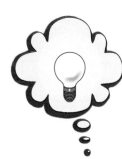

Your sister wants to make a birthday dinner for your dad. She know that he likes ham, red cabbage, tomatoes, and raspberry sherbet. She asks your opinion of the menu. What advice would you give her? How could she improve the menu?

Expanding Your Knowledge

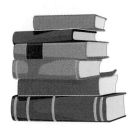

1. Cut out three magazine pictures that show complete meals. Make a poster that explains how the foods in each meal vary in color, shape, size, flavor, texture, and temperature.
2. Plan a menu that could be prepared if you have plenty of time, limited money and skills, and adequate equipment. Alter the menu so that it can be prepared using only a hot plate.
3. Keep a diary of the meals you eat for the next three days. Then analyze each meal. How many servings from each food group did each meal contain? Did the colors, shapes, sizes, flavors, textures, and temperatures of the foods complement each other? What improvements could you make?

4. Visit a supermarket. Find five examples of each type of convenience food. Check the directions on the food packages. How long does it take to prepare each? What skills are needed? What equipment is needed?

5. Conduct a taste test of four brands of canned tuna. Which tastes best? Which looks best? How much does each cost? Which brand would you buy? Why?

6. Interview the manager of your school cafeteria. Find out which convenience foods are used. Ask the manager to describe how convenience foods are prepared.

7. Compare the taste and color of lemonade made from scratch, lemonade from a mix, and canned lemonade. Which requires the least amount of time to prepare? Which costs the most per cup? Which do you prefer? Which would you buy? Why?

8. Write an article for your school newspaper about a new food product. Ask a supermarket manager to tell you which new products were delivered to the store this month. Select one of the new products as the subject of your article. You could write about the taste and cost of the food. You could learn more about the food by writing to the company that made it.

Chapter 12
Smart Shopping

Objective

After reading this chapter, you will be able to

❑ select a food store that meets your needs.

❑ create and use a food shopping plan.

❑ make shopping decisions using unit pricing, nutrition labels, and open dating.

❑ store foods to keep them safe and protect their nutrients and appeal.

❑ explain why food additives are used.

New Terms

organic foods: crops grown on farmland that has not been treated with human-made pesticides or weed killers or fertilized with sewage sludge. Organic meats are from farm animals that received no drugs or hormones to speed their growth rate.

staple foods: foods that stay fresh for a long time, such as flour and sugar.

perishable foods: foods that spoil in a few days.

impulse buying: making an unplanned purchase.

name brands: brands that cost the most because they have fancy packages and are advertised.

store brands: brands sold by supermarket chains.

generic products: products that have plain labels and are not advertised. They are often the least expensive.

unit price: the cost per unit of an item.

food additive: any substance added to foods.

open dating: a system of putting dates on foods to help you to decide which package to buy and which to use first.

universal product code (UPC): a series of black lines, bars, and numbers printed on food labels to identify the product, its manufacturer, its size, and style or form for a computer programmed to reflect the current price of that item.

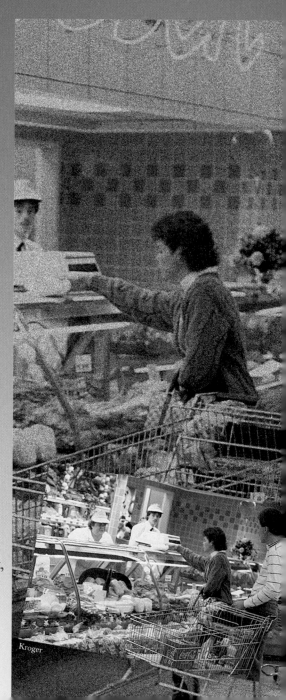

Kroger

Getting ready to shop is like planning a trip! Will you travel to a large supermarket? Maybe you prefer a small specialty shop or a farmers' market. You need to decide where you are going before you leave. Many types of stores sell food. Which one is best for you?

The next part of your travel plans is to decide what you will do when you arrive. On a food shopping trip, you know you'll be buying food. Your trip will go more smoothly if you make careful plans before you leave. That means deciding exactly what you need.

Your shopping list is your ticket to easy travel. It outlines your journey and tells you what you will do. For instance, it may tell you to buy a pound of potatoes or a carton of milk. It also pays to learn some vital travel tips ahead of time. When you get to the store, how will you find the best buy? Which food has the most nutrients? How can you tell if a food is fresh?

Knowing some of the local customs makes travel more enjoyable. Some customs of courteous shoppers are listed in 12-1. Learning some of the local language makes travel easy and enjoyable, too. What is meant by unit pricing, nutrition labeling, and open dating? What is a universal product code?

Supermarket Shoppers' Code

- Handle carts with care. Avoid bumping into other shoppers and displays. Keep aisles clear.
- Avoid unnecessary handling of fresh fruits and vegetables.
- If you knock an item off a shelf, return it to its proper place. If you accidentally break an item, call a clerk so he or she can clean it up.
- If you change your mind about buying an item, return it to its proper place.
- Complete all your shopping before entering the checkout line.
- Learn the rules of the "express line." Usually, it's the number of different items, not the total number of pieces that count. In most stores, six loaves of bread and eight cans of soup are two items.
- Place merchandise on the counter so the cashier can see prices. Keep "two for" items together.
- If you scan the items yourself, follow the directions carefully. Don't forget to scan every item.
- Ask the store to redeem cents-off coupons for only the items you did buy.
- Have your cash, credit card, debit card, check, I.D. card, and coupons ready so you don't delay the checkout line.
- If you take a cart to your car in the parking lot, return it to the area designated for empty carts. Never take a cart off the store's property.

The Confident Consumer, Goodheart-Willcox

12-1 Courtesy and consideration make shopping more pleasant.

When the trip is over, it's time to unpack your bags. You'll need to know how to care for the foods you brought home.

A good plan helps make all of your travels a snap. Smart shoppers know that careful planning pays off. Bon voyage!

Where to Shop?

There are many places to buy food. You can buy food at supermarkets, neighborhood grocery stores, and discount food stores. Other places to buy food are specialty shops, food cooperatives, convenience stores, and farmers' markets.

Each type of food store has good points and drawbacks. Some stores offer more types of food than others. The prices in some stores are higher than in other stores. One store may be closer to your home than others. Some stores may be open when others are closed.

Choosing the best place to shop takes research. You can gather the facts you need by visiting local food stores. While there, check the store's prices, hours, and food choices. Ask yourself the questions in 12-2. The answers can help you pick the store that's right for you. You may decide to shop at more than one store.

Choosing a Food Store Checklist
✓ Do the foods you buy often have good prices?
✓ Is the store in a convenient location?
✓ Are the store's hours convenient for your schedule?
✓ Does the store offer the extra services your family needs, such as check cashing and movie rentals?
✓ Is the store clean and well organized?
✓ Does it offer a variety of fresh foods?
✓ Are the fresh fruits and vegetables kept in chilled cases?
✓ Are the meat and dairy cases kept cold and neat?
✓ Are the shelves neat?
✓ Are there signs on each aisle?
✓ Is the staff helpful?

12-2 When looking for a food store, ask yourself these questions.

Supermarkets

Supermarkets are where many people buy their food. These stores often have lower prices than other types of food stores. That's because they buy such large amounts of food that their suppliers give them low prices. Supermarkets can charge less because the price they pay for food is low. Most supermarkets have sales every week.

Supermarkets may carry 28,000 or more items, 12-3. Many offer special services such as grocery bagging. Some have a drugstore, post office, florist, delicatessen, and bakery inside the store. Most sell nonfood items such as shampoo, greeting cards, and school supplies, too.

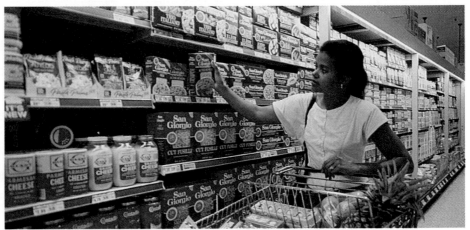

USDA

12-3 There are so many things to look at in a supermarket. If you spent a minute looking at each thing in a supermarket, you would stay in the store for three weeks or more!

Neighborhood Grocery Stores

Neighborhood grocery stores were the first type of food store. They often are called "Mom and Pop Groceries." This is because most of these stores are owned and run by one family.

Neighborhood grocery stores are smaller than supermarkets. They have fewer food choices and higher prices than supermarkets. Many neighborhood grocery stores offer special services. For example, they may deliver your groceries to your home. They often are closer to your home than large supermarkets.

Discount Food Stores

Discount food stores feature low prices. The prices are low because the stores buy large amounts of food and offer few services. Also, most stores are very plain. Many look like warehouses because most products are not put on shelves. They are left in their shipping cartons.

Discount food stores have limited choices. Most carry only foods in cans or boxes. A few carry fresh foods such as fruit and milk. You may find that these stores are a good place to stock up on canned and packaged foods.

Specialty Shops

Specialty shops often feature one type of food. Delicatessens sell mostly cold cuts, cheese, and ready-to-eat foods. Ethnic food stores sell foods that are common in another part of the world, 12-4. Cheese shops, dairies, bakeries, butcher shops, and health food stores are other specialty shops.

12-4 The ethnic food store in this picture sells foods from China.

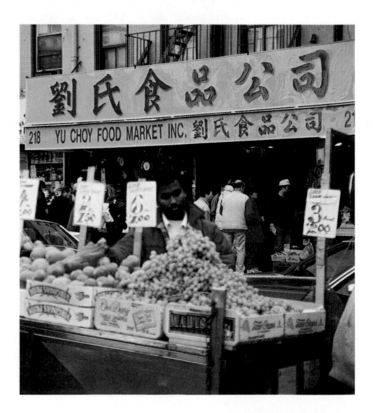

Many specialty shops carry organic foods. ***Organic foods*** include crops grown on farmland that has not been treated with human-made pesticides or weed killers. Also, the farmland cannot be fertilized with sewage sludge. Organic meats are from farm animals that received no drugs or hormones to speed their growth rate. Some people mistakenly think organic foods are more nutritious or safer to eat than other foods. Organic foods tend to be very costly.

The prices in specialty shops often are higher than in other food stores. These shops may sell some foods not found anywhere else. They also may have more types of a food than you would find in any other store. For instance, a cheese shop may have more than a hundred types of cheese.

Food Cooperatives

Food cooperatives form when a group of people get together and buy large amounts of food. They often set up a store much like a discount food store. To buy foods in a food cooperative's store, you must be a member of the group.

The cost of the food sold by food cooperatives is low. This is because the group gets a big discount when they buy a large amount of food. The group keeps prices low by running the store themselves. Each person works a few hours at the store every month. No one gets paid for working in the store. The members trade their time for low food prices.

Food cooperatives have limited food choices. Most foods are canned, dried, or packaged. Food cooperatives seldom have fresh foods or bakeries. They offer few services. For example, you may have to bring your own grocery bags.

Convenience Stores

Convenience stores get their name because they are convenient. They are often located near or in residential areas. They are usually open longer than most other food stores. You pay for this convenience, though. Their prices are higher than supermarket prices. Convenience stores also offer fewer food choices than supermarkets.

Convenience stores may offer extra services. They may sell cold beverages and hot ready-to-eat foods. Some rent movies. Others sell gasoline.

Farmers' Markets

Some communities have a *farmers' market*. See 12-5. Farmers can sell their crops there. Some farmers have their own roadside stands.

At farmers' markets, you can buy fresh fruits, vegetables, and eggs directly from the farm. Most prices are lower than in other food stores. Some farmers' markets are open only during the summer and fall. Most are open only a few hours at a time and have no extra services.

12-5 At farmers' markets you can buy food directly from the farmers.

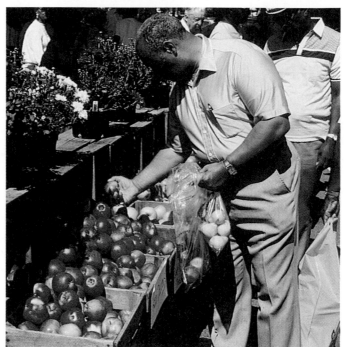

USDA

Ready, Set, Shop

Food stores stock thousands of different items. There are many choices to make. Your shopping trip will be quick and easy if you have a shopping plan.

A *shopping plan* helps you save time, energy, and money. It also helps you reach your food shopping goal. Your goal is to get what you need at the best price.

Get Ready to Save Money _____

It's easy to make a shopping plan when you know what you need. To find out what you need, start by planning your meals. As you plan your meals, watch for ways to save money. Check the newspaper for special sales. Look over any cents-off coupons you have. You may want to change your menus in order to use sale items or coupons.

Supermarkets have sales every week. You can find out about the sales by reading the newspaper on Wednesday or Thursday. See 12-6. You can find cents-off coupons in newspapers, magazines, and food packages. Coupons printed by the makers of food products can be used in any store. Coupons printed in the newspaper often can be used only at the store that put them in the paper. Sales and coupons can save you money if you can use the product.

During sales, you may want to stock up on products you can use. Before stocking up, think about your budget, storage space, and how fast you will use the product. Many people stock up on staple foods when they are on sale. ***Staple foods*** include flour, sugar, and cereals. Staple foods stay fresh for a long time. ***Perishable foods*** spoil in a few days. Fresh fruit, milk, and meat are perishable foods. It's a good idea to buy only the amount of perishable foods you can use quickly. The money you spend is wasted if a food spoils before you can use it.

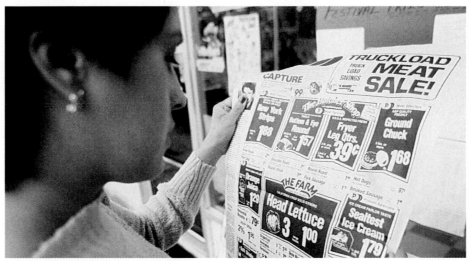

USDA

12-6 Check the paper before shopping to find the best food buys for the week.

Get Set With a Shopping List

Once your menu is set, it's time to make a shopping list. Your list will be your shopping plan. It includes all the items you need to buy.

Begin making your list by reading your menus and recipes. Write every item you need and the amount you need. Check to see if you already have any of the items on your list. If you do, cross them off.

A list helps you to get every item you need. You won't have to run back to the store for something you forgot. Also, a list helps you avoid impulse buying. ***Impulse buying*** is when you buy something that you didn't plan to buy. Impulse items often are costly items you don't really need. They often cause you to go over your budget. Magazines, gum, and candy are common impulse items.

You can save time and energy at the store if you divide your list. You could divide it into groups of foods that are alike. Your list might look like the one in 12-7. You also could list the items you need with the store layout in mind. To do this, list the foods in the order you come to them in the store. You can learn the layout of the store by shopping there a few times.

Grocery List

2	cans peas	1	pound grapes
1	can black beans	2	pounds tomatoes
2	cans soup	1	head lettuce
1	bottle catsup	1	bag carrots
1	jar ice tea mix	1	gallon fat free milk
1	pound rice	1	pound American cheese
5	pounds white flour	16	oz. yogurt
3	boxes macaroni and cheese	12	oz. lean ground beef
2	boxes breakfast cereal	1	pound fresh chicken parts
1	box cookies	1	box fish sticks
2	loaves whole wheat bread	1	box frozen lasagna
1	dozen brown-and-serve rolls	1	bag frozen whole strawberries
1	box of English muffins	1/2	gallon ice cream
4	apples		

12-7 Save time and energy by organizing your shopping list.

When you make your list, try to have alternates in mind. The store may be out of an item you want, or the item may cost too much. For instance, if the store is out of apples, your alternate may be pears. If chicken is too costly, your alternate might be turkey. Planning ahead for alternates makes it easy to change your list. You won't have to waste time at the store trying to think of alternates.

Your Shopping Plan in Action

Once your list is made, it's time to put your shopping plan into action. You'll get all you need if you stick with your plan. It's easier to stick to your plan when you take these actions.

- Try to eat before you shop. You will be less tempted to buy items you don't need. People spend 15 percent more at food stores when they are hungry.
- Try to shop alone. Shoppers often spend more when others shop with them. Others are likely to suggest buying things that aren't on your list.
- Cross items off your list as you go. This way you won't buy things you don't need. Also, you won't forget things you do need.

Selecting Safe Packages

When shopping, select packages that are in good shape. Look for clean, sealed packages. The food in sticky, dirty, or torn packages may not be clean. Avoid cans that are rusty, leaking, or bulging. The food inside is not safe to eat. Food stores often sell dented cans at low prices. If you buy dented cans, choose only cans that are slightly dented. Avoid cans with deep dents or dents on the seams of the cans. These types of dents indicate a can may have a tiny hole where bacteria can enter. Choose frozen foods that are clean and frozen solid. Sticky, stained, or frosty packages are a sign the food thawed and was refrozen. The food may not be the best quality.

It's a good idea to put heavy cans and boxes in your shopping cart first. Just before you check out, put cold foods, such as frozen yogurt, in your cart. Place fragile items, such as bread and fresh fruit, on top. When you put foods in your cart in this order, heavy items won't crush fragile items. Also, cold foods won't get warm.

Comparing Prices _____

As you shop, be sure to compare prices of different brands. See 12-8. Some brands cost more than others. ***Name brands*** cost the most because they have fancy packages and are advertised. The consumer pays the advertising costs through higher prices. ***Store brands*** are sold by the supermarket chain. ***Generic products*** have no brands. They have plain labels and are not advertised. Generic products are often the least expensive.

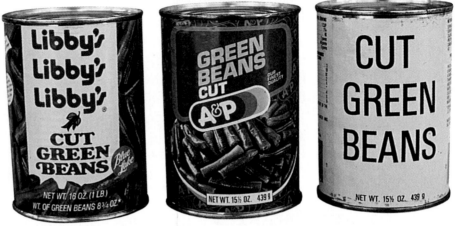

USDA

12-8 Comparing brands can help you find the brand that you prefer and can afford.

Name brand, store brand, and generic products often are very much alike. They usually have the same nutritive value. Their quality might differ. Many name brand foods are high quality. The quality of generic products may not be as high as the others. You will need to try the brands to decide which has the quality and taste you prefer.

When shopping, also compare the prices of sale items to other brands. You may save money by buying a brand other than the one on sale. If you are using cents-off coupons, be sure to compare the price you will pay with the price of other brands. The cents-off price still may be higher than the normal price of other brands.

Unit Pricing

Unit pricing makes it easy to compare prices. The ***unit price*** is the cost of each unit of measure. The unit of measure may be ounces, grams, pounds, quarts, liters, or gallons. Most unit pricing tags are found on the shelf above or below the item, not on the item. The tag lists the item name, brand, package size, total price, and price per unit, 12-9.

Unit pricing tags are very useful when comparing items in different size packages. For instance, apple juice may be sold in 16-, 32-, and 64-ounce cans. If you need 64 ounces, you will want to know which is the best buy. Which would be less expensive—four 16-ounce cans, two 32-ounce cans, or one 64-ounce can?

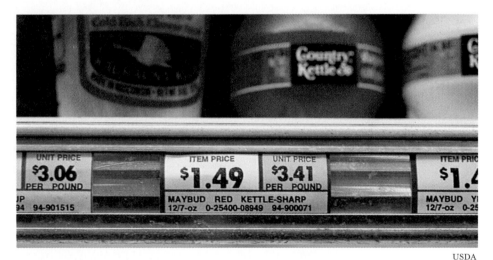

USDA

12-9 The unit pricing tag shows you the cost per unit. You can use this information to find the best buy.

The unit price gives you the answer. It tells you how much each item costs per unit. The unit price of the apple juice is given for one ounce. You can quickly compare unit prices and find the size that costs the least per ounce. Larger packages are often the best buy. They aren't always the wisest buy, though. If the food will spoil before you use it, it would be better to buy a smaller package.

÷ Math in the Kitchen

Computing Unit Prices

The unit price is the price you pay per unit of food. Unit prices make it easy to compare prices at the supermarket. They save you time because someone else did the math for you.

The unit price makes more sense if you know how it is computed. Also, some foods may not have a unit price tag. In that case you will need to compute the unit price. Here's how to compute the unit price.

1. Write the cost of the food.
   Cost of the food = _____

2. Write the type and number of units in the package.
   To find the number and type of units, look at the quantity listed on the package label. For example, a can of soup might contain 12 ounces. The soup has 12 units or ounces.
   The units used for liquid foods often are fluid ounces, liters, or gallons. The units used for dry foods often are ounces, grams, or pounds.

Number and Type of Units in the Package = _____

3. Compute the unit price.
   To do this, divide the cost of the food (Step 1) by the number of units in the package (Step 2).
   The Cost of the Food ÷ Number and Type of Units in the Package = Unit Price
   For example, if:
   Cost of the food = $2.88
   Number and Type of Units in the Package = 12 ounces
   Cost of the Food ÷ Number and Type of Units in the Package = Unit Price
   $2.88 ÷ 12 ounces = 24¢ per ounce

4. Compare the unit prices of the items to find the lowest priced item. You may want to compare the prices of food that use different units of measure. If so, you must convert them to the same unit first. For instance, you may want to compare the price of a gallon of milk with 12 ounces of milk. A gallon is equal to 128 ounces.

Reading Food Labels

Food labels tell you about the food inside a package. You can use labels to find out about ingredients and nutrients in the food. The labels can help you choose the foods you want to buy. The *Food and Drug Administration (FDA)* sets the standards for food labels for all foods except for meat and poultry. The *United States Department of Agriculture (USDA)* sets the standards for meat and poultry labels. Both the FDA and USDA are part of the United States government.

Certain kinds of information are required by law to be on food labels. Every food label must give the following information:

- The name of the food, such as orange juice or corn chips.
- The name and address of the maker, packer, or distributor of the food.
- The amount of food in the package. (The amount might be in ounces, pounds, grams, liters, or gallons.)

Ingredient Labels

Food labels also list the ingredients used to make the food. The ingredients are listed in order of weight. The ingredient used in the largest amount is listed first. The next largest is listed second and so on. The last ingredient is used in the smallest amount. All ingredients, including food additives, used to make the food are included on the ingredient label. See 12-10.

Name of the food

Ingredients (listed in order of weight)

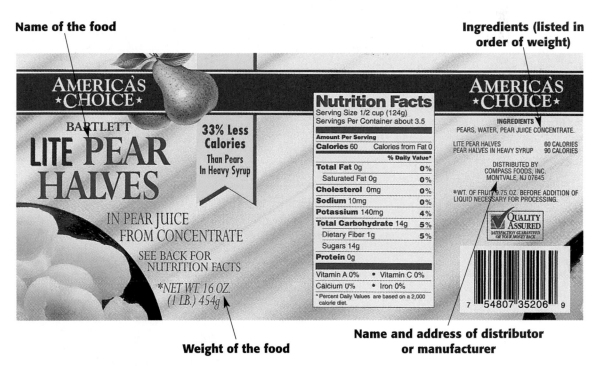

Weight of the food

Name and address of distributor or manufacturer

12-10 A food label gives consumers valuable information.

Food Additives

"Chemicals in my food? No way! I don't want it!" Do you know people who feel this way? It may surprise them to learn that all foods are made of chemicals. Crunchy bread sticks and juicy peaches are made of chemicals. In fact, people are made of chemicals, too! If they don't want to eat chemicals, they won't be able to eat anything.

What they mean is, they don't want to eat foods with additives. Many people think additives are new. They aren't sure what additives do. They wonder if additives are really needed. They want to know if the additives are safe.

Additives aren't new at all. They have been used for thousands of years. Salt and spices were two of the first food additives. These additives are still used today. See 12-11. A *food additive* is any substance that is added to foods. There are four main types of additives:

- *Nutrient additives* make foods more nutritious. Many breads and cereals have added thiamin, riboflavin, niacin, folate, and iron. Milk often has vitamin D added. Some salt has the mineral iodine added.

12-11 Spices have been used for centuries to add flavor and preserve foods.

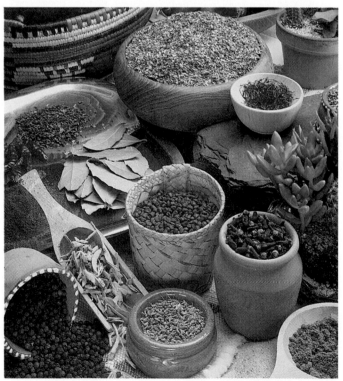

American Spice Trade Association

- *Preservatives* help keep foods fresh longer. They may prevent the growth of mold or bacteria. Without preservatives, some foods would be in short supply. That's because they would spoil before you could use them. For instance, bread would mold before you could eat the whole loaf. Preservatives help keep foods safe to eat, too. An example is the additive that prevents the deadly food poisoning botulism in cold cuts.
- *Color and flavor additives* make foods look and taste more appealing. Red dye is added to canned cherries. Caramel color makes colas look brown. Sucrose is sugar. It makes foods taste sweet. Citric acid gives foods a tart taste.
- *Texture food additives* can make it easier to prepare and process foods. These additives help ingredients blend well or improve the texture of foods. For instance, additives help make ice cream smooth and pickles crunchy. Without these additives, pickles would be limp. Ice cream would feel gritty. Dry mixes would be lumpy.

Laws are designed to protect United States residents from the use of unsafe food additives. The FDA has strict controls on food additives. The FDA must approve every new additive before it can be used. To be approved, an additive must be studied for years. If the studies show the additive works and is safe, the FDA will approve it. If you are concerned about the additives in your food, ingredient labels can help you. You can use them to find out what's in foods. Labels can help you make good food choices.

Nutrition Labels

Nutrition labels report the nutrient content of the food. They can teach you more about what you eat. You can use them to select foods that are good for you. You can use them to find foods that meet your needs. For instance, you may want to eat foods low in fat or high in vitamin C.

To make the most informed choices, you need to learn how to read labels and interpret them. As you can see in 12-12, the first part of the nutrition label reports "Serving Size." This tells you the amount of the food that equals one serving. The next part, "Servings Per Container," tells you how many servings are in the package. How many one-cup servings are in the container on which the label shown in 12-12 appears? If you said two servings, you are right. The label tells you that you could serve two people one cup each of the food.

The next part of the label reports the calories and nutrients in one serving of the food. There are many more nutrients than those that appear on nutrition labels. The nutrients that must appear are those that are of greatest concern to many people in the United States. Remember, many people eat too much fat, saturated fat, cholesterol, sodium, and sugar. Also, many are concerned that they don't get enough dietary fiber, calcium, iron, vitamin A, and vitamin C. You can use nutrition labels to find foods with nutrients in the amounts you need.

The total amount of many nutrients in one serving of the food are listed in grams or milligrams. For example, one serving of the food in 12-12 contains 13 grams of fat and 10 grams of sugar. Many of the nutrients also have a "% Daily Value." The "% Daily Value" tells you how much one serving of the food adds to your daily needs.

Serving Size
The size of one serving of the food.

Servings Per Container
The number of servings of the size given in **Serving Size** above that are in one package of the food.

Calories
The total calories in a single serving. The calories from fat in one serving.

% Daily Value
This shows how the amount of each nutrient in a serving of the food compares to the daily values for a 2,000-calorie diet.

Nutrients
These nutrients must appear on most labels.
Labels on foods that contain few nutrients, like candy and soft drinks, may omit some nutrients. Some food manufacturers list more nutrients.

% Daily Value Footnote
This footnote appears on many labels. It is omitted when there is too little space on the food label to print it. The footnote reports the daily values used to compute the % Daily Values for a 2,000- and 2,500-calorie diet.

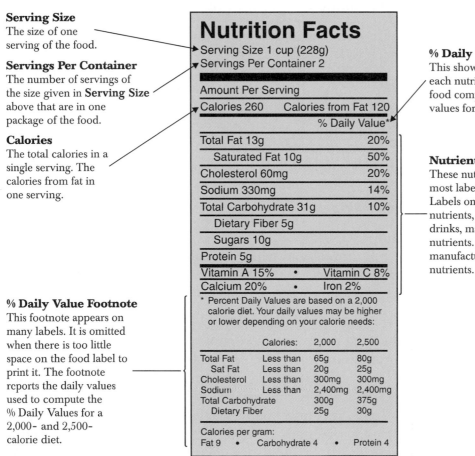

12-12 Nutrition labels follow a format like this.

Some nutrition labels include the Daily Values footnote. This footnote tells you that Daily Values are based on a 2,000-calorie diet. The numbers listed in the column labeled *2,000* were used to figure the % Daily Values. If you need to eat 2,500 calories each day, you can use the column labeled *2,500* to figure your % Daily Values.

Your daily needs may not equal 2,000 or 2,500 calories. However, you can still use the % Daily Values to see how your diet meets advice from nutrition experts. You can use the % Daily Values to see how much one serving of a food adds to your daily diet. Look at the % Daily Value for cholesterol in 12-12. It tells you this food supplies 20% of all the cholesterol nutrition experts believe is healthful to have in one day. You can also use the % Daily Values to compare foods and choose those with nutrients in the amounts you need.

For the most healthful diet, choose foods with high % Daily Values for dietary fiber and total carbohydrate. Also choose foods with high % Daily Values for vitamins A and C, calcium, and iron. Your goal is to reach or go a little over 100% of the Daily Values for these nutrients. Avoid going over 100% of the Daily Values for total fat, saturated fat, cholesterol, and sodium. Getting too much of these nutrients may lead to health problems.

Open Dating

Did you ever notice the dates on food packages? These dates help you to know when a food is freshest. **Open dating** is a system of putting dates on foods to help you to decide which package to buy and which to use first at home. There are three types of dates. They are the freshness date, sell date, and expiration date.

The *freshness date* tells you how long a food will be fresh and tasty. After that date, the product is still safe to eat, but it may not taste as good. Stores often reduce the price of products if their freshness dates have passed. Bread, salad dressing, raisins, and cereal have freshness dates. Examples are "Best before October 7," "Freshest if used by October 7," and "Remains fresh until October 7."

Sell dates also are known as *pull dates*. The sell date is the last day a food should be sold. It is not the last day you should eat it. The food still will be fresh and safe to eat for at least a week after the sell date. You can find sell dates on foods such as yogurt, cheese, milk, and meat. An example is "Sell by August 24." See 12-13.

12-13 Foods with a sell date should not be sold after that date. They will be safe to eat for at least a week after that date.

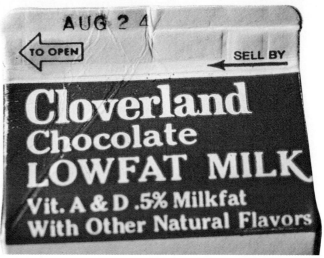

USDA

The *expiration date* is the last day a food should be eaten. It may not be safe to eat if the date has passed. Expiration dates are found on baby formula. Examples are "Use Before March 5" and "Do Not Use After March 5."

Universal Product Codes

The ***universal product code (UPC)*** is a series of black lines, bars, and numbers. It is printed on every food label to identify the type, manufacturer, size, and style or form of the product. See 12-10. The supermarket cashier passes the UPC over the cash register's scanner. The scanner reads the lines and bars. See 12-14. The computer inside the cash register identifies the food and searches its memory for the price. The cash register rings up the sale and totals your order. Your receipt lists the items you bought and their prices.

The UPC saves time and money. The computer uses the UPC to look up the price. Store clerks don't have to put a price tag on every item. One price sign can be posted for each type of item. A drawback to the UPC is that not having a price on an item means it is more difficult for you to check for errors. There are fewer errors at the checkout, though. That's because the cashier doesn't have to keystroke every price.

The UPC also helps the store keep better records. The computer records every sale. The store knows right away when it needs to reorder food items you want.

12-14 The cash register scanner reads the UPC and rings up the item.

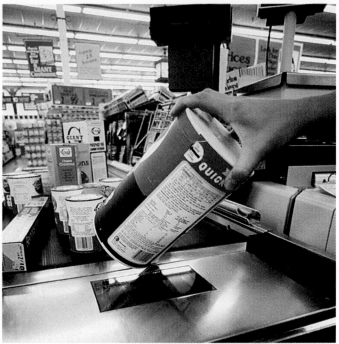

USDA

Storing Foods

After you check out, it's time to head home. Stopping to run other errands on the way home may cause your frozen juice bars to melt and your celery to become limp. You can protect the time, energy, and money you invested in your groceries by going straight home.

Careful storage of food protects its flavor and nutrients. These tips will help you keep your food fresh, tasty, and safe to eat.

- Put refrigerated and frozen foods away as soon as you get home. Keep frozen foods in the freezer until you are ready to use them. They will maintain their quality for many months. Keep refrigerated foods in the refrigerator when you aren't using them. Use refrigerated foods within a week or two.
- Store dry foods, such as flour and cake mixes, in a cool, dry, dark place. Make sure the storage area is clean and free of insects. Once dry foods are opened, store them in airtight containers. See 12-15. They will maintain their quality for a year or more.

12-15 Store dry foods in airtight containers.

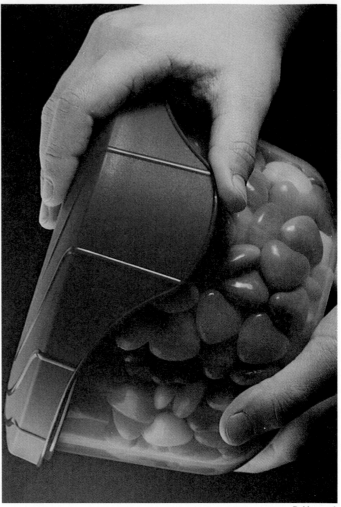

Rubbermaid

- Store unopened canned foods in a cool, dry place. They will maintain their quality for many months. They won't be of top quality if stored more than a year or in a warm place. After opening canned foods, put any unused food in a covered container. Keep the container in the refrigerator and use the food within a few days.
- Don't store foods near the oven or range. The warm temperatures in these areas cause food to lose their quality.
- Don't store foods under the sink. It may get damp in this area. Dampness causes cans to rust. It also attracts insects.

Once your food purchases are made and safely stored, you're ready to make a meal. In the next chapter, you'll discover how to do just that.

Science in the Kitchen

Lights, Flavor, Potato Chips!

Careful storage helps protect the quality of the foods you buy. This experiment will help you see how storage methods affect food quality. You will need six one-pint jars with four lids, aluminum foil, and a medium-sized bag of unopened potato chips.

Begin by covering three jars completely with aluminum foil. No light should show through the jars. Now open the potato chips and divide them into six equal portions. Place one portion in each of the six jars.

Taste one chip from each jar. Rate its flavor using this five-point scale.

1 = dislike very much
2 = dislike
3 = OK – neither like nor dislike
4 = like
5 = like very much

Put lids on two jars that are covered with aluminum foil and on two jars that are not covered. Place one aluminum foil covered jar with a lid and one uncovered jar with a lid on a sunny windowsill. Place the other four jars in a dark cabinet.

Taste the potato chips in each jar every day or so for two weeks. Record your observations each day. Be sure to note which potato chips were most and least crisp. Also rate their flavor using the five-point scale.

When you finish your observations, think about these questions. When did the flavor start to change? When did crispness start to change? What can you conclude about the effect of light and dark on flavor? How did exposure to air affect the chips? Why did the aluminum foil affect the flavor? How are potato chips and other foods packaged? Why do you think they are packaged in this way? How can you use this information?

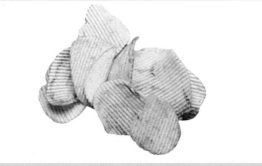

American Heart Association

Discover how storage methods affect the flavor and crispness of potato chips.

In a Nutshell

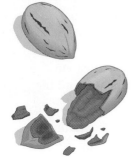

- The types of food stores are supermarkets, neighborhood grocery stores, discount food stores, specialty shops, food cooperatives, convenience stores, and farmers' markets.
- A shopping list helps you get the items you need.
- Name brand, store brand, and generic products have the same nutrients, but their quality and prices often differ.
- Unit pricing tags help you compare the costs of foods in different size packages.
- The food label tells you about the ingredients and nutrients in the food.
- The date on a food package helps you know when the food is fresh.
- The universal product code (UPC) is a series of black lines, bars, and numbers printed on food labels.
- Careful storage of food protects its flavor and nutrients.

In the Know

1. True or false? Prices in neighborhood grocery stores are often lower than prices in supermarkets.
2. List five features to consider when choosing a food store.
3. Give two reasons why you should make a shopping list.
4. Make a shopping list for the recipes in 13-3. Divide the list by the types of foods.
5. True or false? The first ingredient listed on a food label is present in the smallest weight.
6. Name the four types of additives.
7. What is NOT found on a nutrition label?
   A. Price of one serving.
   B. Calories in one serving.
   C. Sodium in one serving.
   D. Size of one serving.
8. It is not safe to eat a food after the _____ date.
   A. pull
   B. freshness
   C. expiration
   D. sell

9. Which is NOT true about a universal product code?
   A. It is a series of black lines, bars, and numbers.
   B. A computer scanner can read it.
   C. It saves time and money.
   D. It tells you a food's cost per unit.
10. The best place to store an unopened can of corn is in _____.
    A. the cabinet above the oven
    B. the refrigerator
    C. a cool, dry cabinet
    D. the cabinet below the sink

What Would You Do?

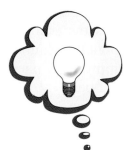

You made a food shopping list. Your sister decided to go shopping with you. She has a cents-off coupon for an item that normally costs $4.19. The coupon will save $1.00. You both agree the coupon makes the item a good buy. However, the item isn't on your shopping list. Should you buy the item? Why or why not?

Expanding Your Knowledge

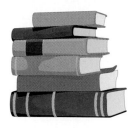

1. Compare prices at different types of food stores. Visit a supermarket, neighborhood grocery store, discount food store, and convenience store. Make a list of the prices for a gallon of milk, can of tuna, loaf of bread, box of cereal, and pound of bananas. Also list the brand names and unit prices. Report your findings to your class.
2. Contact a local food cooperative. Invite someone from the cooperative to visit your class. Make a list of questions to ask the speaker. You could ask these questions. How was the cooperative organized? How is the store stocked? Who can be a member? How do you become a member? Why would someone join the cooperative?
3. Conduct a taste test. Buy three cans of fruit cocktail. Choose a name brand, store brand, and generic product. Compare the labels on each can. Compare the price of each. Then open the cans. Note how the food in each can looks. Do a blindfolded taste test of each product. Compare the taste and texture of each. Which do you prefer? Why?

4. Compare the nutrition labels on orange beverages. You could compare orange soda, orange drink, orange juice, and powdered orange drink mix. Which has the most calories per serving? Which has the most vitamin C? What is the price of a cup of each? Conduct a taste test to compare the color and flavor of each. Which do you prefer? Why?

5. Compare the ingredient labels on shredded wheat, corn flakes, granola, and three other cereals. List the first three ingredients in each cereal. Which has the most sugar? Which have no sugar? Make a poster to report your findings.

6. Plan meals for one week using food advertisements and coupons. Make a shopping list for these meals.

7. Interview the manager of a supermarket that uses cash registers with computer scanners. Ask the manager to demonstrate how the scanner works. Find out why the store uses the scanner. Interview customers to find out how they feel about the scanner.

8. Make a bulletin board on open dating. Use empty food packages with dates on them to illustrate the bulletin board.

9. Learn more about nutrition labeling. Make a video to teach younger children how to use nutrition labeling.

10. Conduct a survey to find out how people use nutrition labeling. You could ask these questions. What information do you look for on nutrition labels? How do you use it? What do you like about the label format? What changes would you make? Using the survey results, create a new label format.

11. Look closely at the food storage areas in your home or in the school lab. What changes should be made? How could you make the changes without spending much money?

12. Visit a supermarket. Find a food item you might buy. Find at least two other brands of the same food item you could buy instead. Compute the unit price of each item. Which is the best buy? Repeat this activity with four more food items.

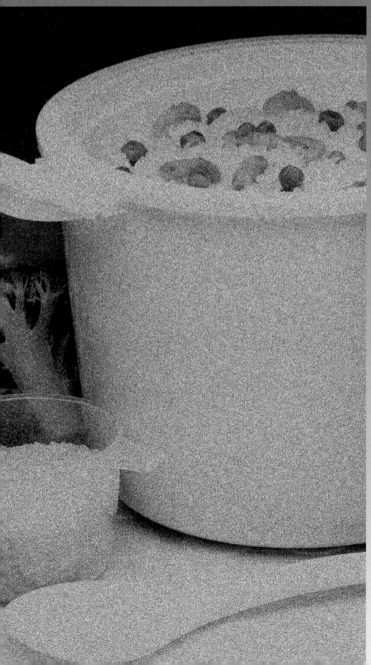

Chapter 13
Ready, Set, Cook!

Objectives

After reading this chapter, you will be able to
- ❏ participate as a team member in the food lab.
- ❏ plan, carry out, and evaluate a work schedule.
- ❏ serve a meal and cleanup afterward.
- ❏ plan a party.

New Terms

work schedule: a plan that lists the time needed to prepare a meal, eat, and cleanup.

dovetail: to do two or more tasks at the same time.

place setting: all the dinnerware, flatware, glassware, and table linen used by one person.

cover: the space needed for one place setting.

R.S.V.P.: an abbreviation written on invitations that means "please reply."

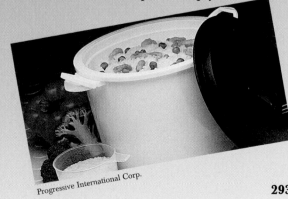

Progressive International Corp.

Imagine you are a master chef. Everyone is depending on you to prepare a delicious meal. How will you ever do it? You've got the menu planned. You selected your recipes and bought all the ingredients. Now, you need to get to work and prepare the meal.

Which recipe should you prepare first? Which should you make next? When should you set the table? Preparing a meal is like solving a puzzle. The puzzle pieces include all the tasks you must complete to prepare, serve, and clean up after the meal. A plan can help you figure out just when each task should be done. If the plan is well thought out and followed carefully, all the puzzle pieces will fall into place. You'll know you've solved the puzzle when the foods in your meal look and taste good and are served on time. With a little planning, a master chef can create a delicious meal. With a little planning, you can create one, too.

Teamwork in the Kitchen

When you put your plan into action, you may be working alone or with others. At school, you will be working on a team. Teams work together to achieve a goal. For example, a football team's goal is to play a good game. When you are on a kitchen team at school, you have a goal, too. Your goal is to prepare food, serve it, eat it, and clean up in the time you have.

Teamwork is important in kitchen labs at school. The labs are small. There are several people on each team. Your time is limited. In order to reach the team's goal, all the team members must work together.

Good team members are ready to do their tasks well and complete them on time. They know that their tasks are vital. If one person doesn't do his or her tasks, it holds back the whole team. Good team members also help other members whenever they can. If you finish your tasks ahead of time, you can help others with their tasks.

The best teams are prepared. Team members know where to find kitchen equipment and how to use it. They know the recipes. They follow the kitchen lab rules, too. A team knows it was a success when the members reach their goal.

Your Team Plan

In order to win the game, a football team makes a plan. A winning kitchen team has a plan, too. This plan is called a work schedule. A ***work schedule*** shows the time needed to prepare the meal, eat, and clean up. It helps you achieve your goal in the time you have.

A work schedule lists the time to begin each task. If it is planned carefully, a work schedule will help you have all the menu items ready at mealtime, 13-1. You'll be able to serve hot foods that are hot and cold foods that are cold. Your work schedule at school also will list who will do each task.

13-1 A carefully planned work schedule helps you have all your menu items ready to serve at mealtime.

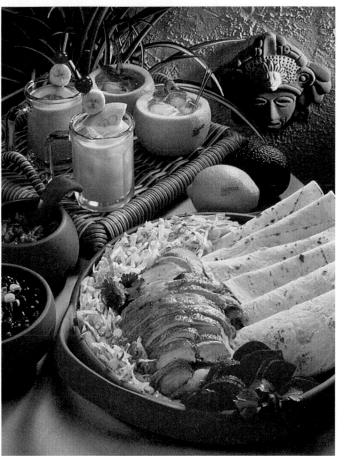

Sunkist Growers, Inc.

13-2 This meal is simple and tasty. It can be prepared and served quickly. Cleanup is fast, too.

M·E·N·U

Peanut Butter Sandwich
Fruit Salad
Oatmeal Cookies
Hot Chocolate

Peanut Butter Sandwich

½ cup peanut butter
8 slices whole wheat bread

1. Spread 2 tablespoons of peanut butter on one side of four slices of bread.
2. Top each slice in Step 1 with a second slice. Cut the sandwiches in half.
3. Serve.

Serves 4

Fruit Salad

1 cup strawberries
1 cup blueberries
2 bananas, peeled

1. Wash the berries. Gently pat dry with paper towels.
2. Slice the strawberries and bananas.
3. Mix the fruit together.
4. Serve right away.

Serves 4

Hot Chocolate

4 cups milk
¼ cup chocolate drink mix

1. Place the ingredients in a saucepan and stir to blend.
2. Heat the chocolate milk until small bubbles form. Stir constantly.
3. Serve immediately.

Serves 4

Oatmeal Cookies

½ cup shortening
1 cup brown sugar
½ cup sugar
1 egg
¼ cup water
1 teaspoon vanilla
3 cups uncooked oats
1 cup flour
½ teaspoon baking soda
1 teaspoon cinnamon
1 cup raisins

1. Preheat oven to 350°F (175°C).
2. Cream the shortening, brown sugar, sugar, egg, water, and vanilla until smooth.
3. Mix the remaining ingredients in a second bowl and add to the shortening mixture.
4. Drop by rounded teaspoonfuls onto a greased cookie sheet. Space the cookies about 1-inch apart.
5. Bake cookies 10 to 12 minutes or until a light imprint remains when you touch them.
6. Cool the cookies on the cookie sheet for 1 minute before placing them on a wire rack to finish cooling.
7. Store the cookies in a tightly covered container.

Makes 5 dozen

13-3 Review your recipes to be sure you have the needed ingredients and equipment.

These are the steps for making a work schedule:

1. Review your menu. It might look like the menu in 13-2. Check each recipe to be sure you have all the equipment and ingredients needed. Look at 13-3. It shows all the recipes used to make the menu in 13-2.
2. List all the tasks that must be done to prepare the meal. The tasks for making the menu in 13-2 are listed in 13-4.
3. Estimate the time you will need to prepare, cook, and serve each recipe. Record these times in a chart like the one in 13-5. As you make the work schedule, note any tasks you can do ahead of time. Also, decide when you should begin making each recipe. Which should be started first? Which should be started next? Which needs to be made at the last minute? Your goal is to have each menu item ready exactly at mealtime.

Tasks

1. Make sandwiches.
   a. Measure the peanut butter and spread it on the bread.
   b. Cut the sandwiches in half and place them on a plate.
2. Prepare the salad.
   a. Measure, wash, and dry the berries.
   b. Peel and slice the bananas and slice the strawberries.
   c. Place the fruit in a bowl and mix it together.
3. Make the cookies.
   a. Measure and combine the ingredients.
   b. Bake and cool the cookies.
   c. Place the cookies on a plate.
4. Make the hot chocolate.
   a. Measure and heat the ingredients.
   b. Pour the hot chocolate into cups.
5. Set the table.
   a. Put placemats on the table.
   b. Arrange the tableware on the placemats.
   c. Place the food on the table.

13-4 Make a list of all the tasks that must be done in order to serve the planned menu.

Preparation Time Chart Mealtime: noon			
Food	**Minutes Needed to Prepare Food**	**Cooking Time (In minutes)**	**Total Time (In minutes)**
Peanut Butter Sandwich	4	-	4
Fruit Salad	9	-	9
Oatmeal Cookies	15	15	30
Hot Chocolate	2	6	8
Get Out Equipment and Ingredients	-	-	3
Set the Table	-	-	5
Serve the Meal	-	-	1
Eat the Meal	-	-	10
Final Cleanup	-	-	5

13-5 These time estimates will help you to see how much time is needed to prepare a menu. The estimates also help you decide which recipes to prepare first.

Math in the Kitchen

Timing Is Everything!

You want to invite several friends over for a cookout next Saturday after the school car wash. Everyone will be hungry after a day of hard work! That's why you'll want to have the meal almost ready to serve when they arrive. A work schedule can help you achieve this goal. Here's what you need to do to have the meal ready on time.

First, plan a menu for a cookout. For example, you could serve hot dogs, corn-on-the-cob, baked beans, fresh strawberries, and juice spritzers. Check a cookbook and food labels to determine how much time each food takes to prepare.

Next, list all the tasks that must be done to prepare the meal. See 13-4. You'll need to decide which task should be done first, second, and so on. Estimate the time needed to prepare, cook, and serve each recipe. Record these times in a chart like the one in 13-5. Remember to note any tasks you can do ahead of time. Also note any tasks that need to be done at the last minute.

Now, make a final work schedule like the one in 13-6. Be sure to begin with the time you want to serve the meal and work backwards. List the time each task is to be done. Be sure to identify any tasks you can dovetail.

You can test your work schedule by trying it out. When the cookout is over, look over your work schedule. How well did it work? Was your meal ready exactly at mealtime? Were hot foods hot at mealtime? Were cold foods cold at mealtime? What changes would you make next time? Why are work schedules important?

4. Make a final work schedule like the one in 13-6. Start with the time you want to serve the meal and work backwards. List the time each task is to be done. Don't forget to leave enough time to eat the meal and clean up. When you make the final work schedule, note where you can take shortcuts. Time-saving equipment and dovetailing are two shortcuts you can use. Microwave ovens and food processors are examples of time-saving equipment. ***Dovetailing*** means to do two or more tasks at the same time. For example, while one food is cooking you could begin making another food. Which tasks are dovetailed in the work schedule in 13-6? As you gain skill, you will be able to use a less detailed work schedule. Some very skilled cooks are able to make a mental work schedule. It's best to write out a work schedule when you are working on a team. A written schedule lets every team member know what to do and when to do it.

Final Work Schedule	
The Day Before	
Time	**Task: Make Cookies**
11:30	Preheat the oven. Get out the needed ingredients and equipment.
11:33	Measure and combine the cookie ingredients.
11:48	Bake the cookies.
	Put away ingredients, begin cleanup.
12:00	Cool the cookies.
12:08	Wrap the cookies.
12:10	Complete cleanup.
12:15	Class ends.
Day Meal Will Be Served	
Time	**Task: Prepare and Serve Meal**
11:30	Set the table.
	Place the cookies on a plate.
11:35	Get out the needed ingredients and equipment.
11:38	Prepare the fruit salad. Place it in a bowl. Chill.
11:47	Make peanut butter sandwiches. Place the sandwiches on a plate.
11:51	Prepare the hot chocolate. Pour the hot chocolate into cups.
11:59	Put the food on the table.
12:00	Mealtime.
12:10	Cleanup.
12:15	Class ends.

13-6 A final work schedule lists the time when each task is to be done.

5. When you make the final work schedule, list the team member who will do each task. Be sure to rotate tasks every time you make a work schedule. Each person should get a chance to cook, serve, and clean up. The same person shouldn't always wash dishes or serve the food.

Getting Ready to Cook

When your work schedule is made, the next step is to get ready to cook. Meal preparation goes faster and more smoothly if you set up the kitchen before starting.

Get out all the equipment and ingredients you will need. This step ensures that you won't have to stop to search for missing ingredients or equipment, 13-7.

Do the preparation steps for all your recipes at once. This includes measuring, washing, peeling, and chopping ingredients. It also includes greasing pans and preheating the oven.

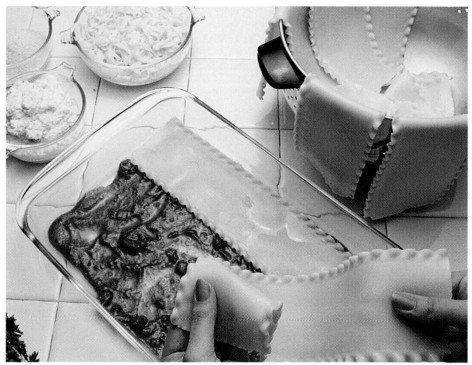

American Heart Association

13-7 Getting out all the ingredients and equipment you need before you start saves time in the kitchen.

Setting the Table

Tableware is arranged on the table in a certain way. This makes it convenient to find the items you need. They are always in the same place.

All the tableware, flatware, glassware, and table linen used by one person is called a ***place setting***. The space needed for a place setting is called a ***cover***. A diagram of how a place setting is arranged is shown in 13-8.

When you set the table, only include the tableware you will need for that meal. For instance, if you aren't serving a salad, don't include a salad plate in the place setting.

Here are some tips to help you set the table.

- Make sure all the tableware is clean.
- Only touch the parts of dishes and utensils that don't come in contact with food.
- Place the plate in the center of the cover.
- Place the plate and flatware one inch from the edge of the table.
- Place the knife to the right of the plate with its blade toward the plate.
- Place the spoons to the right of the knife with their bowls up.

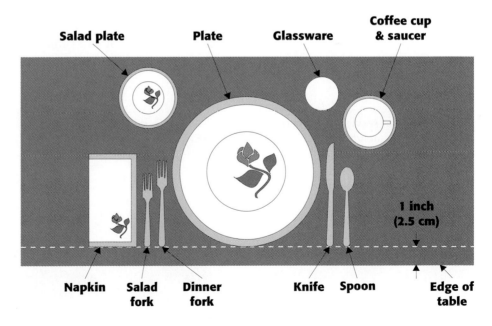

13-8 Tableware should be arranged at each place setting in this way.

- Place forks to the left of the plate with their tines up.
- Place glassware above the knife.
- Place coffee cups to the right of the spoons.
- Place the salad plate to the left of the forks or above them.
- Fold the napkin and place it under the forks, to the left of the forks, on the plate, or in the glass.

Serving Meals

When it's mealtime, all the menu items should be ready to serve. There are four basic ways to serve the meal. These are family style, blue plate style, formal style, and buffet style.

Family Style

Family style is the way meals are served in most homes. In this serving style, the table is set before the meal. All the foods on the menu are put in serving dishes. A serving utensil is placed in each dish. The serving dishes are put on the table. Each person serves his or her own plate then passes the serving dish to the next person.

Blue Plate Style

Meals can be served from the kitchen, too. This serving style is called *blue plate style.* The foods are placed on each person's plate in the kitchen and taken to the table, 13-9. All the tableware is on the table before you are seated except for the plates. Blue plate is a common serving style in restaurants.

13-9 In blue plate service, food is put on the plates in the kitchen.

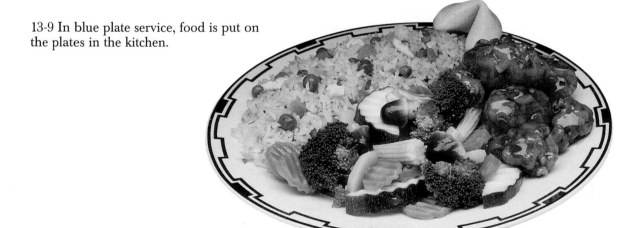

Formal Style

You may be served formal style at banquets or in fancy restaurants. *Formal style* meals are served in courses. A course is one part of the meal. Soup, salad, appetizer, main dish, and dessert each are a course. The main dish course is sometimes called the entree course. In formal style service, the table is set before you are seated. The kitchen staff serves one course at a time. After you eat the course, the tableware you have used is removed. Clean tableware is brought to the table with the next course. This process continues until the whole meal is served.

Buffet Style

Buffet style is used to serve large groups quickly. Each food is placed in a serving dish along with a serving utensil. The serving dishes are placed together on a serving table, 13-10. Tableware is usually stacked at one end of the serving table. With this style, diners pick up the tableware they need then walk around the serving table to serve themselves. They do not eat at the serving table. They may hold their plates or sit at other tables to eat.

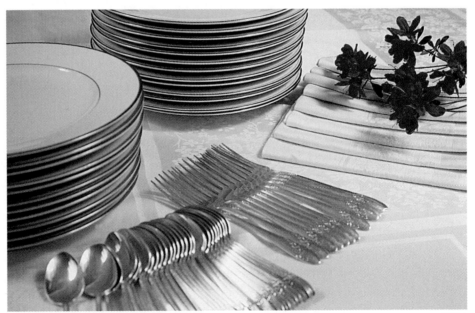

USDA

13-10 When meals are served buffet style, tableware is often placed at one end of the serving table.

Cultures of the World

Sweden, Home of the Smörgåsbord

Sweden is a country in northern Europe. It is so far north, that in the summer, you can see the sun all day and night. In the winter, you may not see the sun at all. As you might guess, it is very cold in Sweden most of the year. Some lakes remain frozen nearly year-round. Only about 10 percent of the land can be used for farming. The rest either has too many mountains or is too cold.

Wheat, oats, barley, and rye are important crops. These grains are used mainly to make breads. The people of Sweden eat breads often. One type is a sweet bread called limpa. Grains are also used to make cakes, sweet pancakes, and other desserts. Desserts are quite popular in Sweden.

Fishing is a very important industry in Sweden. Herring, salmon, and cod are some of the most common fish there. Fish are so popular, they are eaten often. Swedish cooks have many recipes for fish. For example, herring can be pickled, marinated, fried, stewed, or baked.

Sweden is known for its smörgåsbord (SMOR-gus-bored). A smörgåsbord is a table with an assortment of foods intended for a meal. A smörgåsbord often includes several cold dishes like herring, other types of fish, sliced meat, salads, vegetables, cheese, and eggs. One or two hot dishes, such as soup or meatballs, may be included, too.

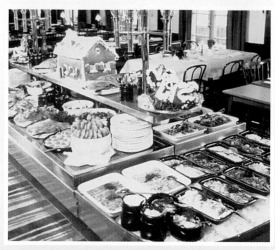

Claes Löfgren

The Swedish word, smörgåsbord, means "bread and butter table." However, a smörgåsbord includes a variety of dishes.

Swedish cooks carefully plan how they will arrange the foods on the smörgåsbord table. They place the dishes so that their colors complement each other. Their careful arrangement makes smörgåsbord tables a delight to see.

Smörgåsbords usually are served buffet style. That is, diners serve themselves at the smörgåsbord table and sit at a different table to eat. The foods served on a smörgåsbord are usually eaten in a certain order. The meal begins with herring. The second course is another type of fish. Cold meats and salads are the third course. Hot dishes are eaten next. The last course is dessert. Cheese or fruit salad are common desserts.

The next time you have a get-together at your house, you could give your meal a Swedish touch. Just arrange your dishes on a serving table and serve the meal smörgåsbord style.

Mealtime Manners

Once the meal is served, it's time to eat. Mealtime is fun when you eat with others. You can talk about your day and share ideas. Mealtimes are most enjoyable when everyone shows respect for each other. You show respect when you behave in a way that makes others feel comfortable and at ease. You make others feel this way when you use good manners, 13-11.

Manners are a way of acting. Manners help everyone feel comfortable, even you! Manners tell you how others expect you to behave at mealtime. Knowing what's expected helps you feel relaxed and sure of yourself. Try using these good manners at every meal.

13-11 Knowing and using good manners helps you feel confident and relaxed at mealtime.

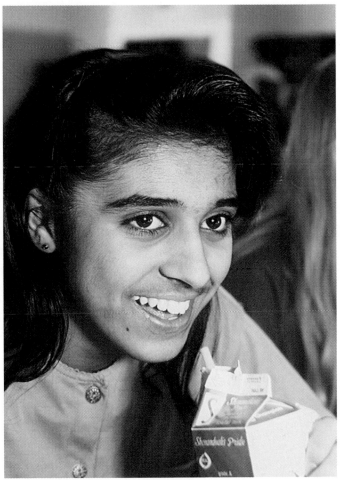

USDA

- Wait until everyone has been served before you start to eat.
- Ask others to pass things you can't reach. Try not to reach in front of people.
- Use one hand to eat and keep the other in your lap. Elbows on the table crowd the person next to you.
- If a food is too hot, wait for it to cool. Don't blow on it.
- Take small sips and bites.
- Chew food with your mouth closed.
- Try not to slurp or smack when you chew.
- Swallow all food before talking or taking a drink.
- Push the last few bites of food onto your fork with a piece of bread or a knife. Don't use your fingers.
- Cut a few pieces of food at a time. Eat the pieces before cutting more.
- Tear bread into smaller pieces. Butter and eat one piece at a time.
- If you get a seed or bone in your mouth, quietly remove it with your fingers. Place it on the side of your plate.
- When you are finished, place the handles of your flatware together and lay them neatly across the plate. Place your napkin on the table.
- Talk about pleasant things. Try to use a soft voice at the table.
- If you aren't sure what to do, watch others.

Cleanup

A neat, clean kitchen saves you time and energy. You are able to quickly find the ingredients and equipment you need. You don't have to waste time looking for them. A clean kitchen also helps protect you from foodborne illness and safety hazards.

It is much easier to work in the kitchen if you clean as you go. When you have a break, wash the equipment you have used. Put away ingredients you have finished using. You can dovetail cleaning with other tasks. For example, you could wash dishes while you wait for a food to bake. When you clean as you go, you will always have clean equipment to use. Also, you won't have to face stacks of dirty dishes, pots, and pans after the meal. If you do not have time to wash equipment as you go, at least put dirty containers in the sink and fill them with water. This will keep food from drying on the containers and make the later cleanup easier.

At the end of a meal, you will need to clear the table. If people are still seated at the table, stand to the left of each person when you clear his or her cover. Remove everyone's plates and flatware first. Then remove the glassware. Pick up the tableware with your left hand. Pass the tableware to your right hand and remove the next person's tableware.

In the kitchen, wrap leftovers and store them. Clean each dish by scraping food scraps into the garbage. It isn't polite to scrape the dishes at the table. Rinse off the dishes, then wash the dishes by hand or put them in the dishwasher.

When you hand wash dishes, start with the tableware that has the fewest food particles on it. In most cases, you should wash the glassware first. Wash the flatware next, then wash the dinnerware. Cooking utensils are washed last. By washing items in this order, your dishwater says cleaner. Be sure to wash each item thoroughly and rinse it in very hot water. If you can, let the items air-dry in a dish drainer. If not, use a clean dishtowel to dry the items.

To clean your kitchen, here's what you need to do.

- Make sure all the equipment you used is clean and dry.
- Return all equipment to its proper place.
- Wipe off counters and tables with a damp sponge or cloth.
- Clean the cooktop.
- Take out the garbage or use the garbage disposal.
- Wash out the sink and dry it.
- Put dishcloths in the laundry area.
- Sweep or vacuum the kitchen and dining areas as needed.

Cleanup is an important part of making a meal. Be sure to allow time for it when you make your work schedule.

Evaluating Your Plan

When the kitchen is cleaned up, you are almost finished. The last thing to do is to think about the meal you made. You can learn a great deal from this.

Look over your menu and work schedule. Ask yourself these questions when the meal and cleanup is complete.

- Did your plan go as you expected?
- What part of your plan worked well?

- Did you have to make any unexpected changes? Why?
- Was the meal served on time?
- Were the hot foods hot and cold foods cold?
- Did everyone enjoy the meal?
- How might you change the plan next time? Why?

Your answers can help you find ways to improve your menus and work schedules. When you make your next menu and work schedule, use what you learned. Your menus and work schedules will get better every time.

Entertaining

Most of the meals you plan, prepare, and serve probably will be for your family. Sometimes, you may invite friends or relatives to a meal. You may even decide to have a party.

Parties are fun for hosts to give and guests to attend. You can put everything you have learned about food preparation and meal planning to work when you entertain others. That's because food is often at the center of many parties. Foods cooked outside on the grill may be the focal point of a Fourth of July get-together. A birthday party may be celebrated with cake, ice cream, and punch.

The goal of get-togethers is to have fun with your guests. To achieve this goal, parties have to be planned carefully. A good party plan can help you feel confident and enthusiastic. That's because by planning ahead, you'll know exactly how much money the party will cost. You'll also know when each party planning task has to be done. So, when party time arrives, all the work will be complete. You'll be able to relax and have a good time with your guests.

Purpose for the Party

The first step is to decide why you want to have a party. Some parties are given to celebrate a special occasion, such as New Year's Eve. Others, such as graduation parties, are given to honor a person. Still other parties simply bring friends and family together to share a festive meal. Knowing why you want to have a party will give you ideas for food, decorations, and entertainment, 13-12. Although, before you choose any of these, you need to decide how much money you can afford to spend.

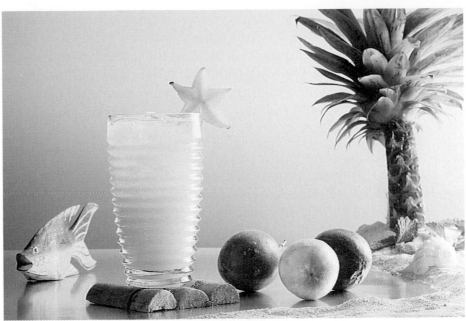

J.R. Brooks & Son

13-12 Choosing a theme can help you plan your party. For example, the menu for a pool party might include refreshing fruits and juices.

Your Party Budget

Most party budgets include these expenses: food, beverages, invitations, decorations, and entertainment. Food often is the most costly part of the budget. Be sure to keep in mind that you don't have to spend a lot of money to have a great party. To stay within your budget, you could plan a menu that uses mostly low-cost ingredients. For instance, pizza and soft drinks make a great, low-cost menu for a graduation party. If you can't afford to serve a whole meal, you could serve snacks.

Your Guest List

Make a list of the people you plan to invite. Your party budget may determine the number of guests you can invite. For instance, if you want to serve a whole meal, but have a limited budget, you'll need to shorten your guest list. Another alternative would be to serve a less costly menu so that you can invite more guests.

The space you have available for entertaining can also affect the size of your guest list. If you have a small space for the party, you'll have to limit your guest list or find another location. For example, you might decide to entertain in a park, restaurant, or community room. Holding a party in locations such as these often increases the cost of the party because you may have to pay rental fees.

When you are selecting a party site, think about how you will arrange the area. Is there space for guests to sit down? Where will you prepare and serve foods? Is there enough room for any entertainment you plan to have? Will you need to rearrange the room for the party? What type of decorations would work best?

Invitations

Once you've made your guest list, it's time to invite your guests. If you are inviting a small group, you could call or ask them in person. If it's a large group, you should send invitations. You can buy invitations or make your own. Invitations can be simple notes or fancy cards. You should invite your guests at least a week or two before the party.

You're Invited to a Party!

Date: Saturday, June 8
Time: 6 to 9 PM
Location: Monroe Wheeler's House
29 First Street
Middletown

It's a pool party!
Bring your swim suit and a towel.
Please R.S.V.P.
555-1234

13-13 An invitation includes all the information guests need to prepare and arrive on time at a party.

The invitations should include the date and time of the party and where it will be held, 13-13. You also may need to include a map or directions to the party site. Include your phone number, too. If you are having a special type of party, such as a costume or pool party, let your guests know.

You also can put *R.S.V.P.* on your invitations. **R.S.V.P.** stands for a French phrase that means "please reply." It tells your guests that they should let you know if they are coming. Knowing the number of guests to expect helps you decide how much food to prepare.

Your Party Menu

The purpose of your party can give you ideas about what to serve. For instance, the menu for a party to celebrate the start of baseball season might feature foods sold at ballparks. You could serve hot dogs, peanuts, and soft drinks. A fancy anniversary party for your parents might include a four-course dinner.

Remember, when planning your menu, there are several other factors to keep in mind, too. You need to consider who will be eating the food and their likes and dislikes. It's a good idea to offer a variety of foods so that everyone will find some foods they like. Also, think about where the food will be prepared and served. For example, if you plan to hold the party in a park, you'll need to choose foods that can be prepared ahead of time at home or cooked on outdoor grills.

When planning your menu, also think about your cooking skills and kitchen equipment. Choose recipes you can prepare easily and successfully with the equipment you have. If you lack a piece of equipment, you may be able to use another item instead. For instance, if you plan to serve punch and don't have a punch bowl, you could serve the punch from a pitcher. You also may decide to rent a punch bowl or borrow one from a friend.

Once the menu is planned, you need to create a food shopping plan and work schedule. These will help you be sure that when your guests begin to arrive, everything will be ready for them.

Party Decorations and Entertainment

Party decorations add a festive look to the party site, 13-14. When planning party decorations, think about the purpose of your party. If you are having a fancy dinner, your decorations might be a centerpiece on the table. For a back-to-school party, you might want to decorate with crepe paper streamers in your school colors. Be sure to include the cost of decorations in your budget. Also, include time on your work schedule to decorate and get the party site ready for guests.

Many parties include entertainment. It could be playing games, listening to music, or dancing. If you're having a beach party, the entertainment may be swimming and playing volleyball. Sometimes the entertainment is just having the chance to have a long conversation with friends. If you need to buy any entertainment supplies, be sure to include that in your budget. Think about how you will keep guests involved and active at the party.

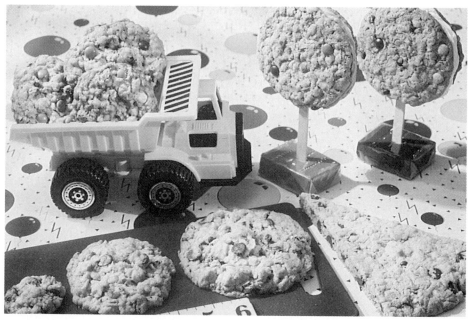

The Quaker Oats Company

13-14 Decorations can help everyone get in the mood to have a good time. This colorful tablecloth and truck would be great decorations for a children's party.

At the Party

There are certain responsibilities party hosts and guests have. By fulfilling your responsibilities as a host or a guest, you do your part in helping make the party a fun time for everyone.

As a host, you should try to spend all your time with your guests. At the beginning of the party, greet guests when they arrive. Make them comfortable by taking their coats and showing them to the area where the party is being held. Move around to different guests and spend time with each of them. Introduce guests who don't know each other. When introducing a person, it's helpful to give some information about each person. For example, to introduce a new student you might say, "This is Sam Jackson. He just moved here from Orlando." If you are introducing an older and younger person, give the older person's name first. You might say, "Mr. Rodriguez, this is Rachel Martin. She is a cheerleader at the high school."

As a guest, you should respond to an invitation right away. Another responsibility is to arrive at the party on time. Arriving early can make it hard for the host to complete last minute preparations. Arriving late may cause the food to get cold and inconvenience other guests. Try to help out the host whenever you can. It's also important to use your best table manners and help keep the party area neat. Be sure to move among the guests and meet new people. You could introduce yourself by saying something like this. "Hi, I'm Olga Anderson. I don't think we've met."

After the Party

When the party's over, there's one last step. It's time to clean up! It'll seem like part of the party if the host gets some friends to help. Start by storing any leftover food. Next, wash dishes and clean the kitchen. Then, clean the party area. Take down the decorations. Put any furniture that was moved back in its former location. Then, sweep or vacuum and empty the trash. Be sure to leave the party area clean and neat. A good cleanup job is one way to get your parents to okay future parties.

In a Nutshell

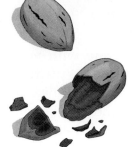

- A kitchen team's goal is to prepare food, serve it, eat it, and clean up in the time you have.
- A work schedule shows the time needed to prepare a meal, eat, and clean up.
- Before cooking, get out all the equipment and ingredients you will need.
- Meals can be served family, blue plate, formal, or buffet style.
- Tableware should be arranged on the table in a certain way to make it convenient to find the items you need.
- Using manners shows that you respect others and want to make them feel comfortable and at ease.
- A neat, clean kitchen saves you time and energy.
- To clear the table, stand to the left of a person and remove the tableware with your left hand.
- After the kitchen is cleaned up, evaluate the meal you made.
- Planning a party includes these tasks: identifying the purpose of the party, setting the budget, making the guest list, sending invitations, planning the menu and preparing the food, decorating the party area, planning the entertainment, and cleaning up afterwards.

In the Know

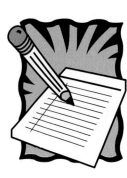

1. True or false? A work schedule lists all the tasks that must be done and when they are to be done.
2. Put the steps for making a work schedule in order.
    A. _____ Make a final work schedule.
    B. _____ List all the tasks that need to be done.
    C. _____ Estimate the time needed to prepare, cook, and serve each recipe.
    D. _____ Review each recipe in your menu.
3. Make a work schedule for an after school snack consisting of cheese, crackers, and lemonade from a mix.
4. You _____ tasks when you do two or more tasks at the same time.

5. In the _____ serving style, one course is served at a time.
   A. blue plate
   B. formal
   C. buffet
   D. family
6. Draw a place setting for the menu in 13-2.
7. _____ are a way of acting that helps everyone feel relaxed.
8. Explain how a neat, clean kitchen can save you time and energy.
9. List the three questions you can ask yourself to evaluate the usefulness of your work schedule.
10. Which of the following expenses are included in most party budgets?
    A. Food.
    B. Invitations.
    C. Decorations.
    D. All of the above.
11. List three responsibilities of party guests.

What Would You Do?

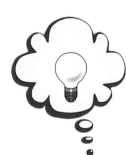

"I really like to cook," said Jamaal. "I don't like to clean up, though. It seems to take longer to clean up after a meal than it took to make the whole meal!" What advice would you give Jamaal? How could he make cleaning go faster?

Expanding Your Knowledge

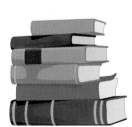

1. Plan a dinner menu. Make a work schedule for this meal. Prepare the meal and evaluate the results.
2. Interview your school cafeteria manager. Find out how the manager plans your school lunches. Take a look at a work schedule the manager uses. How does it differ from the one in 13-6? What are some examples of dovetailing that the manager uses?
3. Write a skit about a meal that was made without a work schedule. Perform the skit. Ask your classmates to describe how the skit would have been different if a work schedule were used.

4. Create a bulletin board called "Dovetailing in the Kitchen." Ask each person in your class to contribute at least one way he or she dovetails tasks. Each student could interview a cook he or she knows to learn new dovetailing ideas.

5. Videotape yourself making a meal at home. Watch the videotape. Note the number of trips you make to the refrigerator, cupboards, and dining area. List ways you could reduce the number of trips you make. List other ways you can save time in the kitchen.

6. Plan a meal for your family. Make a time schedule to follow when preparing all the foods for the meal from scratch. Make a time schedule to follow when preparing the meal using convenience foods. Which meal would you make? Why? How could you adapt this meal to take on a picnic?

7. Create a poster that shows how to arrange the tableware in a place setting.

8. Try a new way to serve a meal at home. For example, if your family usually serves meals family style, you could try blue plate. How does the new style of serving meals compare to the usual way of serving meals? Survey family members to find out what they think about the new serving method.

9. Plan a party to introduce a new exchange student to your friends. You could plan the menu, decorations, entertainment, and design an invitation.

10. Make a pamphlet that describes the responsibilities of party hosts and party guests.

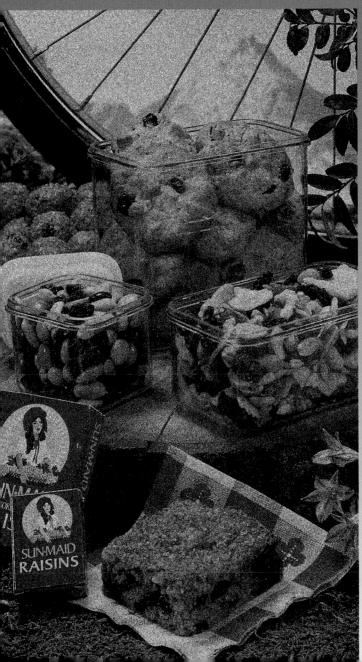

Chapter 14

When You're on the Go

Objectives

After reading this chapter, you will be able to
❏ prepare and store beverages, snacks, one-dish meals, and sandwiches.
❏ pack meals-to-go that are tasty, nutritious, and safe to eat.
❏ choose nutritious meals when eating meals out.

New Term

tip: a sum of money given to restaurant staff to show thanks for good service.

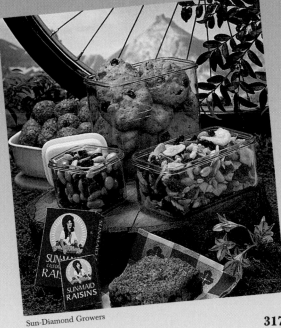

Sun-Diamond Growers

Many people are on the go these days. Their hectic schedules often reduce the time they have available to plan and prepare foods. Some people say they are so busy that they just don't have time to prepare or eat a healthy diet. These people don't realize that it is possible to fit good nutrition into the busiest schedule.

For a fast, nutritious hot meal for the whole family, you could serve a homemade one-dish meal in an hour or less. Between meals, you can whip up many nutritious beverages and snacks in less than five minutes. If you know you're going to be away from home when it's mealtime, you can quickly pack a meal-to-go. For times when you're too busy to make food at home, you may decide to eat out. With all these options, there's no reason to let a hectic schedule deprive you of the food and nutrients you need.

In this chapter, you will discover how to prepare and store beverages, snacks, one-dish meals, meals-to-go, and sandwiches. You'll also learn about eating meals out. Knowing about these types of foods and meals will help you fit good nutrition into the busiest schedule.

Beverages

When you are thirsty, what do you reach for? On cold days, you may prefer piping hot cocoa, hot cider, hot tea, or coffee. On hot days, you might choose chilled juice, frosty lemonade, iced tea, or cold water. Other popular beverage choices are milk, fruit drinks, and soft drinks, 14-1.

Beverages are served along with meals. Beverages can be snacks, too. All beverages help provide the water you need. Some beverages also provide other nutrients. For instance, beverages made with milk supply calcium and protein. Many fruit juices provide vitamin C, 14-2.

Some beverages, such as soft drinks, have a large amount of sugar added to them. They are high in calories and provide almost no vitamins and minerals. Coffee and tea also supply few nutrients and can be high in calories if you add lots of sugar. Cream adds fat and calories to coffee. The most nutritious beverages provide many vitamins and minerals and have little fat and added sugar.

14-1 Cool beverages help quench your thirst on hot days.

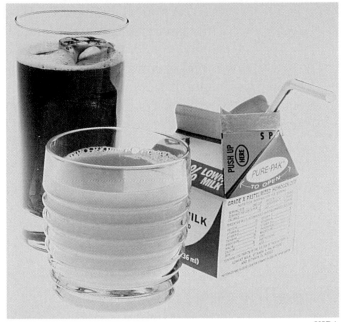

USDA

14-2 Serve orange juice as a beverage to increase your vitamin C intake.

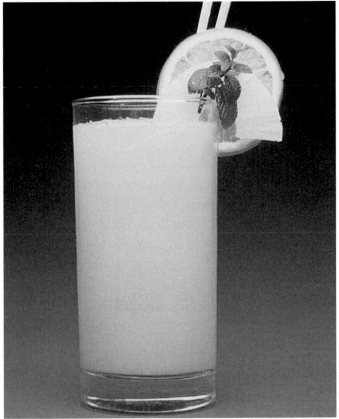

USDA

When planning a meal, choose a beverage that complements the flavors and colors of the foods in the meal. You can improve the nutritional value of the meal by choosing a beverage from a major food group from the Food Guide Pyramid. This is especially important if your meal is missing a food from one of the major food groups. For example, if your meal doesn't have a food from the vegetable group, you could serve carrot juice. If the milk group is missing, you could serve fat free milk. Pineapple juice is a nutritious addition to a meal lacking foods from the fruit group.

Tap water is a readily available, low cost beverage. You can also buy beverages. Food stores sell fresh, canned, bottled, and frozen beverages. Food stores also sell beverage mixes, dried tea leaves, and ground coffee beans. Purchased beverages cost more than tap water.

Preparing Beverages

Most beverages need very little preparation. Tap water requires no preparation. Just pour it in a glass and drink. Fresh, canned, and bottled beverages also do not need preparation. For instance, fresh milk, freshly squeezed orange juice, canned iced tea, and soft drinks are ready to drink when you buy them.

Frozen beverages need some preparation. Frozen juices need to be mixed with water. Frozen milk shakes have to be partly thawed before serving.

Beverage mixes need to be blended with a liquid, usually water. Iced tea mix, lemonade mix, and fruit flavored drink mixes are common mixes that are usually blended with cold water. Instant coffee, flavored coffee mix, and hot chocolate mix are beverage mixes that are usually blended with hot water. The directions on the package tell you how much water to add to the mix.

Most dried tea leaves are sold in a form called tea bags. Tea bags are made by placing dried, chopped tea leaves in a thin bag. Tea is prepared by soaking the tea bags in hot water for a few minutes. The color and flavor of the leaves dissolve and pass into the water. The longer the tea bag is left in the water, the darker the color and stronger the flavor will be. Ground coffee beans are used to brew coffee. When the beans are soaked with hot water, their flavor and color dissolve. This causes the water to become dark brown and flavorful.

Beverages that are served cold can be chilled in the refrigerator before serving. You can keep them cold once they are served by pouring them into ice-filled glassware. You can make them extra cold by pureeing them with ice in a blender. See 14-3.

14-3 To make a frosty beverage, puree 1 cup juice, ½ cup fruit chunks, and 4 ice cubes.

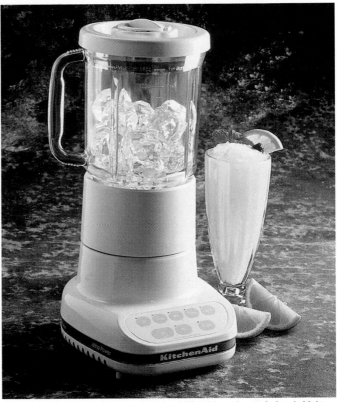

KitchenAid Portable Appliances, St. Joseph, Michigan

Beverages that are served hot need to be heated before they are served. You can heat water, juices, and milk on the cooktop or in a microwave oven. Hot beverages are hot enough when tiny bubbles begin to form and steam starts to form. They do not need to boil. Heating milk requires extra care. Chapter 20 describes how to heat milk correctly.

Coffee is usually made in a coffeemaker. The best coffee results when you use cold water, fresh coffee, and a clean coffeemaker. The directions that come with the coffeemaker will tell you how much coffee and water to use.

Storing Beverages

Fresh beverages should be kept in a closed container in the refrigerator. Use them within a week or so. Canned and bottled beverages can be kept in a cool, dry place for six months or longer. They also can be stored in the refrigerator before they are opened. Once opened, canned and bottled beverages need to be kept refrigerated and used within a week or two. A beverage mix stored in an airtight container that is kept in a cool, dry place will maintain its quality for a year or more. Leftover, prepared beverage mixes should be stored in the refrigerator. Tea bags and ground coffee beans should be placed in airtight containers and stored in a cool, dry place.

Snacks

What do you think of when you hear the word *snack*? Many people only think of chips, cookies, and candy. They don't realize that any food can be a snack. The snacks that are the best choices are those that help you meet your nutrient needs. You get the most nutrients when your snacks come from a variety of foods from the major food groups.

Many people enjoy snacks. Some people eat snacks several times each day. Most small children need snacks because they can eat only small amounts of food at each meal. Mid-morning, mid-afternoon, and bedtime snacks can help children get the nutrients they need. During your teen years, you may need snacks, too. This is because you are growing very rapidly. People who have busy schedules may need snacks to supply nutrients they miss when they skip meals.

To get the most nutrients from your snacks, it's important to plan ahead. First, think about when and where you will snack. Think about the types of snacks you will eat each time. Try to select mostly foods from the major food groups that are rich in vitamins and minerals and low in fat, cholesterol, sugar, and sodium. These tips can help you make the best snack choices.

- To have a sweet snack, carry fresh fruit or dried fruit instead of buying cookies or candy from a vending machine.
- For a crunchy snack, pack carrot sticks or a small box of breakfast cereal instead of buying chips.

Cultures of the World

Snacking: An International Incident

No matter where you go, you'll find people snacking. The snacks people like to eat differ from country to country. This is partly because foods that are available in some regions of the world are not found in other regions. It is also partly because food preferences vary from nation to nation.

Let's take an imaginary trip around the globe to see what teens like you commonly have for snacks. For our first stop, let's head south to Ecuador. There you'll find people snacking on crunchy platano fritos. A platano looks like a large banana. Platano fritos are made by thinly slicing the platano and frying it. This snack looks like banana chips.

Now, let's catch a plane and fly across the Atlantic Ocean to the African country of Ghana. Here, peanuts are a popular snack anytime of the day or night. Next, join a camel caravan and head for Egypt. You can share a snack of falafel with the teens who live there. Falafel is so popular that it is sold in fast-food restaurants. Mashed chickpeas, chili peppers, eggs, garlic, and flour are used to make falafel.

A cruise ship will take us to our next stop, India. In India, everyone enjoys a snack of pani pouri. These treats look like bread bubbles that are about the size of a golf ball. To eat them, punch a hole in them with your finger. Then, fill them with small pieces of potatoes and beans. Next, dip them in a sweet and sour sauce and pop them in your mouth. What a snack!

Now, let's float across Asia in a hot air balloon until we hit China. Here you'll find people snacking on fruit ices. Fruit ices are a lot like a sno-cone, except they are made with chunks of fresh fruit. Fruit ices are very popular on hot summer afternoons.

For our last stop, we'll hop onto a jet. It's destination is the U.S.A. Back home at last! All this traveling has probably made you hungry. Some teens in the United States might choose a slice of apple crumb pie for a snack. Others may prefer crispy, crunchy, carrot sticks. What do you reach for when you want a snack?

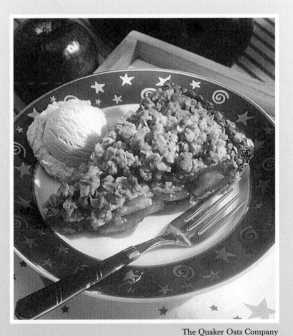

The Quaker Oats Company

Apple pie is just one of the many snacks people in the United States might choose. Can you think of others?

- If you want a cold snack, have frozen, nonfat yogurt or frozen fruit juice bars. You could also freeze washed grapes or a peeled banana.
- Have vegetable juice, fruit juice, or lowfat milk for a liquid snack instead of soft drinks.
- Keep your snacks small so they don't ruin your appetite at mealtime. If a snack is to replace a meal, choose meal-type foods, like sandwiches, salads, and fruits.

Preparing Snacks

Preparing nutritious snacks is quick and easy, 14-4. In fact, many of the most nutritious snacks require little or no preparation. For instance, you only need to open the package to snack on raisins, pretzels, rice cakes, whole-grain crackers, and breakfast cereal.

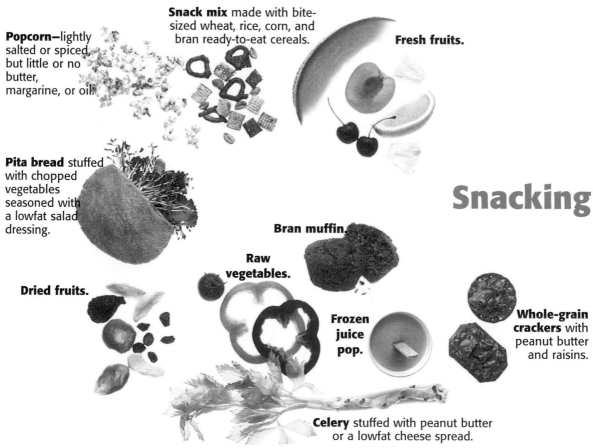

Snack mix made with bite-sized wheat, rice, corn, and bran ready-to-eat cereals.

Popcorn—lightly salted or spiced, but little or no butter, margarine, or oil.

Fresh fruits.

Pita bread stuffed with chopped vegetables seasoned with a lowfat salad dressing.

Snacking

Bran muffin.

Raw vegetables.

Dried fruits.

Frozen juice pop.

Whole-grain crackers with peanut butter and raisins.

Celery stuffed with peanut butter or a lowfat cheese spread.

USDA

14-4 Snacks can come from a variety of foods.

You also don't need to do any preparation to have a snack of lowfat yogurt or cheese slices. For a milk or juice snack, just pour these beverages into glasses. Fresh fruits and vegetables only need to be washed and, perhaps, pared and sliced. Cold hard-cooked eggs, cold fried chicken, and cold pizza can be eaten straight from the refrigerator. Plain popcorn can be popped quickly in a microwave oven or popcorn popper. You can whip up an instant pudding mix by adding cold milk, beating with a mixer, and chilling.

Storing Snacks

To store fresh fruit and vegetable snacks, wrap them or place them in closed containers. Most fresh fruit and vegetable snacks can be safely stored outside the refrigerator. If you plan to store them for more than a few hours, place them in the refrigerator. Fresh fruit and vegetable snacks stay fresher longer if they are refrigerated.

Dried fruit and most bread and cereal snacks should be kept in airtight containers. This storage method will help preserve their freshness and appeal. Snacks that contain milk, eggs, or meat need to be stored in the refrigerator.

One-Dish Meals

Chili, beef stew, tuna casserole, pizza, and tacos are one-dish meals. One-dish meals include foods from several food groups, 14-5. For instance, chili includes foods from the vegetable group and meat

14-5 Which food groups are represented in this meal?

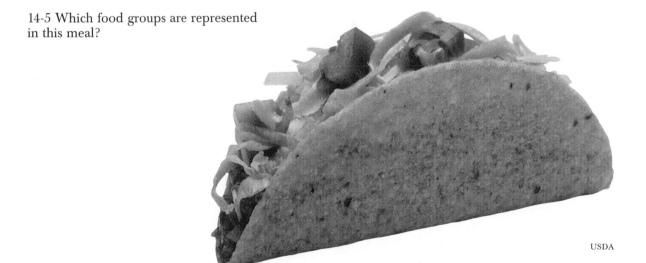

USDA

and beans group. Foods from the vegetable group, grains group, and milk group are used to make pizza. Tuna casserole includes foods from the grains group, meat and beans group, and vegetable group.

To make one-dish meals complete, you'll need to add a beverage. You may need a simple side dish, too. This is because many one-dish meals don't include foods from every major food group. For example, very few one-dish meals include fruits. A side dish that includes the food groups missing in the one-dish meal helps improve the meal's nutritional value. For instance, to add needed nutrients to a tuna casserole meal, serve milk and peach slices with it.

Preparing One-Dish Meals

One-dish meals are a good way to save time in the kitchen. These meals save preparation time because you don't have to prepare each part of the meal separately. All the ingredients are cooked at once. One-dish meals also save cleanup time because there are fewer pots and pans to wash.

14-6 The ingredients for casseroles, such as this turkey strata, can be combined in just a few minutes.

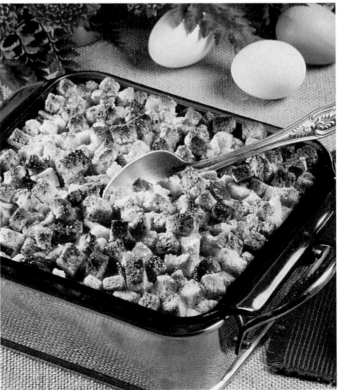

American Egg Board

Most one-dish meals are easy to make. For many stews, you only need to combine the ingredients in a pot and simmer them. For casseroles, you only need to blend or layer the ingredients in a greased pan and bake, 14-6. The chart in 14-7 shows you the formula for creating a casserole or stew. As you can see, almost any food can be part of a one-dish meal.

Creating One-Dish Meals	
Group	**Choices**
1	4 cups cooked rice, pasta, or noodles 4 cups cooked, sliced potatoes
2	2 cups cooked, dry beans 1 cup raw or cooked ground or cubed meat, fish, or poultry
3	2 cups fresh, frozen, or canned (drained) vegetables
4	1 can vegetable soup 1 can cheese soup plus ½ cup liquid* 1 can cream soup plus ½ cup liquid* 1⅔ cups vegetable juice *Liquid can be milk, vegetable juice, or water.
5	½ cup bread or cracker crumbs ½ cup corn flakes ⅓ cup grated cheese 8 uncooked biscuits

Here's how to create a casserole:
1. Using the chart above, choose one food from each of the groups.
2. Grease a three-quart casserole pan.
3. Cover bottom of pan with one of the foods from Group 1.
4. Spread the food from Group 2 over the food already in the pan.
5. Repeat Step 4 for the remaining groups.
6. Bake at 400°F (200°C) for 30 to 40 minutes. The top should be bubbly and brown.
7. Cool 10 minutes and serve.
Serves 6

Here's how to create a stew:
1. Using the chart above, choose one food from Group 1, 2, 3, and 4. You will need to double the amount of ingredients used from Group 4.
2. Place all the ingredients in a four-quart pot.
3. On the cooktop, simmer on medium heat for 30 to 40 minutes. Stir every 10 minutes. Serve immediately.
Serves 6

14-7 Creating one-dish meals is simple and fun.

One-dish meals give you a chance to be creative in the kitchen. That's because it's up to you to choose the foods to use. When choosing foods, think about how they will look and taste together. Pick foods with colors, textures, and flavors that blend well.

One-dish meals are a good way to use leftovers. These meals will save you money if you use leftovers that would have been wasted and thrown away. Remember to only use leftovers that have been safely stored.

Storing One-Dish Meals

One-dish meals need to be covered tightly and refrigerated within two hours after cooking. They become unsafe to eat if they remain at room temperature for more than two hours. One-dish meals that don't contain cream soup can be wrapped tightly and frozen before or after they are cooked. Refrigerated and frozen one-dish meals should be thoroughly heated before they are served.

Meals-to-Go

Many busy families find they aren't always home at mealtime. Every day, thousands of people plan ahead and pack snacks and lunches to carry to school or work. Picnics and potluck dinners are other times people eat homemade food away from home.

There are many advantages to packing meals and snacks to eat away from home. For example, these meals and snacks usually cost less than those you buy in restaurants. Packed foods save you time because you don't have to go to a restaurant and wait for your food to be served. Some people think homemade foods taste better than foods from restaurants of vending machines. When you make your own meal or snack, you have more control over the foods you eat. You can be sure it contains the nutritious foods that you like to eat.

Preparing Meals-to-Go

Almost any food can be part of a meal or snack to be eaten away from home. See 14-8. When you plan these meals and snacks, keep good nutrition in mind. Try to include foods from most of the major food groups. Also try to make the meals and snacks appealing. Include foods with a variety of flavors, colors, and textures.

14-8 Meal-to-go possibilities are almost endless.

Meals-to-Go	
Menu #1 Hot chili Corn bread Apple Iced tea	**Menu #2** Cold chicken Biscuit Carrot sticks Lemonade
Menu #3 Cold cheese pizza Tossed salad Sparkling water	**Menu #4** Meatloaf sandwich Raw cauliflower Grapes Milk
Menu #5 Tuna salad Crackers Celery sticks Chocolate milk	**Menu #6** Macaroni and cheese Cookies Apple juice
Menu #7 Bean burrito Cheese wedge Tomato juice	**Menu #8** Yogurt Banana Muffin Diet soft drink

When packing a meal or snack to go, be sure to wrap foods or pack them in nonbreakable containers, 14-9. This helps to keep foods tasting fresh. For instance, you can keep salads crunchy by storing them in a plastic bag. Add the dressing when you're ready to eat. Also, don't forget to pack napkins and any utensils you will need. For example, you'll need a fork for a salad and a cup to serve a hot beverage.

14-9 Plastic containers preserve the freshness of foods packed to go.

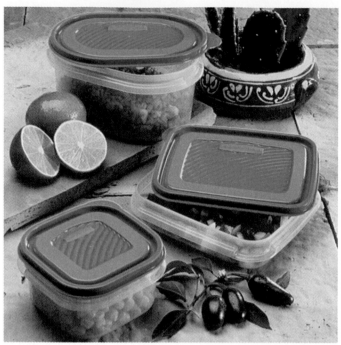

Rubbermaid

 Focus on Nutrition

Eat to Win

After-school activities are one of the reasons why many teens are on the go. These activities may occur at times when

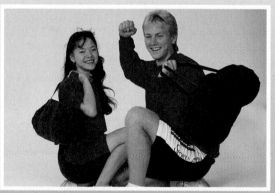

Pineapple Appeal

Teen athletes need a variety of nutritious foods to achieve top performance.

many teens usually eat meals or snacks. For the best nutritional health, teens will need to figure out how to eat and participate, too.

It is especially important for teens who are on sports teams to fit good nutrition into their busy schedules. Each year, coaches and athletes make plans for a winning season. They all know the route to victory includes hours of practice. Many know victory depends on the foods they eat, too.

What Should Athletes Eat?

The best diet for athletes is much like the best diet for nonathletes. It includes foods from all the major food groups each day. The main difference is that athletes need more calories and water than non-athletes. Athletes do not need special foods, supplements, or extra salt.

Calories

Athletes should add more servings of carbohydrate-rich foods to get the extra calories they need. Remember, foods from the grain, fruit, and vegetable groups are rich in carbohydrate.

Some athletes believe that their extra calories should come from protein-rich foods. Protein is important, but not as important as many athletes think. In fact, athletes need only a few grams more protein than nonathletes. Two servings from the meat and beans group and three or four from the milk group provide athletes with more than enough protein. Athletes who eat more servings than these are likely to have a diet that is high in fat.

When training ends, athletes no longer need extra calories. They will gain excess body fat if they don't trim the number of calories eaten to match the calories they burn. Keeping weight under control between seasons makes it easier for athletes to get in shape when the next season begins.

Water

Athletes need to drink an extra quart or more of water daily. This water replaces the water lost in sweat. Drinking too little water can decrease strength and performance. It also can cause the body to become overheated. Athletes who limit water intake aren't likely to win. They also put their lives in danger.

Cool water or fruit juice mixed with water is the best choice. Sports drinks are not needed. These drinks don't make athletes less thirsty or more energetic.

Special Foods and Supplements

Some athletes eat special foods or take protein, vitamin, and mineral supplements. They believe these will help to make them star athletes. However, no food or supplement gives athletes extra energy, strength, or power. Also, protein supplements or extra protein from food will not make muscles larger or stronger. Exercise is the only way to safely increase the size and strength of muscles.

Salt

Did you ever notice that sweat tastes salty? That's because sweat contains the minerals that make salt. Sodium is one of these minerals. Athletes lose more sodium than usual when they sweat a lot. The lost sodium is quickly replaced by foods and beverages in athletes' diets. Athletes do not need salt pills or sodium tablets. In fact, salt pills and sodium tablets can be very harmful.

What's the Best Pre-event Meal to Eat?

The best meals to eat before an athletic event contain mostly carbohydrate-rich foods. These meals should be low in fat because the body takes longer to digest fat than carbohydrate. These meals also should contain plenty of water and fruit juice.

Athletes should plan to eat at least three hours before an event. This gives the body enough time to digest the food. By eating a nutritious diet, athletes are ready when event time finally arrives. Good nutrition combined with practice helps an athlete have the best performance possible.

Keeping Meals-to-Go Safe to Eat

Meals- and snacks-to-go should be safe to eat, too. Safety starts at home with clean kitchen equipment. Safety counts after you hit the road, too. Keeping foods safe to eat means keeping cold foods cold and hot foods hot. You can keep cold foods safe by chilling them well before packing the meal or snack. Then, store cold foods in an insulated container until you are ready to serve them. Keep the container in a cool place. Don't set it next to a heater or in sunlight. You can keep the container cold by putting a cold pack in it. You can make your own cold pack by putting ice cubes in a zip-top bag or a plastic container that seals tightly. If you can, store the insulated container in a refrigerator until lunchtime.

Keep hot liquids safe by carrying them in a vacuum bottle. Vacuum bottles are ideal for carrying chili, stews, soups, and hot cocoa. The liquid stays hot longer if you preheat the bottle. You can preheat it by filling it with very hot water. Let it stand a few minutes then pour out the water. Pour in the hot liquid right away and close the bottle. The food will stay hot and safe to eat for a few hours.

You can also use vacuum bottles to keep cold beverages cold. Another way to keep beverages cold is to freeze them in a plastic bottle that has a tight-fitting lid. Don't fill the bottle all the way to the top because liquids expand when they freeze. Keep the liquid an inch or two below the top of the bottle. If the bottle is filled up, the freezing beverage will force the top off the bottle. Frozen beverages help keep the rest of your meal cool and will be thawed enough to drink in three or four hours.

Sandwiches

Sandwiches are one of the most popular foods for meals-to-go, 14-10. They are said to have been invented over 200 years ago by the Earl of Sandwich. He was so busy playing cards that he didn't want to stop for dinner. He asked his cook to bring him some meat and bread. He picked up the meat with the bread and ate it without stopping the game. The sandwich was born!

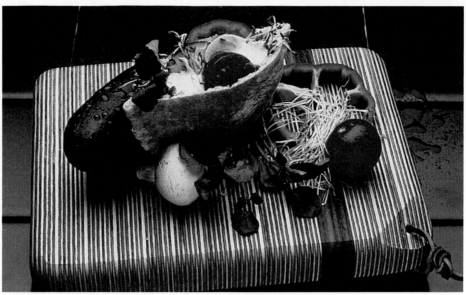

USDA

14-10 Sandwiches were one of the first meals-to-go. People have enjoyed them ever since the Earl of Sandwich invented them in the 1700s.

Preparing Sandwiches

There are many sandwich choices. You can put most anything between two slices of bread. You can use any type of bread. See 14-11. The nutrients in your sandwich will depend on the ingredients used.

To make a sandwich meal complete, just add a beverage and soup or a piece of fresh fruit. If you need to boost the calories, add a second sandwich or some cookies.

Storing Sandwiches

If you won't be eating your sandwich right away, wrap it tightly in plastic wrap or foil. This will keep it fresh. This will help to prevent the bread from becoming hard and stale.

Spreading butter, margarine, peanut butter, or mayonnaise on the bread will keep it from getting soggy. These spreads add extra fat and calories to the sandwich. You also can wrap the bread, filling, and extras separately. Your sandwich won't get soggy if you put it together just before eating it.

Building a Sandwich			
Bread			
bagel biscuit crackers English muffin French bread	hard roll hot dog bun Italian bread onion roll pita bread	pumpernickel bread raisin bread rice cake rye bread	sourdough bread sub roll tortilla waffles whole wheat bread
Protein Fillings		**Extras**	
American cheese Cheddar cheese chicken breast chicken salad egg salad fish sticks ham hamburger patty mashed beans	meat loaf peanut butter roast beef salami sardines Swiss cheese tofu tuna salad turkey	bananas bean sprouts grated carrots cucumber slices green pepper slices guacamole hot pepper sauce honey jelly	lettuce mushrooms mustard olives onion slices pickle relish pineapple slices raisins spinach tomatoes
1. Start with the kind of bread you want for your creation. 2. Choose a protein filling. 3. Dress it up with extras.			

14-11 You can use your creativity when building a sandwich.

Sandwiches made ahead of time that contain meat, cheese, or eggs should be kept in the refrigerator or in an insulated container. If your sandwich doesn't contain eggs, mayonnaise, or uncooked vegetables, you can freeze it. Frozen sandwiches thaw in three or four hours, just in time for lunch.

Eating Out

People eat out for many reasons. Some eat out for a change of pace. Others eat out for fun and entertainment. Many people eat out because they don't have the time or energy to prepare a meal. Eating out does save preparation time, but more time is usually spent at the table. When eating out, you need to allow time to be seated, place your order, get your food, eat, and pay the bill.

The cost of eating out depends on where you eat and what you order. However, it almost always costs more to eat out than to eat at home. That's because when you eat out, the price of the food includes more than just the cost of the food itself. The price also includes a small part of the restaurant's rent and electricity, staff's wages, and supplies, such as menus and napkins.

Eating Out Know-How

All types of restaurants have several similarities. For example, certain events, such as making your food selections and paying your bill, occur every time you eat out. Knowing what to expect when you eat in a restaurant helps you feel comfortable and confident.

Placing an Order

A menu is a list of all the foods and beverages a restaurant sells. It also lists the price of each food and beverage. The menu may be one large poster that's hung up in the restaurant for everyone to see. The menu also may be printed and given to each person. After reviewing the menu, you may have a question about a menu item. For example, you may want to know how the item is prepared. The person waiting on you is there to help you. He or she should be able to answer your questions or to find out the answers to your questions.

Place your order by telling the server what you would like to eat. Speak clearly and slowly so that your order is correctly placed. Be sure to state your choices for optional items. For example, you may have a choice of baked potato toppings. If you are ordering a meal that is served in courses, state your food choices in the sequence they will be served. That is, begin by stating the appetizer you want. Then, name the salad and entree you want. Dessert orders often are taken after you have finished the entree.

Paying the Check

Diners are given a bill that states the cost of the meal. This bill is often referred to as a restaurant check. In some restaurants, you pay a cashier before eating. In others, the food server puts the check on your table after you finish eating. Review your check carefully to be certain that the charges are correct. If there is a charge you do not understand, politely ask the person waiting on you to explain it.

Checks brought to the table may be placed on the table, on a tray, or in a small folder. In some restaurants, you pay a cashier as you leave. In others, your food server takes your payment and returns your change.

Before leaving your table, it is a custom to leave a **tip** for the service received. A tip is also called a *gratuity*. It is left to show thanks for good service. For average service, an appropriate tip is about 15 to 20 percent of the total bill. You may want to leave a larger tip if the restaurant staff gave you special service.

Restaurant Manners

Restaurant meals are the most enjoyable when every diner looks neat and uses good manners. By being neat and using good manners, diners show respect for each other and for the restaurant staff. Good manners help others feel comfortable and at ease. Try to use all the good manners listed in Chapter 13 every time you eat out.

Occasionally, you may have a problem with your food or service when you eat out. The food server may have forgotten to bring your beverage. Perhaps your salad has the wrong dressing on it. If you have a problem, quietly ask your server to correct it. Try not to disturb other diners. If the food server isn't able to correct the problem, ask to see the manager. In most cases, the restaurant staff will do their best to be sure you enjoy your meal.

Types of Restaurants

There are many different types of restaurants. They range from casual to formal. Some have fancy decorations. Others are plain. Some feature a wide variety of foods. Others have a limited menu. Some are inexpensive. Others are very costly.

Fast-food restaurants offer fast service at fairly low prices, 14-12. There are several reasons why service is fast. One reason is that the menu choices are limited and many foods are fried. Frying cooks foods quickly. Another reason is that fast-food restaurants are self-service. Customers place their order, pay, receive their food, and leave or carry the food to a table. When they finish eating, customers dispose of their trash and leave. Self-service helps to keep prices low. The large volume of food these restaurants sell also helps keep prices low. Fast-food restaurants don't have table service, so tipping isn't necessary.

Math in the Kitchen

Estimating Tips

When you eat at full-service restaurants, it is a custom in most countries, including the United States, to leave a tip. It is appropriate to leave 15 to 20 percent of your total bill. To leave a 15 percent tip means to leave 15 cents for every dollar you spend. To leave a 20 percent tip means to leave 20 cents for every dollar you spend. Does that mean you should take a calculator with you when you eat out? You could, but you won't need to if you know how to estimate the tip in your head.

Here's one way to estimate a 15 percent tip:

Step 1. Look at the total cost of the meal.

Step 2. Round to the nearest dollar.

Step 3. Multiply the rounded number of total dollars by 0.15.

Example: Suppose the bill for you and a friend adds up to $9.20.

Step 1. Total Cost = $9.20

Step 2. Rounded Cost = $9.00

Step 3. $9.00 x 0.15 = $1.35

The tip for you and your friend would be $1.35.

Here's another way to estimate a tip.

Step 1. Look at the total cost of the meal.

Step 2. Determine what 10 percent of the bill would be.
An easy method to determine this is to move the decimal one place to the right.
For example: $ 9.20
So, 10 percent of the bill equals $0.92 (or 92 cents).

Step 3. Determine what 5 percent of the bill would be by dividing 10 percent of the bill in half.
$0.92 ÷ 2 = $0.46 (or 46 cents).

Step 4. Compute the total tip by adding Step 2 (10 percent of the bill) to Step 3 (5 percent of the bill). Remember, 10 percent + 5 percent = 15 percent. Your tip would be $0.92 + $0.46 = $1.38. Diners usually round their tip up or down to the nearest nickel or dime.

Notice that the two methods give similar answers. They differ because the first method rounds the total bill and the second method does not. However, the differences between the two are very small.

Some people prefer one method over the other. You should practice both to determine which you like best. By practicing, you'll feel more confident when you go out to eat. To practice, make a list of five bills you might pay in a restaurant. Compute a tip for each of the bills using both of the methods.

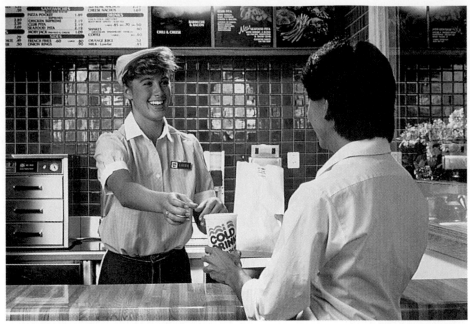

Jack In The Box

14-12 Fast-food restaurants offer quick service.

Cafeterias display a wide variety of prepared foods along a serving line. Customers select the foods and beverages they want and place them on their trays, 14-13. Each food is served in individual portions and priced separately. Customers pay for their food at the end of the serving line. Then, the food is carried to a table and eaten. In some cafeterias, the customer takes the dirty dishes to a central cleaning area. In others, restaurant staff clear the table. Cafeterias, like fast-food restaurants, have fairly low prices. The service is fast because the foods are prepared in advance. Cafeterias usually don't have servers who deliver food to your table, but restaurant staff may refill coffee and tea and clear dirty dishes. If so, a tip of about 10 percent of the food bill is appropriate.

Full-service restaurants have table service. In some full-service restaurants, diners seat themselves. In others, a host takes diners to a table. When seated, diners are given menus. After a few minutes, a food server comes to the table and takes the diners' orders. Foods are served in courses in many full-service restaurants. Appetizers are served first. Salad comes next, then comes the entree. Dessert is served last. Beverages often are brought to the table after the order is placed. When the meal is over, the food server brings the check, 14-14.

14-13 At a cafeteria, diners serve themselves.

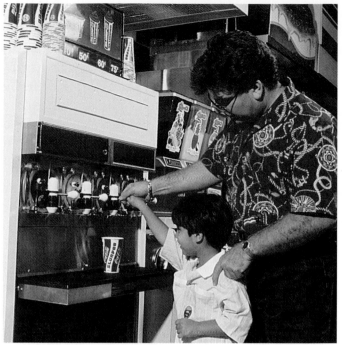

Parker Hannifin Corporation

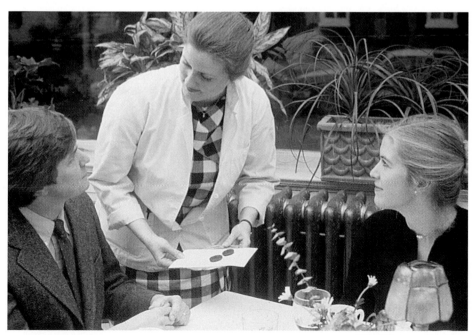

National Restaurant Association

14-14 At a full-service restaurant, a server presents a check to diners at the end of the meal.

It usually takes more time and costs more to eat at full-service restaurants than at fast-food restaurants or cafeterias. It takes longer to eat at full-service restaurants because most of the foods are not prepared until they are ordered. However, because many of the foods are prepared to order, you can ask that foods be made a little differently than the menu specifies. The price is higher in full-service restaurants because customers receive more service from restaurant staff than they do in fast-food restaurants or cafeterias.

Full-service restaurants that are formal tend to be more expensive than those that are casual. This is because most formal restaurants feature high-quality foods and service. For instance, foods served at formal restaurants usually are prepared by highly skilled chefs. In addition, the ingredients used are often of the freshest, highest quality. Some diners also tend to tip a bit more in formal restaurants than they would in other restaurants.

Fast-food restaurants, cafeterias, and full-service restaurants aren't the only places you might go to eat out. Anytime you eat somewhere other than at home, you are eating out. You are eating out when you eat in your school cafeteria. You also may eat out at a concession stand at the movies, at a cookie vendor in the mall, or from a vending machine.

Wherever you go to eat out, keep good nutrition in mind when selecting the foods you want to eat. Try to focus on foods from the major food groups. Also, try to keep fat and sugar intake down. You can do this by trading off high-fat and high-sugar foods with foods lower in fat and sugar. For instance, bring along a piece fruit instead of ordering pie at a fast-food restaurant. At vending machines, skip the candy and chips. Instead, try choosing nonfat yogurt, frozen fruit bars, raisins, pretzels, and fat free milk.

As you can see, no matter how busy you are, good nutrition can fit into your schedule. Many nutritious snacks and beverages can be prepared in just a few minutes. One-dish meals are easily prepared in less than an hour. In the next chapters, you'll learn how to prepare even more types of foods.

In a Nutshell

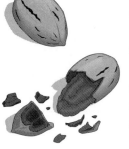

- Beverages add nutrients, flavor, and color to meals and snacks.
- Most beverages require little preparation and can be easily stored.
- The best snack choices are foods that add needed nutrients to your diet.
- One-dish meals include foods from several food groups.
- One-dish meals save preparation and clean-up time.
- When you pack foods to eat away from home, keep them safe by storing them in an insulated container until serving time.
- Keep sandwiches fresh by wrapping them tightly in plastic wrap or foil.
- Many people eat out because they don't have the time or energy to prepare a meal.
- It almost always costs more to eat out than to eat at home.
- Good manners help make restaurant meals enjoyable for all diners.
- Speed of service and cost vary depending on the type of restaurant.

In the Know

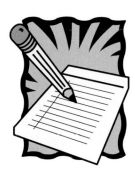

1. Name two beverages that would add needed nutrients to a meal of waffles topped with peanut butter, raisins, and bananas.
2. True or false? Beverage mixes should be kept in an open container in the refrigerator.
3. List two nutritious snacks from each of the major food groups that you could eat when you are in a hurry.
4. Beef stew is made with beef and vegetables. Which foods would be the best choices to add to make this meal complete?
   A. Green beans and biscuits.
   B. Corn bread, fresh blueberries, and tomato juice.
   C. Dinner rolls, melon wedge, and milk.
   D. Corn, peas, and rice.
5. True or false? One-dish meals are time consuming to make.
6. Explain how to store one-dish meals.
7. A _____ _____ keeps chili taken to school for lunch hot and safe to eat.
8. Create a menu for a meal-to-go. Explain how you will keep it fresh and safe to eat.

9. In restaurants, it is a custom to leave a ___ to show thanks for good service.
10. Which type of restaurant displays a wide variety of prepared foods along a serving line?
     A. Fancy, full-service restaurant.
     B. Cafeteria.
     C. Fast-food restaurant.
     D. Casual, full-service restaurant.

What Would You Do?

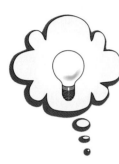

You and your friends are talking after school. Shawna was eating her third candy bar for the day. "I know what a nutritious meal is, I just don't have time to prepare and eat one," she said. "I know what you mean," said Tom. "It takes too long to make something nutritious every time I get hungry. Besides, I feel fine most of the time. Why worry about what I eat?" What advice would you give your friends?

Expanding Your Knowledge

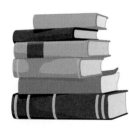

1. Conduct a beverage taste test. Select several forms of the same beverage. For example, you could try freshly squeezed, canned, and frozen orange juice. Set up a taste panel to compare the flavor, smell, texture, and color of the forms. Also compare the time needed to prepare each form.
2. Investigate snacks that are popular in other areas of the world. Write the recipes for the snacks on cards. Create a bulletin board that uses a world map to show where the snacks are popular. Use yarn or string to connect the recipe cards with their countries of origin.
3. Write a television commercial designed to sell fruits as a snack. Videotape your commercial and show it to young children.
4. Conduct a snack survey. Begin by brainstorming to identify questions to ask. For instance, you might ask people: What are your favorite snacks? Do you eat them often? Do you want to change any snacking habits? Why do you think certain snacks are more popular than others? What influences you to eat the snacks you do? Develop a form to collect the survey information. Interview 15 people. Report your findings to your class.

5. Create a one-dish meal using the information in 14-7. Describe the dish's flavor and appearance. Would you make the dish again? Why or why not?

6. Design a poster about sandwiches. Include tips for making them. Illustrate the poster with drawings or pictures from magazines. Display the poster in your classroom or school cafeteria.

7. Invite friends over to make a monster sandwich. Select two protein fillings and four extras from 14-11. Make the sandwich using a large, uncut loaf of bread. Slice the bread lengthwise into three pieces. On the bottom slice, arrange the protein fillings. Place the middle bread slice on the protein filling. Arrange the extras. Top with the remaining bread slice. Use a serrated knife to cut the sandwich crosswise into one-inch thick pieces.

8. Plan a picnic. What foods would you take? How would you prepare them? How will you keep them fresh and safe to eat?

9. Role-play eating out at a full-service restaurant. Have a friend act as the server. Practice placing an order, paying the check, and computing a tip.

Chapter 15
Fabulous Fruits

Objectives

After reading this chapter, you will be able to
- ❏ identify types of fruit.
- ❏ describe how to buy and store fruit.
- ❏ prepare fruit dishes to maintain nutrients, colors, flavors, and textures.

New Terms

drupes: a type of fruit that has one large pit or seed and grows on trees.

pomes: a type of fruit that has a core that contains seeds and grows on trees.

citrus fruit: a type of fruit that has a leathery skin, many segments filled with juicy pellets, and grows on trees.

berries: small, juicy fruits that contain many tiny seeds.

melons: large, moist fruits that grow on vines and contain seeds. They have a thick skin that may be smooth or rough.

tropical fruit: a type of fruit that grows only in warm, sunny climates.

produce: fresh fruits and vegetables.

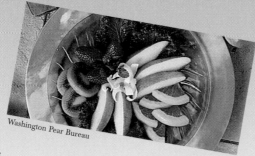

Washington Pear Bureau

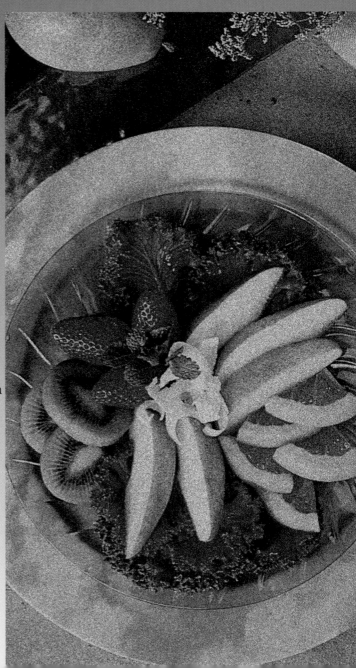

344

Fruits grow all over the world. They are part of every nation's cuisine. Imagine jetting around the globe, tasting fruits as you go. You could stop off in Germany for a tasty apple strudel. Then hop over to Egypt for some sweet figs and dates. You'll find coconut milk on the menu when you arrive in Thailand. On your way home, take a break in Fiji and savor a juicy pineapple.

Fruits are one of the great gifts of nature. Their colors, flavors, scents, and textures tempt the appetite. Fruits make meals and snacks more inviting. Many are good sources of fiber and vitamins A and C. All fruits, except avocados and coconuts, are low in fat and calories.

➕ Health Alert

Science Solves Vitamin C Mystery!

You may have heard that vitamin C cures colds. Does it? Scientists have been working hard to answer that question. Now they have an answer. How did they find the answer? They set up many experiments. Here's what the scientists did to make sure their experiments gave them the right answer.

1. They asked many people to participate. In each experiment, the people were very much alike.
   - Their age and gender were the same. For example, one experiment studied teen boys. Another studied only adult women.
   - Their health and diets were similar. If some got more colds or ate more vitamin C-rich foods, the experiments would be unfair.

2. They divided the people into two groups.
   - Group A got a vitamin C pill.
   - Group B got a pill that looked like Group A's pill. However, Group B's pill didn't contain any vitamin C.

The people did not know if they had the pill with vitamin C or not. Knowing if the pill contained vitamin C would make an experiment unfair. (When you know you are getting vitamin C and believe it will cure your cold, you may underestimate how bad your cold is. Also, you may get better much faster. Wanting to get better is an important part of healing.)

3. They asked a person who wasn't involved with the experiment to give out the pills. Only this person knew who got the vitamin C pills. This person kept a list of the people in Groups A and B. The list was given to the scientists after the experiment ended. During the experiment, the scientists did not know who was taking the vitamin C pills. If they knew who was taking the vitamin C pills, they may have been swayed.

After analyzing the results of many experiments, scientists found the answer. Large doses of vitamin C have almost no effect on colds. Remember, though, vitamin C is needed for good health. You can get plenty of vitamin C from fruits and vegetables.

Types of Fruits

A fruit is a plant's seed envelope. This soft, juicy part holds the plant's seeds. Some fruits, such as plums and mangos, have large seeds that are not eaten. Kiwifruit, berries, and figs have many tiny seeds. The tiny seeds are easy to chew, so they are eaten along with the fruit.

Most fruits taste sweet. They get sweeter as they ripen. Avocados and breadfruit are not sweet. Avocados taste nutty. Breadfruit tastes bland like rice.

Fruit may grow on trees, vines, or bushes. There are six types of fruit: drupes, pomes, citrus fruits, melons, berries, and tropical fruits.

Drupes

A *drupe* is a fruit with one large pit or seed, 15-1. Drupes grow on trees. Cherries and peaches are drupes. The skin on drupes can be eaten, but some people prefer to pare fuzzy peaches.

15-1 Drupes have one large pit or seed. Nectarines are drupes.

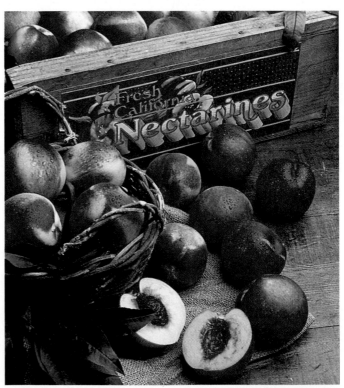

California Tree Fruit Agreement

The best drupes smell sweet and are plump and juicy. Ripe drupes give a little when squeezed gently. Wrinkled drupes are dry and mealy. Soft drupes are bruised or too ripe. Hard ones are not yet ripe.

You can ripen drupes by keeping them at room temperature for a few days. Very hard drupes may not ripen properly at home.

Peaches and other dark yellow drupes are rich in vitamin A. How many of these drupes have you tried?

- Apricots
- Cherries
- Nectarines
- Peaches
- Plums

Pomes

Pomes have cores that contain seeds. Pomes grow on trees. Apples, pears, and quinces are pomes. Their smooth skin can be eaten, 15-2.

The best pomes are firm and smell good. Pomes that are wrinkled or feel spongy are old and dried out. Ripe pears should give a little when squeezed gently. Rough squeezing causes bruises and harms the fruit. You can ripen pears at home at room temperature.

15-2 Pomes have cores that contain seeds.

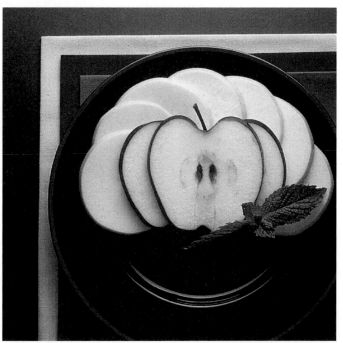

Washington Apple Commission

There are many varieties of apples and pears. How many have you tried?

- Golden Delicious apples
- Granny Smith apples
- McIntosh apples
- Rome apples

- Anjou pears
- Bartlett pears
- Bosc pears
- Comice pears

Citrus

Citrus fruits have a shiny, tough, leathery skin. Often the skin is brightly colored, but some types of oranges look brown or green when they are ripe. The skin of citrus fruits usually isn't eaten. Citrus fruits have many segments that are filled with juicy pellets. The segments also may contain seeds, 15-3.

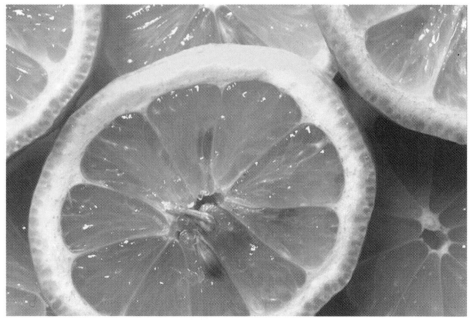

Corel Fruits & Vegetables

15-3 Citrus fruits contain segments with many juicy pellets.

Citrus fruits grow on trees, 15-4. Citrus fruits cannot ripen after being picked. The best citrus fruits are not spotted or wrinkled. They are firm and heavy. Heavy fruits usually are more juicy than lighter fruits.

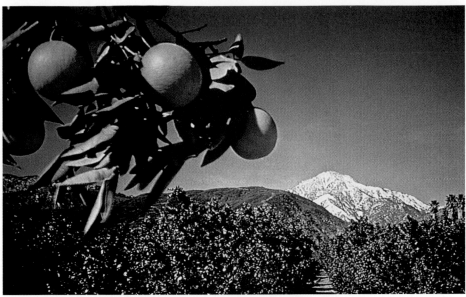

Sunkist Growers, Inc.
15-4 Citrus fruits grow on trees. They are rich sources of vitamin C.

Citrus fruits are rich sources of vitamin C. Some taste sweet. Others, such as kumquats, taste sour. How many of these citrus fruits have you tried?

- Pink grapefruit
- Kumquats
- Lemons
- Limes
- Blood oranges
- Mandarin oranges
- Navel oranges
- Temple oranges
- Valencia oranges
- Tangelos
- Tangerines
- Ugli fruit

Berries

Berries are small, juicy fruits, 15-5. They contain many tiny seeds. Most grow on bushes, but mulberries grow on trees. Grapes and strawberries grow on vines.

The best berries are plump, juicy, sweet, and brightly colored. Berries stop ripening once they are picked, so be sure to buy ripe berries. Unripe berries are sour, pale, and hard.

Berries are fragile and bruise easily. Soft or moldy berries have spoiled. When buying, check the bottom of the box. Berry juice stains mean some berries were crushed.

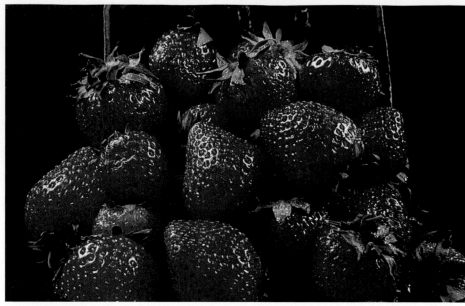

USDA

15-5 The best berries are bright, plump, and juicy. When shopping, avoid green, mashed, or moldy berries.

Most berries are good sources of vitamin C. How many of these berries have you tried?

- Blackberries
- Blueberries
- Boysenberries
- Cranberries
- Currants
- Dewberries

- Gooseberries
- Grapes
- Loganberries
- Mulberries
- Raspberries
- Strawberries

Melons

Melons are large, moist fruits that grow on vines and contain seeds. They have a thick skin that may be smooth or rough. Most have a hollow center full of seeds. Watermelon is an exception. It is not hollow and its seeds are scattered throughout the melon, 15-6.

Ripe melons have a faint, sweet smell and feel firm. When tapped gently, a ripe melon makes a hollow sound. Melons that are too ripe smell sour and may be soft or wrinkled. Melons, except watermelon, can be ripened at home.

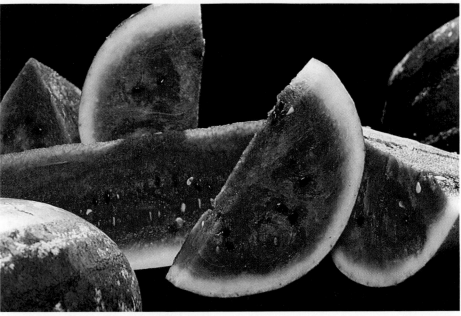

USDA

15-6 Melons are large, moist fruits that grow on vines.

Cantaloupes and other melons with a deep yellow color are rich in vitamin A. They are also a good source of vitamin C. How many of these melons have you tried?

- Cantaloupe
- Casaba
- Crenshaw
- Honeydew
- Musk

- Persian
- Santa Claus
- Sugar Baby
- Watermelon
- Yellow watermelon

Tropical Fruit

Tropical fruits grow only in warm, sunny climates. Many grow on trees, 15-7. Some, such as avocados and pineapples, need to be pared.

The best tropical fruits are firm and free of spots and bruises. Dates and figs may be wrinkled. Other tropical fruits that are wrinkled are old and too ripe.

15-7 How many of these tropical fruits can you name?

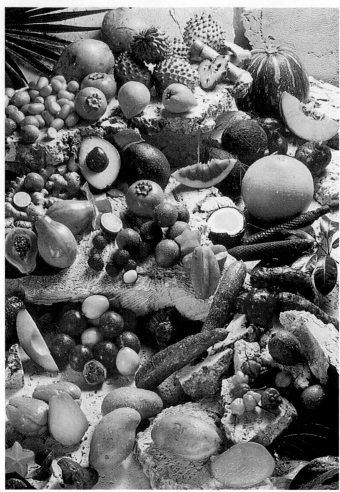

J. R. Brooks & Son

Papayas, mangos, kiwifruit, and avocados can be ripened at home. They are ripe if they give a little when squeezed gently. Bananas can be ripened at home, too. Ripe bananas are golden yellow and speckled with brown spots.

How many of these tropical fruits have you tried?

- Avocados
- Bananas
- Breadfruit
- Carambola (star fruit)
- Coconuts
- Dates
- Figs
- Guavas

- Kiwifruit
- Lychees
- Mangos
- Papaya
- Passion fruit
- Pineapple
- Plantains
- Pomegranates

Cultures of the World

A Taste of the Caribbean

The Caribbean Sea stretches from Florida to South America. There are more than 30 islands there. The islanders have a wide range of languages and cultures. The islands were settled by the Spanish, British, French, and Dutch. Africans were taken there to work on the farms. These settlers mixed their cuisines with those of the tribes living there. This blending became the cuisine of the islands.

Fish is a large part of the diet. It is used to make many dishes. Sopito (soh-PEE-toh) is a tasty soup made with fish and coconut.

The sunny climate is ideal for growing fruits and vegetables. Many foods are grown for export. The main crops are sugar cane, pineapple, bananas, coconuts, and citrus fruits. Cocoa, coffee, nutmeg, and ginger are other major crops.

Plantains, bananas, coconut, beans, peanuts, and rice are often eaten. Plantains look like large bananas. They are starchy, not sweet. Plantains may be roasted, sautéed, baked, or boiled.

Bananas are one of the most popular fruits in the Caribbean. Islanders eat them ripe or unripe. They eat them raw or cooked. Bananas may be eaten alone or added to other foods. Bananas with ice

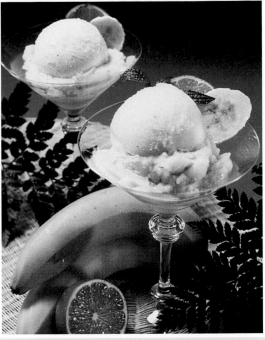

The International Banana Association

Bananas and citrus fruits are often used to make desserts in the Caribbean Islands.

cream is a popular dessert. Bananes au coco (BAH-nahns ah coh-coh) is another way bananas are served. This dish is made by splitting a banana lengthwise. Then, it's topped with a mixture of coconut, brown sugar, and butter and baked. It's so easy to prepare! This delicious dessert is served in many Caribbean Island homes. You could serve this delicious dessert in your home, too.

Buying and Storing Fruits

Fruits sold in supermarkets may be fresh, frozen, canned, or dried. Which type you choose depends on how you plan to use it and its availability.

Focus on Food

The Juicy Facts

A juice is a juice. Or, is it? Many beverages are made with fruits. Some contain fruit juice. Others don't contain any fruit juice at all! The label on the juice container will let you know what you're getting. Many fruit drinks have added sugar and water. Fruit drinks cost less than juice, but they may not be as good for you. Read the label to judge the nutritive value.

Keep these juice names in mind when you shop:

- *Fresh juice* is the liquid from squeezed fresh fruit.
- *Frozen juice concentrate* is fresh juice with most of its water removed. Sometimes sugar is added.
- *Juice made from concentrate* is made by adding water to frozen juice concentrate. The added water replaces the water that was removed to make the concentrate.
- *Fruit nectar* is fruit juice and pureed fruit. Water and sugar are added, too.
- *Fruit juice drink* is made by adding water and sugar to small amounts of juice. The percent of juice in the drink is indicated on the label.

- *Fruit drink* may have natural juice flavor, but it may not contain any real fruit juice. It may be just water, sugar, and artificial flavors.
- *Fruit ades* contain water and sugar. Some contain juice, others contain only fruit flavoring.

Fruit juice is a tasty beverage. Your best bet for good nutrition is fresh fruit juice, frozen fruit juice concentrate, or fruit juice made from concentrate.

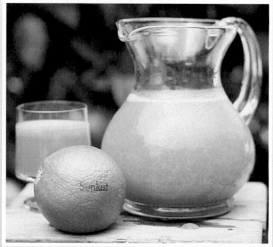

Sunkist Growers, Inc.

Fruit juice is the most nutritious choice when choosing between a fruit juice and a fruit drink.

Calorie Facts			
Juice (one cup)	**Calories**	**Fruit**	**Calories**
apple juice	120	1 medium apple	80
cranberry juice cocktail	145	1 cup cranberries	46
grape juice	140	25 grapes	95
orange juice	110	1 orange	60

Keep in mind that juice often has more calories than a serving of fresh fruit.

Fresh Fruit

Fresh fruit is found in the produce section of the grocery store, 15-8. ***Produce*** means fresh fruits and vegetables.

Produce is seasonal. Some fruits, such as strawberries, ripen in spring. Others, such as cherries, are in season during the summer. Apples are harvested in the fall. During the winter, citrus fruits grow in warm regions. Fruits are often the best during their peak growing season. Prices are usually lowest then, too.

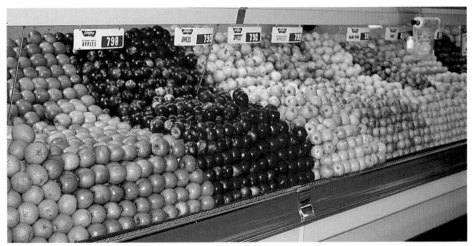

Washington Apple Commission

15-8 Fresh fruits and vegetables are found in the produce area of supermarkets.

Rapid shipping makes it possible to buy produce when it's out of season in your area. Refrigerated planes, railroad cars, trucks, and ships bring fruit from distant places. Fruit shipped from far away may not taste as sweet as locally grown, in-season fruit. Shipping adds to its cost, too.

Fresh fruits need little preparation. You can just wash and eat most of them. If you are making a fruit dish, you may need to peel the fruit or cut it into pieces. Some supermarkets sell ready-to-eat fruit salads. These salads save you time, but they often cost more than fruit salad made at home.

Buying Fresh Fruit

The best fresh fruit

- feels heavy and firm
- has no cuts, bruises, or decay
- smells pleasant
- isn't sticky, wrinkled, or moldy.

Fruit that feels light or looks wrinkled has been stored too long. It has lost its juicy freshness. Damaged fruit has cuts, bruises, or decay. The damaged parts should be removed and thrown away. Fresh fruit is too ripe when it is soft, moldy, sticky, or smells sour.

Fresh melons, drupes, and pears can be ripened at home. If you won't need them for a few days, choose slightly underripe fruits. Leave them at room temperature to ripen.

Storing Fresh Fruit

Fresh fruits are fragile and bruise easily. That is why they must be handled gently. Rough handling causes bruises that lead to decay. Decayed parts must be removed and thrown away.

Wash fruit in cool running water just before eating or preparing it to remove dirt and insect spray. You should even wash fruits like oranges and melons that have rinds or skins you are going to remove. Do not wash fruits before storing them.

Cover cut fruit with plastic wrap. Plastic wrap protects the fruit. It keeps the fruit from drying out, turning brown, and rotting.

Store fresh fruits in the refrigerator's crisper or in plastic bags. This helps them stay fresh longer and retain their flavors. It also keeps them from picking up the flavors of other foods in the refrigerator. Most fresh fruits will last a week or two in the refrigerator. Some fruits, such as apples and citrus fruits, can be stored for a month or more. Berries decay fast and don't store well. Keep them in the refrigerator and use within a day or two.

Refrigerate fresh melons, drupes, and pears only if they are ripe. Cold prevents ripening. Bananas should not be refrigerated because the cold causes them to spoil quickly.

Canned Fruit

Canned fruits need no preparation. They can be served right out of the can. Canned fruits can be added to soups, desserts, salads, and other recipes. Canned fruits often cost less than frozen, dried, and fresh fruits that are out of season.

Buying Canned Fruit

There are many canned fruit choices. It is important to read the can's label to be sure you get what you need. When buying canned fruit, ask yourself

- Do I need fruit that is whole, halved, sliced, chopped, or crushed?
- Do I want fruit canned in water, juice, or syrup?

Your choice will depend on how you plan to use the fruit. Crushed pineapple in juice is fine for pineapple-upside down cake. Pineapple rings in syrup work well to garnish a ham.

The choice also depends on cost. Whole fruits are more costly than pieces. Fruit canned in water or juice may cost more than fruit canned in syrup.

Storing Canned Fruit

Store unopened canned fruit in a cool, dry place. The fruit will maintain its quality for a year. Canned fruit won't be top quality if it is stored longer or in a warm place. If fruit smells sour when the can is opened, it has spoiled. Fruit in a dented, rusty, leaking, or bulging can is not safe to eat. Throw the fruit away so no one, including pets, can eat it.

After opening a can, place any unused fruit in a covered container. Store the fruit in the refrigerator and use it within a few days.

Frozen Fruit

Frozen fruit is more like fresh in color, texture, and flavor than canned or dried fruit. It is a good choice when fresh fruit is not available. Frozen fruit is quick and easy to prepare. It doesn't need to be washed or peeled. Just thaw it and eat or use in cooking.

It is more costly to ship and store frozen fruit than canned or dried fruit. Therefore, frozen fruit may cost more than other forms of fruits.

Buying Frozen Fruit

Some frozen fruits, such as raspberries, are sold whole. Others, such as melon balls and sliced peaches, are sold in pieces. Some frozen fruits have sugar added to them. Read the package label to see that you are getting what you want.

Select frozen fruit packages that are clean and solidly frozen. Soft packages tell you the temperature of the freezer is too high. Sticky or stained packages are a sign that fruit thawed and was refrozen. Soft, sticky, or stained packages mean that fruit may not be the best quality.

Storing Frozen Fruit

Store frozen fruit in the coldest part of your freezer. When stored at 0°F (-18°C), fruits maintain their quality for 8 to 12 months. It's best to use frozen juices in 4 to 6 months. Once frozen fruits are thawed, do not refreeze them because they will become mushy. Refreezing may also make fruits unsafe to eat.

Dried Fruit

Dried fruit is convenient. You can eat it right out of the package or it can be cooked. This lightweight food is ideal for camping and hiking trips. Some common dried fruits are raisins, dried plums (prunes), currants, cherries, and apricots.

The main difference between fresh and dried fruit is water. Dried fruits have much less water, so they weigh less. See 15-9. The water (and weight) can be returned to dried fruit by soaking it in hot water for a few minutes.

Dried fruit is a good buy when you think about how much fresh fruit was used to make it. For example, it takes four to five pounds of fresh grapes to make one pound of raisins.

Choosing Dried Fruit

When buying dried fruit, look for clean, sealed packages. If a package is sticky or torn, the fruit inside may not be clean. Some stores sell dried fruit in large bins. When buying dried fruit from bins, be sure the bins are clean and free of insects.

15-9 Dried fruit has less water than fresh fruit. This lightweight snack is easy to carry in packed lunches and picnics.

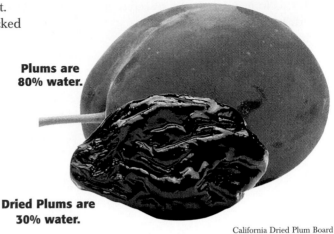

Plums are 80% water.

Dried Plums are 30% water.

California Dried Plum Board

Storing Dried Fruit

Dried fruit is easy to store. Place it in an airtight container and store in a cool, dry place. When the weather is warm and humid, put the container in the refrigerator. Dried fruits will maintain their quality for many months.

Fruit as Any Part of the Meal

Fruits are great any time of the day. They can be served at every meal as any part of the meal. You can serve them raw or cooked. The choices are endless, 15-10. Fruits can be

- washed and eaten raw (melon wedge)
- squeezed to make juice (orange juice)
- pureed to make a chilled soup (strawberry yogurt soup)
- dried to make fruit leather (pear leather)
- diced and added to a salad (Waldorf salad)
- simmered to make a sauce for a main dish (raspberry sauce for lamb chops)
- marinated to make an ice cream topping (cherries Jubilee)
- baked in pies, breads, and cobblers (orange nut bread)
- broiled to make a warm side dish (broiled peach half)
- deep-fried to make fritters (apple fritters)
- candied to garnish a main dish (candied orange peel for baked chicken)

What are some other ways you could prepare fruits?

15-10 This fruit drink can be served as a dessert. It could also be a snack or part of a light lunch.

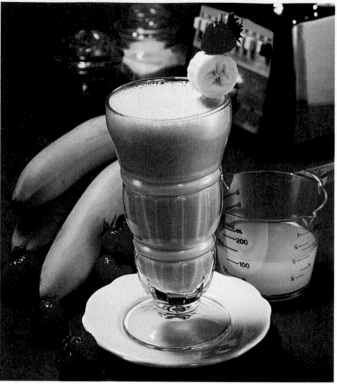

The International Banana Association

Preparing Fruits

Fruits often require very little preparation. Preparation usually depends upon the type of fruit you are using.

Preparing Fresh Fruit

Fresh fruits need to be washed. Washing removes dust, bacteria, and insect spray. Some fruits, such as bananas and avocados, must be peeled. Many fruits, like bananas and apples, turn brown when they are peeled and sliced. Oxygen reacts with the fruit and causes this browning to occur. To stop the browning, you can heat the fruit. You can also stop the browning by sprinkling the fruit with an acid such as orange or lemon juice. Another way to prevent browning is to cover the fruit with salted or sugared water.

Preparing Canned Fruit

Preparing canned fruit can be as simple as chilling the can, opening it, and eating. You can also add the fruit to a recipe. Drain the juice unless your recipe calls for it. Save the juice for a nutritious snack.

Preparing Frozen Fruit

Frozen fruit is ready to eat when it is partly thawed. It will have a better texture than completely thawed frozen fruit. Frozen fruit juice concentrate doesn't need to be thawed before mixing it.

Preparing Dried Fruit

Dried fruit is ready to eat. You can eat it from the box or add it to a recipe. To stew it, soak it in water and simmer slowly. If you want to add sugar, do it at the end of cooking. Dried fruit may not soften and absorb water as well if sugar is added during cooking.

Cooking Fruits

Cooking makes the flavor of a fruit milder. Colors change, too. Apples become soft and golden. Strawberries get pinker. Cooking also makes fruit easier to digest. Any fruit can be cooked, but a few fruits must be cooked. Plantains and breadfruit require cooking. Overcooked fruits are mushy and bland. They lose their appeal and some nutrients. To preserve the nutrients, colors, textures, and flavors of fruits

- Cook fruits with the skin on. The skin helps the fruit retain its nutrients. Be sure to pierce the skin several times if you are cooking unpared fruit in a microwave oven. If the skin must be removed, pare thinly. Most nutrients are right under the skin.
- Cook fruits in a small amount of water. Water-soluble vitamins leak out of the fruit into the water. The more water used, the more vitamins that will be lost. Water also dilutes the flavor of the fruit.
- Cook fruits quickly and gently. Long cooking and high heat destroy some vitamins. Cooking too long makes fruit mushy. It also causes the fruit to lose its color and shape. Steaming and cooking in a microwave oven help to preserve the quality and nutrients in fruits.

- Preserve the shapes of fruits. Fruit will keep its shape if you leave its skin on. Adding sugar to the cooking water also will help preserve its shape. For example, if you are stewing apples, add sugar to the cooking water to retain the fruit's shape. When no sugar is added to the cooking water, the fruit breaks apart. Add sugar after cooking the fruit if you are making a smooth applesauce.

Fruit Desserts

Fruits make excellent desserts. They are a sweet, low-calorie way to end a meal, 15-11. Canned, dried, frozen, or fresh fruits can be used. They may be served warm or cold.

Fruit desserts can be as simple as a fruit salad or a baked apple filled with cinnamon and raisins. Other ideas include

- fruit kebabs
- peach slices over ice cream
- pineapple chunks in yogurt
- a melon half filled with cherries
- blueberries and milk
- applesauce and raisins
- frozen grapes
- frozen orange juice bars

Fruits are also used to make pies, cakes, and cookies. These desserts have added sugar and fat. They will have more calories than the desserts listed above.

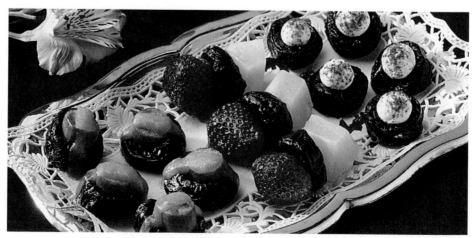

Sun-Diamond Growers

15-11 Fruits are a sweet, nutritious way to end a meal.

The best fruit desserts are tasty and nutritious. They are prepared in ways that protect the appeal and nutrients of the fruit.

Delicious fruits are just one part of a nutritious diet. In the next chapter, you'll discover how vegetables add variety and interest to your diet.

In a Nutshell

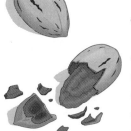

- Fruits are rich sources of fiber and vitamins A and C. Almost all fruits are low in fat and calories.
- Drupes, pomes, citrus, berries, melons, and tropical are types of fruit.
- Canned, frozen, dried, and fresh fruits are sold year-round.
- Fruits are quick and easy to prepare.
- Proper storage protects the flavor, texture, and nutrients of fruits.
- Fruits can be served at all meals as any part of the meal.
- Carefully prepared fruits have pleasing colors, flavors, and textures. Their nutrients are preserved.

In the Know

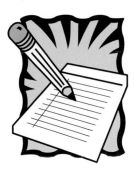

1. List the six types of fruit. Name one fruit from each group.
2. A _____ is a fruit that grows on trees and has one large pit or seed.
3. True or false? The best fresh fruits smell pleasant and aren't sticky or wrinkled.
4. Match each fruit with the storage method that will best preserve its quality.

   ___ fresh strawberries
   ___ bananas
   ___ underripe pears
   ___ canned peaches
   ___ raisins

   A. store at room temperature
   B. store unopened in a cool, dry place
   C. store at room temperature until ripe, then refrigerate
   D. place in an airtight container and store in a cool, dry place
   E. store unwashed in the refrigerator

5. Which type of fruit is most like fresh fruit?
   A. Canned.
   B. Frozen.
   C. Dried.

6. List three steps you can take when cooking fruits to preserve their nutrients, colors, textures, and flavors.
7. True or false? When no sugar is added to the cooking water, the fruit breaks apart.
8. True or false? Long cooking times and high temperatures help retain the nutrients in fruits.

What Would You Do?

Your sister enjoys fruit and eats several pieces each day. Next week, she leaves for college. Her dorm is near a grocery store. She won't have a refrigerator in her room and she doesn't know how she will be able to keep fruit in her room. What advice can you give her? Your brother is going camping this weekend and wants to take fruit along. What advice would you give him?

Expanding Your Knowledge

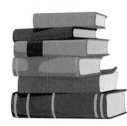

1. Interview friends and family. Ask them to describe their favorite fruit dishes. Write down their recipes. On the back of the recipe card, explain why the dish was a favorite one. Try as many recipes as you can. Write your reaction on the back of each recipe card.
2. Have a fruit tasting party. Select several fruits you have never tried. Make an information card for each fruit that includes: the name of the fruit, its origin, when it's in season, and its calorie content. Wash the fruits and cut them into bite-sized pieces. Place the information cards next to the fruits. Ask everyone to describe the taste of each fruit. Write taste descriptions on the back of the card for each fruit.
3. Select several varieties of the same fruit. For example, you could choose Bartlett, Bosc, Comice, and Anjou pears. Set up a taste panel to compare the flavors, smells, textures, and colors of the varieties.
4. Prepare cold peach soup using fresh, canned, dried, and frozen fruit. (You can use pineapple instead of peaches.) Pour each variation into a dish. Cover the dish and label with the variation letter. Chill 24 hours. Set up a taste test to compare each variation.

Compare the tastes, colors, and textures of the four samples.

A. Puree 1 cup plain yogurt, 2 tablespoons pineapple juice, and ½ cup fresh, pared peaches.

B. Puree 1 cup plain yogurt, 2 tablespoons pineapple juice, and ½ cup canned, drained peaches.

C. Puree 1 cup plain yogurt, 2 tablespoons pineapple juice, and ½ cup partly thawed, frozen peaches.

D. Simmer 1 cup water and ¼ cup of dried peaches in a saucepan for 10 minutes. Cool five minutes and drain. Puree 1 cup plain yogurt, 2 tablespoons pineapple juice, and simmered peaches.

5. Sugar can be added before or after cooking fruit. The texture of the cooked fruit depends on when the sugar is added. Compare the textures, tastes, and colors of these two applesauce variations. (You also can use pears or nectarines.)

Applesauce A

1. Peel and core 2 medium apples. Cut into ¼-inch slices.
2. Heat ¼ cup water in a saucepan to boiling.
3. Add apples.
4. Cover the pan. Reduce heat to medium. Simmer for 7 to 10 minutes.
5. Remove from heat.
6. Mix in 3 tablespoons sugar.
7. Pour into a serving dish and allow to cool.

Applesauce B

Follow the directions for Applesauce A above, EXCEPT add apples and 3 tablespoons of sugar in Step 3. Omit Step 6.

6. Create a menu for one day that includes at least one type of fruit at each meal. Use at least three fruits and prepare them in different ways. Compare the cost of using fresh, frozen, canned, and dried fruits in each recipe. Predict how the taste, color, and texture would differ if you used fresh, frozen, canned, and dried fruits.

7. Fruit grows all over the world. Design a bulletin board that uses a map to show the country where fruit recipes originated. For example, you could include a recipe for fruit chutney from India.

8. Write and produce a commercial to sell a fruit. Include interesting facts, nutrient information, and suggestions for choosing and preparing the fruit. Videotape the advertisements to show to classmates or younger children.

Chapter 16
Versatile Vegetables

Objectives

After reading this chapter, you will be able to
- ❏ identify types of vegetables.
- ❏ select high-quality vegetables.
- ❏ describe how to store vegetables.
- ❏ preserve the colors, flavors, textures, and nutrients of vegetables during cooking.

New Terms

bulb: a short, rounded bud that has a very short stem covered with overlapping leaves.
tuber: the swollen portion of a plant's underground stem.

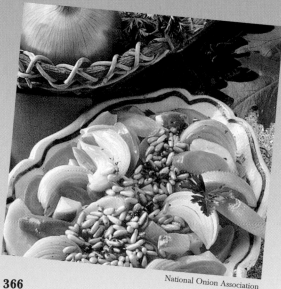

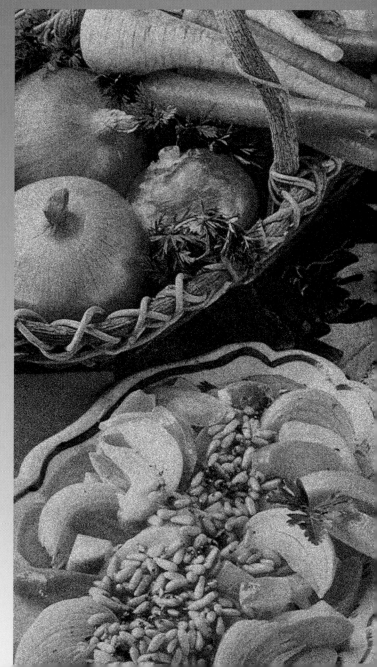

366

National Onion Association

Imagine walking through the produce section of your supermarket. You can see the bright red peppers and yellow squash. Think of the sound crunchy carrots make when you eat them. You can taste the sweetness of corn on the cob. You can smell the strong scent of garlic. You can feel the skin of smooth eggplant or fuzzy okra.

Vegetables appeal to every sense and add interest to meals. They are rich sources of vitamins, minerals, and fiber. Vegetables are low in calories and fat, too.

Types of Vegetables

You can group vegetables by color, flavor, or texture. An easy way to group them is by the parts of the plant you eat. When you eat lettuce, you are munching leaves. You nibble flowers when you eat broccoli. Vegetables may be roots, bulbs, tubers, fruits, seeds, or stems, too.

Leaf Vegetables

Leaves capture the sun's energy and make food for the plant. The freshest leaf vegetables are crisp, clean, and tightly bunched. They are not spotted, yellow, or wilted. Small leaves are tender. Larger ones are tough and woody, 16-1.

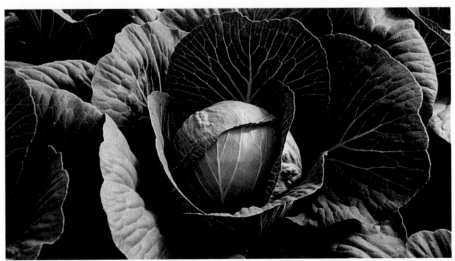

USDA

16-1 Cabbage is a leaf vegetable. The best leaf vegetables are crisp and clean.

Science in the Kitchen

Biotechnology

Biotechnology can help improve the quality of the food supply. *Bio* is short for biology. It refers to living plants and animals. *Technology* refers to the processes used to create new structures. Thus, *biotechnology* means using biological processes to create plants and animals with new traits. For example, scientists use biotechnology to develop plants that resist insects. That means less insecticide needs to be used, which helps protect the environment. Scientists use biotechnology to raise the nutrient levels in foods. They have produced a type of rice that is packed with vitamin A. This rice will help prevent blindness in thousands of children living in poor countries. Scientists use biotechnology to increase the amount of food a plant can produce. This will help lower food prices and provide more food to poor countries. Scientists can also use biotechnology to create vegetables that stay fresh longer than others.

Biotechnology is also called *genetic engineering*. Genetic engineering allows scientists to move specific genes from one plant or animal to another. A *gene* is a unit of information that can be passed to an offspring. All the characteristics of all plants and animals are stored in their genes. Genes determine if a carrot will be long or short. They also determine whether a cow will have spots or be one color.

Some people think biotechnology is new. In reality, biotechnology began long ago. For centuries, farmers have manipulated the genes of animals and plants. For instance, they have bred pigs to be leaner. Corn is another example. Wild, native corn has only two or three kernels on each ear. After many years of careful breeding, corncobs now have hundreds of juicy kernels.

Early biotechnology was slow. Scientists could not carefully control which genes were transferred. They did not always get the results they wanted, either. Scientific advances since 1970 have allowed scientists to speed up the process of changing the characteristics of plants and animals. Scientists can now move the gene for a desired trait from one plant or animal to another. For instance, to protect potatoes from beetles, scientists have inserted a gene found in a bacterium into potatoes.

Some people worry about risks caused by moving genes among plants and animals. In the United States, government agencies work together to ensure that foods produced through biotechnology are safe. For instance, the Food and Drug Administration (FDA) judges the safety and nutrition of foods produced by biotechnology. Foods that could cause an allergic reaction must include this information on their labels. Foods that have altered nutrient levels must be labeled, too. By learning more about biotechnology, you will be able to make wise choices about foods produced with this technology.

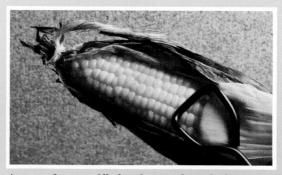

An ear of corn is filled with sweet kernels due to biotechnology.

Leaves that are dark green, such as collard greens and spinach, are high in vitamins A and C and folate. They are also good sources of calcium and iron. The darker the green color, the more nutrients leaf vegetables are likely to have. For instance, collard greens supply more nutrients than iceberg lettuce. How many of these leaf vegetables have you tried?

- Arugula
- Brussels sprouts
- Cabbage
- Collard greens
- Dandelion greens
- Endive
- Escarole
- Kale
- Lettuce
- Mache
- Mustard greens
- Parsley
- Romaine
- Radicchio
- Spinach
- Watercress

Stem Vegetables

Stems support the plant. The best quality stem vegetables have crisp, straight stalks. Slim stalks are more tender than wide ones, 16-2.

How many of these stem vegetables have you tried?

- Asparagus
- Bamboo shoots
- Bok choy
- Celery
- Kohlrabi
- Rhubarb

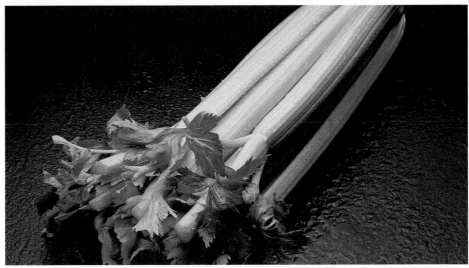

American Celery Council

16-2 The freshest stem vegetables are crisp and crunchy. Slim stalks are the most tender.

Root Vegetables

Roots are a pathway for nutrients from the soil to the plant. Roots also anchor the plant. Hard, smooth root vegetables are the best choice. Wrinkles mean the vegetables are old and dried out. Small root vegetables are the most tender, 16-3.

How many of these root vegetables have you tried?

- Beets
- Carrots
- Daikons
- Jicamas
- Parsnips
- Radishes

- Rutabagas
- Salsify
- Sweet potatoes
- Taros
- Turnips
- Yuca roots

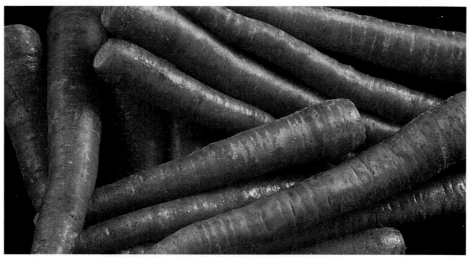

USDA

16-3 The best root vegetables are firm and smooth.

Bulb Vegetables

Bulbs are short, rounded buds that grow underground. They have a very short stem covered with overlapping leaves. Bulbs store food for the plant. The best bulbs are dry and firm. If they are soft, the plant used the stored food before you did, 16-4.

How many of these bulb vegetables have you tried?

- Garlic
- Leeks

- Onions
- Shallots

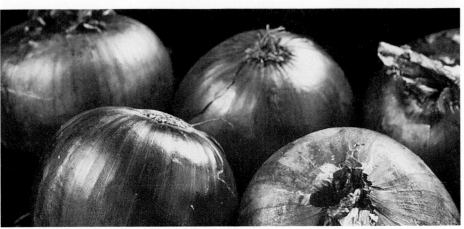

USDA

16-4 Look for firm, dry bulb vegetables. Soft bulb vegetables are old.

Tubers

Tubers grow underground. They are a part of the underground stem that swells to store food. New plants use the stored food until they can make their own. Look for firm tubers that are free of bruises and decay. Shriveled or sprouted tubers are old.

Potatoes are the best known tuber, 16-5. Have you ever tried another tuber called a Jerusalem artichoke?

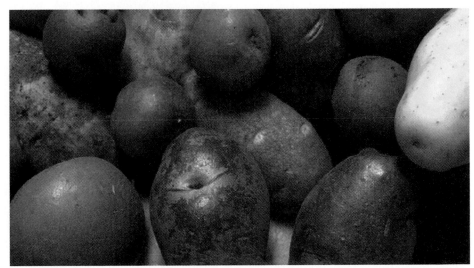

Corel Fruits & Vegetables

16-5 Most of the potatoes sold in the United States are brown or red. Did you know that potatoes come in many other colors?

Focus on Food

Are Potatoes Really Fattening?

A medium-sized potato has about 90 calories and almost no fat. The calories

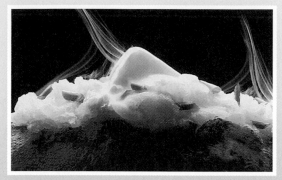

Idaho Potato Commission

Plain potatoes are low in fat and calories. When you add butter or other toppings, you add calories.

and fat in bananas and apples are about the same as potatoes. Why do people think potatoes are fattening and not bananas and apples? It's because potatoes often are fried or served with extras. The oil from frying and the extra ingredients add calories. Look at the list below to see how the calories rise.

baked potato, plain	90 calories
boiled potato, plain	90 calories
baked potato with 1 tablespoon sour cream	115 calories
boiled potato with $1\frac{1}{4}$ cup cheese sauce	165 calories
baked potato with 1 tablespoon butter or margarine	190 calories
25 potato chips	265 calories
1 cup hash browns	340 calories
25 French fries	400 calories

16-6 An artichoke is a flower vegetable. Crisp, firm flowers are the best quality.

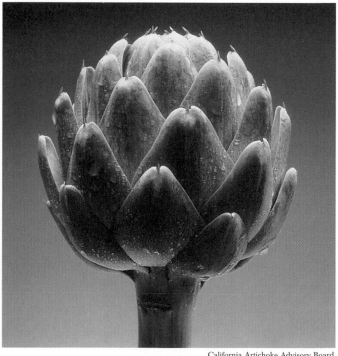

California Artichoke Advisory Board

Flower Vegetables

Flowers are the plant's blooms. The best quality flowers are crisp and firm. Look for closed flower clusters on broccoli and cauliflower. Yellow buds mean broccoli is old and strongly flavored, 16-6.

How many flower vegetables have you tried?

- Artichoke
- Broccoflower
- Broccoli
- Cauliflower

Fruit Vegetables

Fruit vegetables are not as sweet and juicy as fruits. They are called fruit vegetables because they contain the seeds of the vegetables. The freshest fruit vegetables are firm and heavy. They have no spots, wrinkles, or bruises, 16-7.

16-7 Fruit vegetables contain the seeds of the plant. Note the many tiny seeds inside these tomatoes and cucumbers.

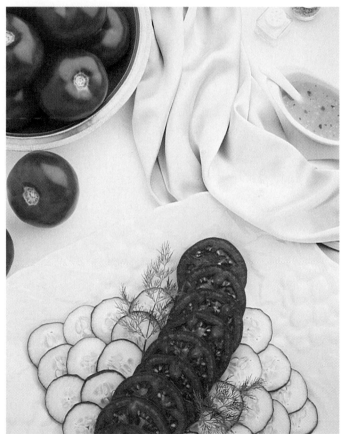

Florida Tomato Committee

How many of these fruit vegetables have you tried?

- Cucumbers
- Eggplant
- Okra

- Peppers
- Tomatillo
- Tomatoes

Seed Vegetables

Some vegetables grow from seeds. Seed vegetables are best when they are freshly picked. They lose their crispness and flavor quickly. Small seeds have the best flavor, 16-8.

How many of these seed vegetables have you tried?

- Corn
- Green beans
- Green peas

- Snow peas
- Wax beans
- Yardlong beans

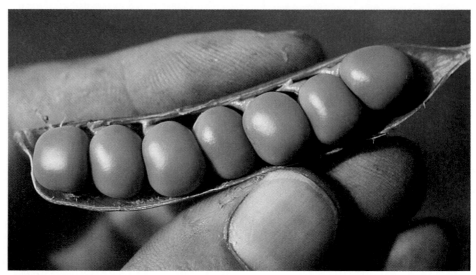

USDA

16-8 Seed vegetables have the best flavor when they are fresh.

Buying and Storing Vegetables

Vegetables can be purchased in four forms: fresh, frozen, canned, and dried. These forms are sold in supermarkets year-round.

Fresh Vegetables

Fresh vegetables are more plentiful and less costly when they are in season in your region. You may be able to buy locally-grown vegetables at a nearby farmer's market. At other times, refrigerated planes, ships, trucks, and trains bring fresh vegetables from all over the world to your supermarket. Transporting vegetables from other areas increases the price of fresh vegetables.

Fresh vegetables need more preparation than other forms. They must be washed under cold, running water to remove dirt and insect spray. You may want to peel, slice, and cook them. Some supermarkets sell pre-washed salad greens, shredded cabbage, and pared carrots. These foods save time but often cost more than plain fresh vegetables.

Buying Fresh Vegetables

The best quality fresh vegetables are crisp and not wilted or wrinkled. They are also brightly colored and firm, not soft. They are free of cuts, bruises, and decay, too, 16-9.

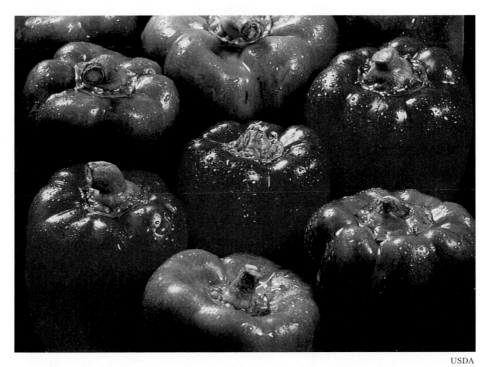

USDA

16-9 These fresh peppers are of top quality. Note their bright colors.

Vegetables that are limp, pale, or soft have been either stored too long or stored incorrectly. All damaged parts should be removed and thrown away.

Storing Fresh Vegetables

Keep leaf, stem, seed, fruit, and flower vegetables fresh by storing them in the refrigerator. An airtight container or the vegetable drawer of the refrigerator will help prevent wilting. Fresh vegetables stay fresh longer if you do not wash them before storing. Too much moisture can cause spoilage. Use fresh vegetables within a week or two. They lose vitamins, color, and flavor as they age.

Store bulb, tuber, and root vegetables in a cool, dark, and dry place, 16-10. They will stay fresh for three months or more. Pumpkins, winter squash, and other vegetables with hard skin can be stored this way, too.

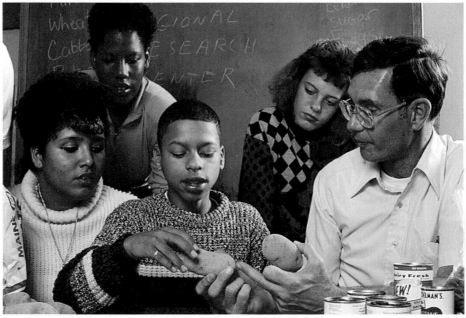

USDA

16-10 Learning how to store fresh vegetables properly can help you preserve their quality.

Science in the Kitchen

Munchy, Crunchy Vegetables

Fresh vegetables contain a large amount of water. As they age, the water dries out and vegetables become limp or wrinkled. They lose their crispness. Proper storage methods can help slow water loss and slow down aging.

This experiment will help you to identify storage methods that slow vegetable aging and prevent water loss. For this experiment, you'll need eight celery stalks, plastic wrap, two plates, and a refrigerator. First, wash all eight celery stalks and separate them into four groups having two celery stalks each. Wrap one group of two stalks tightly in plastic wrap and place them in the refrigerator. Wrap the second group of stalks tightly in plastic wrap and place them on the countertop. Place the third group of stalks unwrapped on a plate in the refrigerator. Place the fourth group of stalks unwrapped on a plate and leave it on the countertop.

Wait 24 hours. Then, taste the stalks from each group. (Be sure to wash the celery in the fourth group again before tasting it.) How did the celery in each group taste? What was the texture like? How did it look? Which celery stalk stayed the crispest? Which looked best? Why? What effect did the plastic wrap have on the celery? How can you use the information gained from this experiment?

Canned Vegetables

Canned vegetables are cooked during the canning process. There is no need to wash, peel, or slice them. They can be served right from the can, heated, or used as an ingredient. Canned vegetables are good for soups, casseroles, and side dishes. They usually cost less than fresh and frozen vegetables.

Buying Canned Vegetables

Canned vegetables may be whole or chopped. Some have sauces or butter added. Plain, chopped styles are the least costly. The style of canned vegetable you choose will depend on how you plan to use the vegetable. For example, whole asparagus stalks make an attractive side dish. Chopped asparagus is fine for stews and casseroles. Remember to select cans that are not dented, rusty, swollen, or leaking.

Storing Canned Vegetables

Store canned vegetables in a cool, dry place. Carefully stored canned vegetables will maintain their quality for a year. After that, they are safe to eat, but their quality and nutrient value will be lower. If the vegetable smells or looks odd when the can is opened, it has spoiled and isn't safe to eat. Spoiled vegetables should be discarded.

Once opened, place any unused portion of canned vegetables in a covered container. Store the container in the refrigerator and use within a few days.

Frozen Vegetables

Frozen vegetables are ready to cook. All the cleaning, trimming, and paring has been done. They were blanched before being frozen, so they cook faster than fresh vegetables. Frozen vegetables may cost more than canned.

Buying Frozen Vegetables

Frozen vegetables are a good choice when fresh vegetables are not available. Their color, flavor, and texture are more like fresh than canned or dried.

There are many frozen vegetable choices. You can buy one vegetable or a mixture of several vegetables. Some vegetables are whole, others are cut into pieces. They may be frozen plain, in sauce, or combined with other foods to make a main dish such as beef stew. Some frozen vegetables come in a special plastic pouch or a microwaveable dish. Plain, cut-up vegetables cost the least. Sauces and special features add to the price.

Before buying, read the label to be certain you are getting what you want and need. Check the directions on the package and compare preparation times. Consider the cost of various brands and forms. Frozen vegetables in soft or stained packages have thawed at some time. They may not be safe to eat.

Storing Frozen Vegetables

Frozen vegetables will last in the freezer for six to eight months. Keep them solidly frozen until you are ready to prepare them. Once thawed, do not refreeze them because the quality will be decreased.

Dried Vegetables

Dried vegetables are made by removing the water from fresh vegetables. Water is added back when the vegetables are prepared. Most dried vegetables are legumes. Supermarkets may sell dried vegetable soups, onions, tomatoes, potatoes, and herbs such as parsley.

Dried vegetables are lightweight and easy to transport. They take up less storage space than other forms and often cost less.

Dried peas and beans take longer to prepare than most vegetables. Dried beans need to be soaked for an hour or more before cooking. Other dried vegetables, such as potato flakes, require little preparation time and energy.

Buying Dried Vegetables

Select clean, sealed packages. Vegetables in torn or open packages may be dirty. If you are buying dried vegetables from a bin, make sure the bin is clean and free of insects.

Storing Dried Vegetables

Store dried vegetables in an airtight container in a cool, dry place. They will keep for six months or more. When it is hot and humid, store the container of dried vegetables in the refrigerator.

Vegetables as Any Part of the Meal

Vegetables are versatile. They can be served at any meal as any part of the meal. You could serve vegetables as a

- beverage (tomato juice, carrot juice)
- salad (celery sticks and dip, coleslaw, tossed salad)
- soup (chilled cucumber soup, lentil soup, onion soup)
- main dish (spinach omelet, bean tortilla, stuffed peppers)
- side dish (cauliflower with cheese sauce, baked squash, corn on the cob)
- bread (zucchini bread, potato pancakes)
- garnish (red pepper strips, radish roses)
- dessert (carrot cake, pumpkin pie)

Focus on Food

Herbs and Spices

Open a jar of cinnamon and sniff it. Does it remind you of cinnamon rolls or pumpkin pies? When you smell oregano, do you think of pizza? Cinnamon and oregano are *seasoners.* They add fragrance and flavor to foods. There are five types of seasoners: spices, herbs, aromatic seeds, seasonings, and vegetable spices.

Spices are bits of bark, fruits, flowers, and roots. For example, cinnamon is from bark. Nutmeg and pepper are from the fruit. Saffron is from the flower. Ginger is from the root. *Herbs* are leaves from certain shrubs. Bay leaves, dill weed, parsley, sage, and basil are herbs. *Aromatic seeds* are seeds that are tasty or scented. Examples are caraway seeds, celery seeds, mustard seeds, poppy seeds, and sesame seeds. *Seasonings* are a blend of two or more spices, herbs, or seeds. Salt may be added, too. Pumpkin pie spice, chili powder, curry powder, and poultry seasoning are examples. *Vegetable spices* are

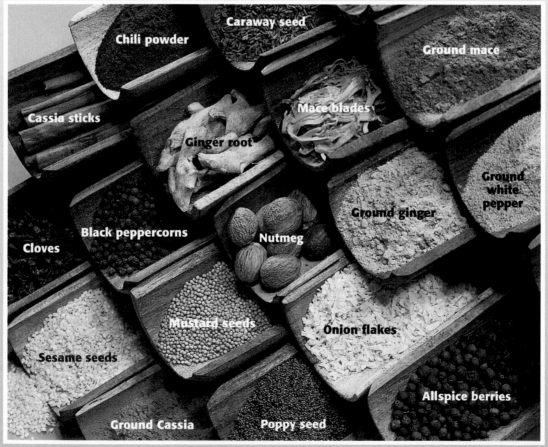

American Spice Trade Association

How many of these seasoners have you tried?

strongly flavored vegetables. Small amounts of vegetable spices add flavor to other foods. Garlic, onion, chili peppers, and horseradish are examples.

For thousands of years, seasoners have been used in cooking. Years ago, they had other uses, too. Egyptians used spices to prepare the cloth in which mummies were wrapped. The Greeks used seasoners as medicines. Some used cinnamon as perfume. The Romans thought that a hat made of bay leaves protected the wearer from lightning. Today, some people use herbs as dietary supplements.

Until recent times, spices were in short supply. They had to be carried by camels over long routes from China and India to Europe. Travel was very slow and dangerous. This made the small amount of spices that were available very costly. Spices were as valuable as gold.

Spice traders made fortunes. They kept the source of spices a secret for years. It was Marco Polo who unlocked their secret. After spending 30 years traveling through Asia, he wrote a book about his adventures. In 1298, he told the world that spices were grown in India, China, and on islands in the Pacific Ocean.

People who read Marco Polo's book wanted to visit the lands he described in his book. For many, the travel was too long and dangerous. Christopher Columbus and others tried to find a safer, faster route.

Today, it is easy to transport spices around the world. Planes, ships, trains, and trucks bring spices to your supermarket. The price is much lower than it was years ago. A pound of ginger no longer is worth as a much as a sheep. It doesn't take seven fat oxen to buy a pound of nutmeg.

Even though seasoners are much less costly today, you will want to protect your investment. You can do this by:

- buying small amounts. Seasoners tend to lose their flavor quickly. You can tell if they are still tasty by sniffing them. Seasoners with a faint scent will have little flavor.
- storing dried seasoners in a tightly closed container in a cool, dry place. Sunlight, heat, and air cause seasoners to quickly lose their flavor.
- storing fresh herbs in a covered container in the refrigerator. Before storing, wrap fresh herbs in a paper towel and put them in a plastic bag.

Vegetables make meals more exciting. They add color, flavor, and texture. When planning meals, try to include two or more vegetables.

Choose vegetables that blend well with the colors of the other foods being served. A meal of mashed potatoes, cauliflower, ham, and milk looks dull. Tomatoes and red cabbage would clash with the pink ham. Corn and broccoli complement the ham and make the meal more attractive.

Tasty meals have several flavors that mix well. Either too many strong flavors or too many mild flavors can be unappealing. It is a good idea to limit strong-flavored vegetables to one per meal, 16-11. For instance, serving Brussels sprouts, garlic, and turnips in the same meal might overwhelm your taste buds.

Vegetable Flavors	
Strong-Flavored Vegetables	**Mild-Flavored Vegetables**
Brussels sprouts cabbage cauliflower garlic onion rutabaga turnips	beans carrots corn lettuce peas squash tomatoes

16-11 Select vegetables that blend well with the flavors of the meal. Serve only one strongly-flavored vegetable in a meal.

The most appetizing meals include foods with different textures. Crisp spinach leaves, smooth sweet potatoes, and firm, raw squash slices add pleasant contrasts.

Another way to make meals more exciting is to dress up vegetables. They can be served with cheese sauce, lemon juice, chili sauce, soy sauce, or honey. You also can dress up vegetables with crumbled bacon bits, sliced hard cooked eggs, toasted nuts, or a sprinkle of garlic.

Preparing Vegetables

Vegetables can be deep-fried, sautéed, stir-fried, steamed, baked, broiled, grilled, or cooked in a microwave oven. Sometimes they are served raw. They can be served plain or with sauces, herbs, or spices. The goal is to serve attractive, nutritious, and tasty vegetables.

Cultures of the World

Sunny Greece

Greece is a beautiful country with a long history. There are many ancient structures in Greece. For example, the Parthenon was built nearly 2,500 years ago.

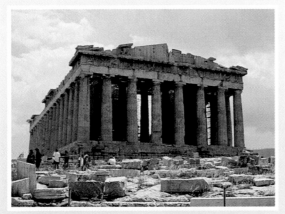

Abercrombie & Kent International

This is the Parthenon in Athens, Greece. The culture of Greece is rich in both its history and cuisine.

Greece is located on the north side of the Mediterranean Sea. It has a long coastline and hundreds of islands. The sea is a major source of food. Greek dishes use many types of fish, shrimp, and squid. Sheep, pigs, and goats thrive in the mountains of Greece. These animals provide milk, yogurt, cheese, and meat.

The rocky, rugged mountains of Greece make farming difficult. Grape vines, citrus trees, and olive trees grow well, though. Olives and olive oil have been part of Greek cooking since ancient times. It is said that Athena, a Greek goddess, brought olive trees to Greece.

Herbs and spices are common in Greek cooking. They bring out the natural flavors of food. Cinnamon, basil, dill, bay leaves, garlic, and oregano are added to many recipes.

Tomatoes, green peppers, zucchini, garlic, and eggplant are found in many Greek dishes. The fertile valleys and warm climate of Greece are ideal for growing vegetables.

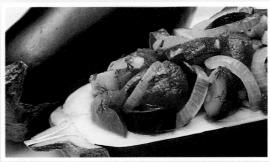

American Heart Association

Eggplant and other vegetables are used in many popular dishes in Greece.

Eggplant is one of the most popular vegetables in Greece. It is served mashed, stuffed, and sliced. Cooks often add it to other foods. Moussaka (moo-sah-KAH) is a rich eggplant casserole. It is a well-known Greek dish.

In Greece, people get together at mealtime to talk and have fun. Meals are informal and not rushed. They are festive times shared with friends and family. Life centers on the dinner table. A typical Greek dinner might include moussaka and whole wheat rolls. Many Greek cookbooks are available. You could use one to plan a festive Greek meal for your family.

Fresh Vegetables

Fresh vegetables need to be washed to remove dust, bacteria, and insect spray. Depending on your recipe, you may need to pare, chop, or cook fresh vegetables. Some vegetables, like eggplant and potatoes, darken when they are peeled and sliced. You can keep them from turning brown by heating them, sprinkling them with an acid, such as lemon juice or vinegar, or soaking them in water.

Canned Vegetables

Canned vegetables can be eaten right from the can, chilled, or heated. Canned vegetables also can be used as an ingredient in a recipe.

Frozen Vegetables

Frozen vegetables can be served as a side dish or added to a recipe. Frozen vegetables usually aren't thawed before they are prepared.

Dried Vegetables

Most dried vegetables need to be soaked in liquid to soften them. Some, like dried beans and potatoes, need to be cooked after they are soaked. Others, such as dried tomatoes and onions, don't have to be cooked. Still others, like dried herbs, don't need to be soaked or cooked. Your recipe will tell you how to prepare dried vegetables.

Cooking Vegetables

Cooking makes vegetables easier to chew. It also makes flavors mellow and colors change.

Properly cooked vegetables have bright colors, pleasant flavors, and firm textures, 16-12. Overcooked vegetables are mushy and dull. Some become bland when overcooked, while others become bitter. Overcooked vegetables also have lost many nutrients.

16-12 The vegetables in this picture were cooked properly. They are colorful and appetizing.

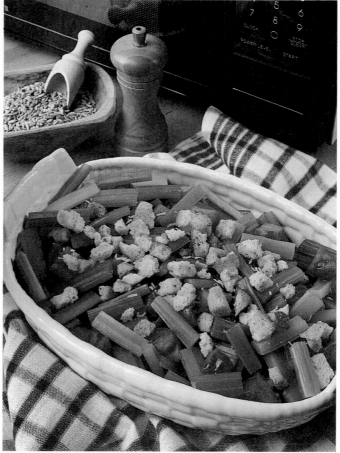

American Celery Council

Heat causes green vegetables to fade. They turn brownish green when overcooked. When yellow vegetables are overcooked, the water turns yellow or orange, and the vegetable becomes pale. When white vegetables are overcooked, they turn yellow or gray. When some red vegetables are cooked in water that contains minerals, they turn purple or purplish green. Adding a little vinegar or lemon juice to the cooking water will keep these vegetables bright.

Here's how to protect the looks and nutrients of vegetables:

1. Most nutrients are just under the skin, so
   - pare thinly
   - cook the vegetable in its skin
2. Nutrients and flavor can leak into the water, so
   - cook whole or in large pieces
   - cook in a small amount of water
   - avoid soaking vegetables in water

3. Heat destroys nutrients and causes colors to be drab, so
   - do not overcook
   - shorten cooking time by adding vegetables to boiling water and using a lid
   - choose fast, gentle cooking methods, such as steaming, stir-frying, and cooking in a microwave oven, to keep vegetable colors bright

Vegetables are an important part of your diet. In the next chapter, you'll discover how vegetables, along with fruits and other foods, can be used to create super salads.

In a Nutshell

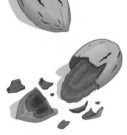

- Vegetables are rich sources of many nutrients. They are low in calories and fat.
- Vegetables may be leaves, stems, roots, bulbs, tubers, flowers, fruits, or seeds.
- Fresh, frozen, canned, and dried vegetables are available year-round.
- Careful storage protects the color, flavor, texture, and nutrients of vegetables.
- Vegetables add variety to meals.
- Properly cooked vegetables have bright colors, pleasant flavors, and firm textures.

In the Know

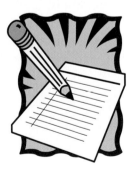

1. Match the vegetable with the part of the plant you can eat.
   ___ cabbage   A. stem
   ___ asparagus   B. root
   ___ carrot   C. flower
   ___ garlic   D. fruit
   ___ broccoli   E. tuber
   ___ potato   F. bulb
   ___ corn   G. leaf
   ___ tomato   H. seed

2. A _____ is the part of a plant's underground stem that swells to store food.

3. Which is *not* a characteristic of high-quality fresh vegetables?
   A. Crisp.
   B. Not wilted.
   C. Pale color.
   D. Firm.

4. Match each fresh vegetable with the storage method that will best preserve its quality. (HINT: Some letters may be used more than once.)

   ___ corn
   ___ lettuce
   ___ potatoes
   ___ pumpkins

   A. store on the kitchen counter
   B. wash and store in the refrigerator
   C. store in a cool, dark, and dry place
   D. store unwashed in the refrigerator

5. True or false? Leftover portions of canned vegetables should be placed in an airtight container and stored at room temperature.

6. Which changes occur when vegetables are cooked?
   A. They become easier to chew.
   B. Flavors mellow.
   C. Colors change.
   D. All of the above.

7. Describe two ways to preserve the nutrients in vegetables when you cook them.

What Would You Do?

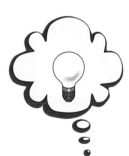

Your mother likes to buy fresh vegetables. Now that she has a new job, she doesn't have time to wash, peel, slice, and cook them. Your family doesn't like canned vegetables. Your mother is afraid she will only have time to serve vegetables on the weekends. What suggestions could you give her?

Expanding Your Knowledge

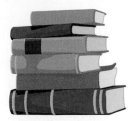

1. Design a poster that describes the types of vegetables. Use drawings or magazine pictures to illustrate the poster.
2. Prepare a tray of raw vegetables you have never tried. Add interest by using variety in the way you cut the vegetables. Try pepper rings, turnip sticks, squash wedges, and radish roses.
3. Select an unfamiliar vegetable and find out its origin and nutrient content. Find three recipes for preparing it. Prepare one of the recipes.
4. Set up a taste panel to compare the flavor, smell, texture, and color of different forms of the same vegetable. For example: tomatoes (fresh, canned, juice, sun-dried); carrots (fresh, canned, frozen, juice); or cucumbers (fresh, pickled—sweet and dill).
5. Visit a supermarket. Make a list of all the forms of vegetables sold and the price per selling unit. Examine the fresh vegetables. Do they have the qualities described in the chapter? Which vegetables were available in the most forms? Which form was the best buy?
6. Invite a produce manager from a local supermarket to come to class. Prepare a list of questions to ask. You could ask: How is the produce section organized? How is the produce kept fresh? Where is the produce grown? How is it shipped to the store? How can shoppers help the supermarket keep produce prices down?
7. Prepare each of six spinach leaves in one of the following ways and serve each on a white plate. Compare the taste, color, and texture of the six samples.
    A. ½ cup boiling water, a lid on the pan, cook 2 minutes.
    B. ½ cup boiling water, a lid on the pan, cook 10 minutes.
    C. ½ cup boiling water, no lid on the pan, cook 2 minutes.
    D. ½ cup boiling water, 1 teaspoon vinegar, a lid on the pan, cook 2 minutes.
    E. 2 cups boiling water, a lid on the pan, cook 2 minutes.
    F. 1 tablespoon of water in microwave-safe dish covered with plastic wrap that is vented, microwave for 1 minute.
8. Create a dinner menu that includes at least two vegetables. Compare the time, energy, and cost of using fresh, frozen in a sauce, canned, and dried vegetables for the meal.

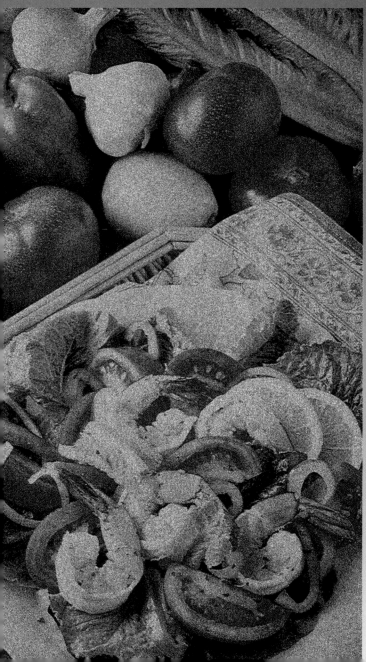

Chapter 17
Salad Success

Objectives

After reading this chapter, you will be able to
- ❏ name the types of salads.
- ❏ identify the parts of a salad.
- ❏ explain how to prepare salad ingredients and assemble a salad.

New Terms

gelatin: a powdered protein substance that, when mixed with liquid, forms a firm, jelly-like consistency.
emulsifier: an ingredient that causes oil to mix with water.
emulsion: a mixture of oil and water.

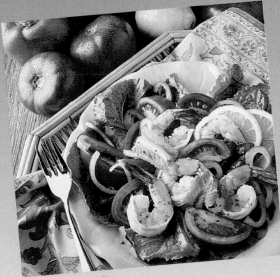

Florida Tomato Committee

389

Does the word "salad" make visions of rabbit food dance in your head? Does the thought of eating a salad make you want to say "What's up, Doc?" If so, you may not realize that a salad can contain almost any food. A salad can be just vegetables. It also can include meat, fruits, grains, or some of each.

Salad ingredients are the oldest known foods. Prehistoric people gathered leafy plants, nuts, and berries. These same ingredients are used in many salads today.

Salads can be served anytime. They are ideal side dishes, appetizers, main dishes, snacks, and even desserts! Salads are easy to make at home. Some supermarkets and delicatessens sell salads that are ready to eat.

Salads can add many nutrients to your diet. The nutrients they provide will depend on the ingredients used. For instance, salads made with vegetables will contain vitamins A and C. Salads that include meat provide protein. Salads made with grains provide fiber, protein, and B vitamins.

Types of Salads

Salads bring together the flavors, textures, and colors of many foods. Some salads have one ingredient. Others have many. The ingredients may be cooked or raw. Most salads are served cold, but some are served hot. Many are served with a dressing.

Salads are grouped by the ingredients used to make them. The five types of salads are: vegetable, fruit, protein, grain, and gelatin.

Vegetable Salads

Vegetable salads contain mostly vegetables. Any frozen, canned, dried, or raw vegetable can be used. These salads boost the nutrients in your diet while adding only a few calories, 17-1.

Vegetable salads make good appetizers or side dishes. In the United States, these salads are usually eaten before the main dish. In Europe, vegetable salads are often served just before dessert.

Vegetables Add Nutrients			
Vegetable	**Calories**	**% of daily need for vitamin A**	**% of daily need for vitamin C**
Broccoli-1 spear	40	47%	235%
Cabbage-1 cup	15	2%	55%
Carrot-1	30	400%	12%
Cauliflower-1 cup	25	1%	120%
Dandelion greens-1 cup	35	250%	32%
Iceberg lettuce-¼ head	20	9%	8%
Peppers (sweet, red)-1	20	85%	235%
Peppers (sweet, green)-1	20	8%	160%
Spinach-1 cup	10	74%	25%
Tomato-1	25	28%	37%

17-1 Vegetables can add a nutritional boost to salads.

Vegetable salads may be as simple as sliced cucumbers or as fancy as a Caesar salad, 17-2. How many of these vegetable salads have you tried?

- Caesar salad (romaine, garlic, and cheese)
- Carrot salad (carrots, raisins, and mayonnaise)
- Coleslaw (cabbage, carrots, spices, and vinegar)
- Potato salad (potatoes, celery, mayonnaise)
- Spinach salad (spinach and mushrooms)
- Tossed salad (pieces of raw vegetables)

17-2 Vegetable salads add vitamin A and C to your diet.

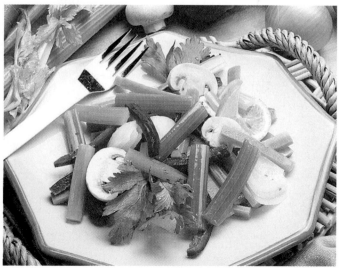

American Celery Council

Fruit Salads

Fruit salads add color, sweetness, and juiciness to meals. They also add many vitamins and few calories. A citrus cup, for example, has less than 100 calories. It meets your daily need for vitamin C.

Fruit salads make good appetizers, side dishes, and desserts, 17-3. They become a main dish when served with meat, cheese, or yogurt.

Any fresh, frozen, canned, or dried fruit can be used. Whipped cream, a fruit sauce, or yogurt dressing is served with some fruit salads. Most of these salads are served chilled. Some are frozen.

Popular fruit salads are

- Ambrosia (orange segments and coconut)
- Waldorf salad (apples, raisins, nuts, and mayonnaise)
- Citrus cup (segments of citrus fruit)
- Fruit cocktail (chunks of fruit in juice or syrup)

17-3 Fruit salads make delicious side dishes.

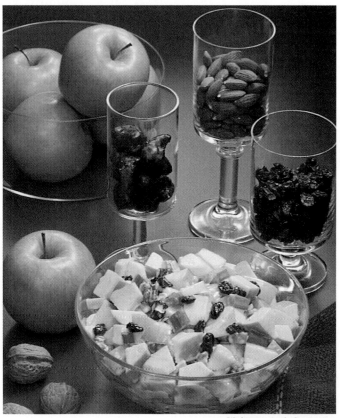

Washington Apple Commission

Protein Salads

Protein salads contain a protein-rich food and fruits, vegetables, or grains. Protein salads usually are served as a main dish. Smaller portions can be an appetizer or a side dish. A main dish protein salad includes at least one of the foods listed in 17-4.

Protein Salads	
Protein-Rich Food	**Amount Needed for One Serving as a Main Dish**
Meat Ground beef, ham, pork, sausage	⅓ cup
Seafood Crab, salmon, sardines, shrimp, tuna	⅓ cup
Poultry Chicken, duck, goose, turkey	⅓ cup
Lunch meats Smoked turkey breast, pepperoni, pastrami	2 ounces
Eggs	1 egg
Cheese American, Cheddar, cottage cheese, Swiss	2 ounces
Legumes Chickpeas, kidney beans, peanuts	½ cup
Nuts Cashews, macadamia nuts, pecans, walnuts	¼ cup
Seeds Poppy seeds, sesame seeds, sunflower seeds	¼ cup

17-4 Protein salads all have at least one protein-rich food. To make a protein salad, you could include any of these protein-rich foods in the amount listed.

Protein salads may be prepared by tossing the ingredients with a dressing, 17-5. Chicken salad and tuna salad are made in this way. These salads make tasty sandwich fillings. They also can be served on a bed of raw vegetables.

Some protein salads are made by laying the protein-rich food atop the other ingredients. A chef's salad is prepared this way. It has egg slices and meat and cheese strips laid on a bed of cold, crisp vegetables.

17-5 Salads are more than just rabbit food. This egg salad is a main dish salad. For a complete meal, just add bread and a beverage.

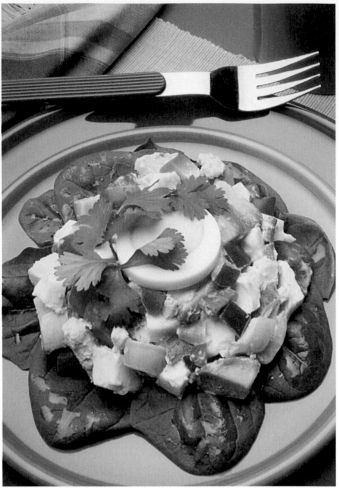

American Egg Board

Most protein salads are chilled. A few, such as Mexican fajitas, are served hot. Fajitas are made by sautéing strips of meat, onions, and green peppers. Fajitas are served in a tortilla.

Hearty protein salads are a meal in themselves. Just add bread and a beverage and you've got a complete meal. How many protein salads have you tried?

- Crab salad (crab, onions, and mayonnaise)
- Antipasto salad (sliced meats, hot peppers, lettuce, and tomatoes)
- Taco salad (tortilla chips, lettuce, tomatoes, cheese, and beans or meat)
- Turkey salad (turkey chunks, celery, and mayonnaise)

Grain Salads

Grain salads can include rice, wheat, corn, or any other grain. These salads may contain vegetables, fruits, and protein-rich foods, too. Macaroni salad and taboulleh (tah-BOO-lee) are grain salads, 17-6.

Grain salads make tasty side dishes or appetizers. They are a great way to use leftover rice and noodles. Each serving of a grain salad has about ¾ cup of cooked grain. Some popular choices for grain salads are chow mein noodles, corn chips, pasta, popcorn, rice, macaroni, and noodles.

Grain salads add texture and flavor to meals. They also add vitamins, minerals, and fiber. Most grain salads are served chilled. Have you tried any of these grain salads?

- Macaroni salad (macaroni, celery, olives, and mayonnaise)
- Pasta salad (pasta, tomatoes, broccoli, and salad dressing)
- Taboulleh (cracked wheat, herbs, lemon juice, and olive oil)

17-6 Grain salads add variety and nutrients to meals.

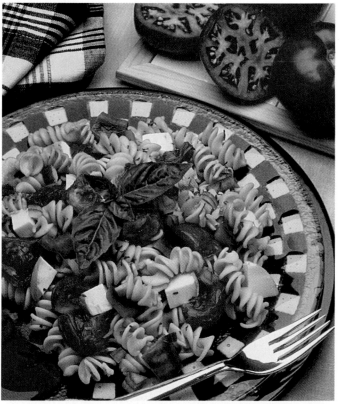

Florida Tomato Committee

Gelatin Salads

Gelatin salads are a special way of making vegetable, fruit, protein, and grain salads. Gelatin salads are often prepared in a mold. They always include gelatin and liquid, 17-7.

17-7 Cool, refreshing molded salads are made with gelatin and a liquid. This molded salad combines the flavors of cranberries and oranges.

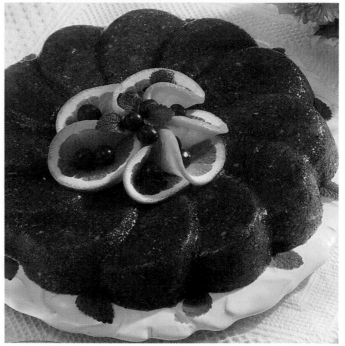

Wilton Enterprises

Gelatin is a powdered protein ingredient that has no color or taste. It dissolves in hot liquid. As the liquid cools, the gelatin absorbs the liquid and thickens, forming a firm, jelly-like consistency. Heat causes the gelatin to become liquid again. Therefore, all gelatin salads must be kept cold and served chilled.

There are two types of gelatin: unflavored gelatin and flavored, sweetened gelatin. Unflavored gelatin is used to make gelatin main dish or side dish salads. Gelatin dessert salads can be prepared with either type of gelatin.

Almost any liquid can be used to make these cool, refreshing salads. Some examples are broth, vegetable juice, milk, water, fruit juice, ginger ale, and lemonade. Broth, vegetable juice, or milk is used in gelatin main dishes and side dishes. Gelatin dessert salads are made with milk, water, or sweet liquids such as fruit juice.

Two popular gelatin side dish salads are tomato aspic and sunshine salad. The main ingredients of aspic are unflavored gelatin and tomato juice. Sunshine salad is made with orange juice, unflavored gelatin, and pineapple.

Lemon chicken salad is a gelatin main dish salad. It is made with diced chicken, rice, and lemon flavored gelatin.

Gelatin dessert salads usually include fruit. Bavarian cream is a gelatin dessert salad. It is made by blending whipped cream and fruit pieces into a gelatin, milk, and egg mixture.

A mold holds the gelatin salad's ingredients until the gelatin thickens the liquid. Molds can be any shape or size. An ice tray, pan, or bowl can be used as a mold. Special shapes, such as rings and hearts, can be purchased.

Building a Salad

The best salads have ingredients that complement each other. Their colors, textures, and flavors blend to create a tasty dish. The most appealing salads have

- only one or two strong flavors
- some crisp textures and some soft textures
- contrasting colors

Salad Blueprint

A blueprint is a building plan. The blueprint for salads has four parts: base, body, dressing, and garnish. All salads have a body. Some salads omit the base, dressing, garnish, or all three.

Base

The base is the foundation or bottom layer of a salad. It is the first thing placed on the serving dish. The other parts of the salad are built on the base, 17-8. Some common salad bases are

- green leafy vegetables
- a scooped out tomato
- a cantaloupe half or a hollowed out watermelon
- a pineapple or an avocado half
- a tortilla or slice of bread
- chow mein noodles

17-8 Lettuce forms the base for this avocado salad.

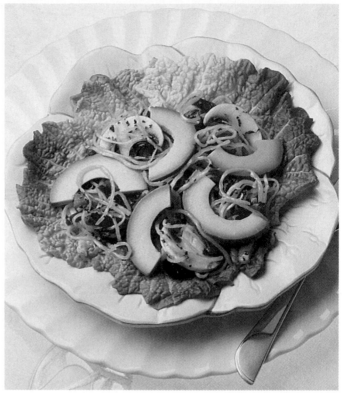

California Avocado Commission

The base makes the salad look more interesting. It can add color, flavor, or texture. A scoop of tuna salad on a plate is more colorful when served in a tomato. A base of corn chips adds texture and flavor to a taco salad. A watermelon carved to look like a basket makes an appealing fruit salad base. The base's color, flavor, and texture should blend with the body and dressing.

Many salad bases, such as lettuce leaves, are eaten. Some bases, such as watermelon rinds, are not eaten. If the base is eaten, it adds nutrients to the salad.

Some salads omit the base. For example, a fruit salad can be served in a bowl. Ham salad may be placed right on a plate. Few gelatin salads have a base.

Body

The body is the main part of the salad. It may be vegetables, fruits, protein foods, grains, or a combination. The body is arranged on the base.

All salads have a body. For example, the body of egg salad includes eggs and mayonnaise. The body of a spinach salad has spinach and mushrooms. The body of a gelatin salad includes gelatin and liquid.

Most of the nutrients in a salad come from the body. The ingredients in the body also affect taste, texture, and eye appeal of a salad.

Dressings

Dressings are sauces added to salads. They blend with the salad base and body to create a unified dish. The dressing is added last.

Salad dressings add flavor. The flavors range from mild mayonnaise to spicy Russian dressing. They also can be a sweet fruit sauce or whipped cream.

Many dressings add fat and calories, too. Oil, mayonnaise, and creamy ingredients are rich in fat. The fat makes them high in calories. Dressings made without fat-rich ingredients, such as fruit juices, have fewer calories.

Salad dressings may be mixed with the body of the salad or poured on top. Pasta salad and egg salad are made by blending the dressing with other ingredients. The dressing is drizzled over the body of tossed salads and chef's salads.

Some salads are served without dressings. Citrus cups and other fruit salads often do not have a dressing. Few gelatin salads have dressings.

Dressings can be made at home or bought at the supermarket. Salad dressings are sold as dried mixes and in bottles ready to serve.

Salad dressings can be as simple as lemon juice. Some are complex mixtures of herbs, spices, eggs, and cream. The three basic types of dressings are French, mayonnaise, and cooked.

French dressing is made with salad oil, vinegar or lemon juice, mustard, and paprika. Salad oil does not mix with ingredients that are mostly water like vinegar and lemon juice. To help oil and water blend, an emulsifier is used. An ***emulsifier*** mixes well with both oil and water. It causes ingredients that are oils to mix with those that are mostly water. Mustard, paprika, and egg yolks are emulsifiers.

Emulsifiers cause salad dressings to become emulsions. An *emulsion* is made when an emulsifier is used to blend oil with ingredients that are mostly water. French dressing is a *temporary emulsion.* Shaking causes the oil and water ingredients to mix. They separate again in a few minutes.

Many salad dressings are based on French dressing. Italian, poppy seed, Russian, and vinaigrette are all types of French dressings.

Mayonnaise is made with oil, egg yolks, and vinegar or lemon juice. This dressing is a *permanent emulsion.* Its ingredients do not separate. They stay mixed.

Cheese, chili sauce, onion, and other ingredients are added to mayonnaise to make other dressings. Some of these dressings are blue cheese, creamy garlic, cucumber, and thousand island.

Cooked dressings are made with vinegar or fruit juice and flour, cornstarch, or egg yolks. Cooked dressings do not contain fat or oil. They are lower in calories than French and mayonnaise dressings. Cooked dressings made with juice are good on fruit salads. Those made with vinegar are tasty toppings for grain, vegetable, and protein salads.

Other dressings are made with yogurt, sour cream, and whipped cream. See 17-9. Many flavors can be created by mixing in herbs, spices, and fruit purees. Lowfat yogurt mixed with pureed berries is a low-calorie topping for fruit salad. A blend of sour cream and chopped onions adds flavor to protein salads.

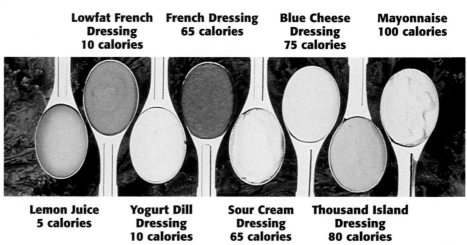

Lowfat French Dressing 10 calories   **French Dressing** 65 calories   **Blue Cheese Dressing** 75 calories   **Mayonnaise** 100 calories

Lemon Juice 5 calories   **Yogurt Dill Dressing** 10 calories   **Sour Cream Dressing** 65 calories   **Thousand Island Dressing** 80 calories

USDA

17-9 There are many salad dressing choices. The calories in a tabelspoon of dressing vary greatly.

Science in the Kitchen

Mixing the Unmixable?

Oil and water don't mix, or do they? They can mix when an emulsifier is used. Emulsifiers mix with both water and oil. This experiment will show you how an emulsifier works.

To start, place 1 tablespoon of vegetable oil and 1 tablespoon of water in a jar. Stir the oil and water rapidly with a spoon. What happens? Now, tighten the lid and shake the jar rapidly for one minute. Describe what happens. Place the jar on a table and determine how long it takes for the oil and water to separate again.

To see the effects of an emulsifier, open the jar and add 1 teaspoon of mustard. Tighten the lid and shake the jar for a minute. What happened this time? How long did it take for the oil and water to separate? Mustard helps oil and water form a temporary emulsion. It's temporary because the oil and water slowly separate over time.

A permanent emulsion does not separate. It's a little trickier to make a permanent emulsion. If you follow these directions very carefully, you can create the permanent emulsion called mayonnaise. Place ¼ cup thawed egg substitute, 1 teaspoon dry mustard, ¼ teaspoon paprika, and 1 tablespoon of lemon juice (or vinegar) in a bowl. Using an electric mixer, beat on high speed for 1 minute.

Now, add 1 teaspoon of oil and beat for 30 seconds. Repeat this step 11 more times. Next, add 2 teaspoons of oil and beat for 30 seconds. Repeat this step 11 more times. Then, add 1 tablespoon of oil and beat for 30 seconds. Repeat this step three more times. Finally, slowly stir in 1 tablespoon of lemon juice. How does the mayonnaise look and taste? How does the mayonnaise you made compare to the mayonnaise you buy?

Salad dressings that contain eggs, milk, cream, or yogurt will spoil at room temperature. They should be kept in the refrigerator. Unopened bottled dressings and dried packets can be kept in a cool, dry place. Once they are opened, store them in the refrigerator.

Hold the Dressing!

The best salads have just enough dressing to lightly coat salad body ingredients. To cut down on salad dressing calories, try the "dab and stab" method:

1. Put a little dressing in a cup.
2. Dab your fork into the dressing.
3. Stab your salad.

If you want more than a dab and are concerned about fat and calories, you have a few options.

- Try a lowfat, low-calorie bottled dressing.
- Use plain vinegar, lemon juice, or chili sauce.
- Make a dressing with lowfat yogurt.
- Make a cooked dressing.

Garnish

Some salads have a fourth part, a garnish. The garnish adds eye appeal. It may add flavor and texture, too. Some garnishes are bacon bits, bean sprouts, carrot curls, croutons, and grated egg yolk. Other garnishes are potato sticks, nasturtium blossoms, nuts, and sesame seeds.

Focus on Food

Flower Petals in My Salad!

Flowers add flavor, color, and beauty to foods. You can float petals on beverages or soups. Flowers can be added to sauces and desserts. Flowers make a fresh, appealing garnish. They are especially tasty in salads.

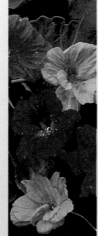

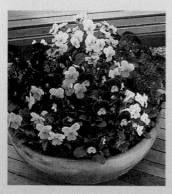

People of many cultures have eaten flowers for centuries. For example:

- The ancient Chinese thought chrysanthemums helped them have longer, healthier lives. These flower petals are added to Chinese foods today.
- In the 15th century, cooks often used violets in soups and sauces.
- Fried squash blossoms are a tasty Native American treat.
- The British enjoy tea made from tiny flowers called chamomile.
- Grocers in Holland stock dried marigold petals. These flowers

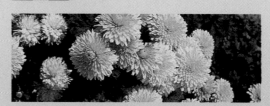

Flowers and Their Flavors		
Flower	**Flavor**	**How to Use**
Carnation	spicy	mix with butter or cream cheese and serve on bread, add to salads and stuffed peppers
Chrysanthemum	slightly bitter	float on soup, add to rice dishes and salads
Dandelion	mild	add to salads and omelets
Geranium	mildly sweet	add to salads
Hollyhock	very mild	add to sandwiches and salads
Marigolds	mild	add to chowders, cookies, custards, muffins, salads, rice dishes, broth, and sandwiches
Nasturtium	peppery	add to salads, omelets, soups, vegetable dishes, sandwiches, and sauces
Petunia	sweet	add to desserts
Rose petals	mild	add to salads, float on soups
Violet	sweet	add to desserts, jellies, sauces, sandwiches, salads, and soups, mix with cream cheese and serve on bread

Flowers can add interest to meals.

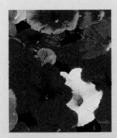

are the secret to the flavor and color of Dutch soups.

Before eating any flower, it is important to know that it is safe to eat. Some types of flowers are poisonous. The chart above names flowers that are tasty and safe to eat. Be certain that you can identify the flower before eating it. Also, only use flowers that have not been sprayed with pesticides. Always wash the flowers before using them.

For the most tasty and beautiful flowers:

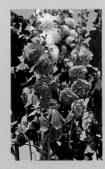

- Remove white tips on petals and stems. These taste bitter.

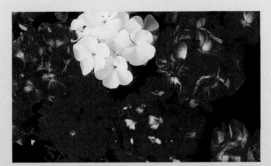

- Lay the flowers on a damp paper towel. Place in a plastic bag and store in the refrigerator.
- If flowers are limp, refresh them by dipping them in ice water.
- When using flowers in a recipe, do not use metal pans or utensils. The metal will darken the flowers.
- Add flowers to salads after adding dressing. The dressing causes them to wilt.

Preparing Salad Ingredients

Salad ingredients may be raw or cooked. They can be fresh, frozen, canned, or dried. The best ingredients are clean, tasty, and good for you.

Fruits and Vegetables

Wash fresh produce to remove dirt and insect spray, 17-10. Using cool, running water keeps produce from becoming water-logged and soggy. To wash iceberg lettuce, begin by removing the core. Loosen the core by hitting it on the kitchen counter. Next, grasp the core and pull it out. Then, let water run into the hole where the core was. Drain the head by placing it in a colander core side down.

Be sure to dry fruits and vegetables thoroughly. Dressing clings better to dry ingredients. Dry fresh produce by placing it between paper towels or clean dishtowels and patting gently. You can also use

17-10 Before using fresh vegetables in a salad, be sure to wash them to remove dust and pesticides.

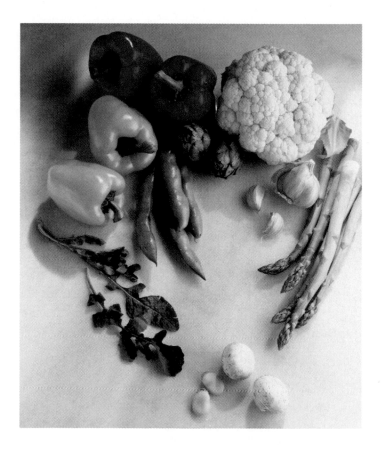

a salad spinner to dry fresh produce. A salad spinner has an inner basket that spins rapidly, causing the water to spray off the produce.

Cut salad ingredients into bite-sized pieces. To add interest, cut ingredients into a variety of shapes. You could serve melon balls, kiwi fruit wedges, and banana circles. Tear or cut salad greens into small pieces. Shred, slice, or steam carrots and other hard vegetables. This makes them softer and easier to chew.

Fruits that darken, such as avocados and apples, should be dipped in lemon juice. This will keep them from turning brown. Also, the edges of salad greens won't darken if you tear or cut them just before serving.

Prewashed and cut vegetables can save time when making salads, but they usually cost more than other produce. Before buying them, check to see that they are bright and crisp. Rinse and dry them again before you use them.

Most salad recipes tell you to drain the liquid from canned fruits and vegetables before using them as ingredients. Chill the canned food unless the salad is to be served hot or at room temperature.

Frozen fruits and vegetables have the best textures when they are partly thawed. Wipe off any ice crystals. If these foods are part of a hot salad, prepare them according to the recipe.

Soak dried vegetables for salads in hot water for a few minutes. They will absorb water and soften. Raisins and other dried fruits usually do not need to be soaked.

Protein-Rich Foods

Any cooking method can be used to prepare protein-rich foods for salads. Unless the salad is to be served hot, chill the protein-rich foods after cooking them. Nuts, seeds, luncheon meats, and canned protein foods do not require cooking.

Grain

Some grains need to be cooked before use in salads. Follow the package directions to prepare dried grains. If the grain was cooked in water, drain it well. Chill grains to be used in cold salads.

Ready-to-eat breads and canned grain foods, such as croutons and chow mein noodles, need no cooking. You can use them right from the package.

Assembling Salads

Many salads are best if they are assembled just before serving, 17-11. However, the body of most grain, protein, and gelatin salads should be made at least several hours before serving time. To assemble salads, begin with the base and then add the body. Add the dressing and any garnish last.

It is easy to assemble an attractive salad. Arrange it as though you were painting a picture. Think of the ingredients as the colors on an artist's palette.

Fruit and Vegetable Salads

The best fresh fruit and vegetable salads are prepared as close to serving time as possible. It is possible to prepare the ingredients up to a day in advance. If you must make a salad ahead of time, place the clean, dry ingredients in plastic bags. Refrigerate and assemble the salad just before serving. Always wait until the last minute to add the dressing. Adding the dressing too early will cause the ingredients to wilt and be limp.

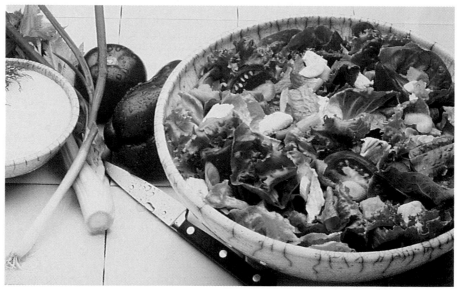

USDA

17-11 The best fresh fruit and vegetable salads are served as soon as they are made.

Protein and Grain Salads

The body of many protein and grain salads can be prepared up to a day ahead of time. Salads made by tossing the ingredients with the dressing are more tasty when made a day in advance. Turkey salad and ham salad are examples. They need time to develop their flavors. Keep them in a covered container in the refrigerator. Place on a base just before serving.

Protein salads that are served hot, such as fajitas, are best when made and assembled just before serving. The same is true for protein salads that contain fresh produce or crisp grain foods, such as taco chips.

Gelatin Salads

Gelatin salads must be made in advance. Gelatin needs a few hours in the refrigerator to thicken.

The best gelatin salads are firm and tender. Their texture depends on the amount of gelatin, liquid, and other foods used. Gelatin salads will be tough and rubbery if you use too much gelatin or too little liquid. Gelatin will be weak and break apart if you add too many solid ingredients or use too much liquid. To get the right amount of liquid, measure carefully. Also, drain foods well before adding them to gelatin. Some fruits contain a substance that won't allow the gelatin to thicken. These include fresh or frozen pineapple, kiwifruit, figs, and papaya. These fruits can be used if they are blanched or canned.

A few minutes before serving time, remove the salad from its mold. To do this:

1. Dip the mold in warm water. Hot water will melt the gelatin.
2. Loosen the edge of the salad with the tip of a knife.
3. Rinse the serving plate in cold water and do not dry it. This allows you to move the salad if it is not centered on the plate.
4. Place the plate on top of the mold. Hold the plate and mold tightly and turn them over together. The plate should then be on the bottom.
5. Shake the mold gently. Lift it off.

Add the dressing at the last minute. You may prefer to serve the dressing on the side.

Salad Bars

A salad bar offers a variety of foods that can be used to make a salad. You can use the ingredients provided to create a special salad just for you, 17-12.

Lettuce, spinach, and other salad greens are included on salad bars. Most salad bars also include several types of raw fruits and vegetables. For instance, you might find orange segments, pineapple chunks, tomato wedges, and cucumber wheels. An assortment of dressings are included, too. Some salad bars also offer garnishes. Croutons, grated cheese, bacon bits, sunflower seeds, and alfalfa spouts are popular salad bar garnishes. Already prepared salads, such as tuna salad, pasta salad, and gelatin salads, may be part of a salad bar, too. If protein-rich foods are included, the salad bar can make a complete meal.

You'll find salad bars in some restaurants and school cafeterias. You can even set up a salad bar at home for a special family dinner or a party. The best salad bars offer a variety of colorful, nutritious, and tasty salad ingredients.

These tips can help you create an appealing salad bar. Be sure to carefully wash and dry all raw fruits and vegetables. To prevent browning, slice fresh fruits and vegetables as close to serving time as

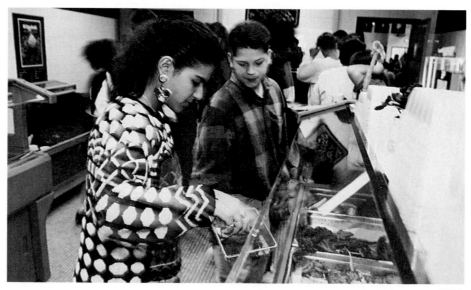

USDA

17-12 Salad bars give you a chance to create your own salad masterpiece.

Cultures of the World

Tempting Thailand Cuisine

Thailand is in Southeast Asia. It is near the equator. This hot and rainy country has a long coastline. Fish farms are common in Thailand. The farmers feed fish or shrimp. When the seafood is large enough, the fish farmers harvest and sell it.

Rice is the main crop in this part of the world. It thrives in hot, humid weather. This grain grows in very wet fields called paddies. Rice is served at every meal.

Thailand is known for its exotic fruits. In most Thai markets, you can find rambutans (RAM-boou-tans) and durians (DER-ee-ans). Rambutans are hairy red fruits. Durians look like large melons with spikes. It is said that elephants enjoy eating this strongly scented fruit.

Thailand is one of the largest coconut growers in the world. In one area, monkeys are taught to pick coconuts. A well trained monkey can pick 500 coconuts a day! This fruit is used in many Thai foods. Coconut milk is a favorite drink.

Thai lunches and dinners include soup, fish or chicken, salad, vegetables, and rice. Fruits end the meal. Until recently, foods were eaten with the hands. Today, forks and spoons are used.

Thais value fresh ingredients. Most people shop every day at outdoor markets. In some rural areas, the market is in boats. The sellers float down the river, stopping at each house to sell their goods. Thai markets are a saladmaker's dream. There are many fresh fruit and vegetable choices.

Thai salads are some of the most beautiful and delicious salads in the world. These tasty salads are called yams. They may be spicy hot, salty, sweet, or sour. Yam neua is a tasty Thai beef salad. Mien Kham is a salad made with coconut, peanuts, shrimp, and lettuce. Som Tam is a popular vegetable salad that is often served with chicken and rice. The next time you are responsible for making a salad, think about serving one from Thailand.

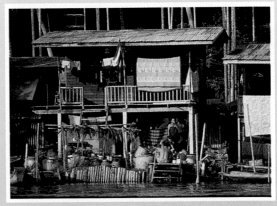

Abercrombie & Kent International

In Thailand, a variety of fruits and vegetables can be purchased from a floating market.

possible. Add interest by cutting fruits and vegetables in different shapes. When it's time to serve your salad bar, you'll want to keep the ingredients fresh and cold. You can do this by setting the bowls in a pan filled with ice cubes. If you keep these tips in mind, you'll be assured of salad success!

In a Nutshell

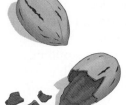

- Salads can be served as side dishes, appetizers, main dishes, snacks, and desserts.
- The best salad ingredients are fresh, clean, tasty, and nutritious.
- There are five types of salads: vegetable, fruit, protein, grain, and gelatin.
- The colors, textures, and flavors of salad ingredients should complement each other.
- A salad usually has four parts: base, body, dressing, and garnish.
- There are three types of salad dressings: French, mayonnaise, and cooked.
- French dressing and mayonnaise are emulsions.

In the Know

1. List the five types of salads. Name one salad from each group.
2. Which of the following is an example of a main dish salad?
   A. Bavarian cream.
   B. Taco salad.
   C. Waldorf salad.
   D. Taboulleh.
3. Name two types of ingredients always used to make gelatin.
4. The ___ serves as a salad's foundation.
   A. base
   B. body
   C. dressing
   D. garnish
5. All salads have a _____.
   A. dressing
   B. body
   C. garnish
   D. base
6. Which ingredient can help oil and water to mix, forming an emulsion?
   A. Egg yolks.
   B. Paprika.
   C. Mustard.
   D. All of the above.
7. True or false? Mayonnaise is a temporary emulsion.

8. Explain why it is important to dry all fresh salad ingredients.
9. True or false? To remove a gelatin salad from its mold, dip it in warm water.

What Would You Do?

You and some friends decide to get together Saturday evening. The time is set for one hour after the school football game ends. You agree to bring a cold, crisp salad. After the game, you plan to go home and change clothes. You are afraid there won't be enough time to make a salad and get to your friend's house on time. What could you do to achieve all your goals?

Expanding Your Knowledge

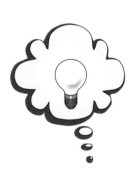

1. Use cookbooks to research salad recipes. Use this information to plan a salad party. Ask each friend to bring a different salad. While you eat, have each person describe how the salad was made.
2. Teach younger brothers and sisters how to make a tossed salad. Be sure to show them how to wash, dry, and cut the vegetables. Explain how they can make tasty, appealing salads.
3. Interview a restaurant owner about salads. You could ask: What types of salads do you serve? How do you keep them fresh and tasty? Are salads popular menu items? Do patrons seem to order more salads today than they did five years ago? What knowledge and skills does a saladmaker in a restaurant need?

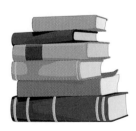

4. Create a salad collage using magazine pictures. You may want to limit your collage to one type of salad, such as vegetable salads or dessert salads.
5. The length of time a dressing is in contact with ingredients affects the texture of the salad. Compare the texture of lettuce leaves using the following variations after 1 minute, 5 minutes, 15 minutes, and 30 minutes. How can you use this information?
Variation A:
Wash and dry one leaf and place it on a saucer.
Variation B:
Wash and dry one leaf and place it on a saucer. Top with one teaspoon of salad dressing.
Variation C:
Wash a lettuce leaf. Do not dry it. Place it on a saucer. Top with one teaspoon of salad dressing.

6. The amount of liquid and gelatin used in a gelatin salad affects its texture and flavor. The type of liquid used can also affect texture and flavor. Compare the texture and taste of these gelatins.

Gelatin A:
2 3-ounce boxes of fruit-flavored gelatin
½ cup boiling water
½ cup cold water

Gelatin B:
1 3-ounce box of fruit-flavored gelatin
1 cup boiling water
1 cup cold water

Gelatin C:
1 3-ounce box of fruit-flavored gelatin
2 cups boiling water
2 cups cold water

Gelatin D:
1 3-ounce box of fruit-flavored gelatin
1 cup boiling water
1 cup cold pineapple juice made from frozen concentrate
Prepare each gelatin in a separate bowl labeled *A, B, C,* or *D.*
Use these directions for all four gelatins.
1. Add boiling water to gelatin. Stir 2 minutes.
2. Add cold water or juice.
3. Chill 2 hours or overnight.

7. There are many different green, leafy vegetables. Select six to ten green, leafy vegetables and set up a taste panel. Ask each person to write down at least five words that describe each green, leafy vegetable. They could describe the color, flavor, shape, and texture of the vegetable.

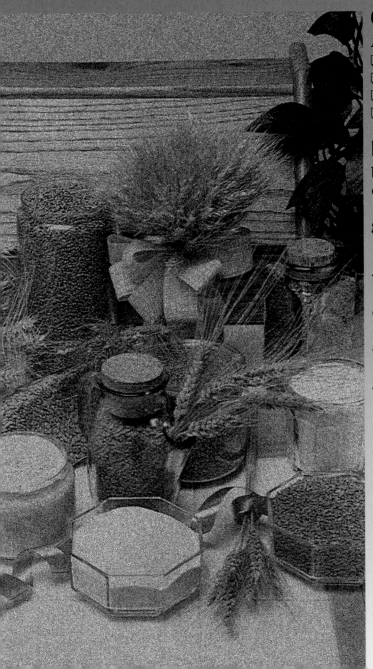

Chapter 18

Super Cereals

Objectives

After reading this chapter, you will be able to
- [ ] describe the variety of grains available.
- [ ] select grain products in the supermarket.
- [ ] store grain products to protect their quality.
- [ ] prepare grain products.

New Terms

bran: a grain kernel's tough outer coat.

endosperm: the largest part of a grain kernel. It contains mostly starch.

germ: the smallest part of a grain kernel. It contains most of the kernel's nutrients. A new plant sprouts from the germ.

whole grain foods: cereal foods that include all three parts of the grain kernel.

enriched: foods that have nutrients lost during processing added back to them.

al dente: pasta that is cooked until it is tender but firm.

gelatinization: a process that occurs when starch granules absorb water, swell, and cause a liquid to get thicker.

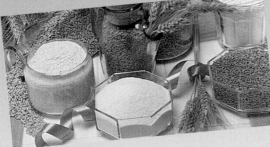

Wheat Foods Council

What comes to mind when you hear the word *cereal?* Is it breakfast? Is it snap, crackle, and pop? You may be surprised to learn that you eat cereal at almost every meal. Corn flakes, spaghetti, bread, fried rice, pizza crust, and popcorn all are cereals.

Humans have relied on cereal foods throughout history. In fact, cereals are so important that bread is often called the "staff of life." This name refers to the vital role cereal plays in nourishing people.

Cereals grow all over the world. Over 80 percent of the people on earth get most of their nutrients and calories from cereals. These low-cost foods are good sources of protein, starch, fiber, B vitamins, and iron.

Cereals are also called grains. They are the seeds of tall grasses. Seeds are called kernels, too. See 18-1.

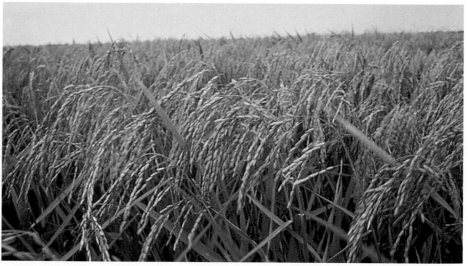

USA Rice Council

18-1 Grains are tall grasses.

What's in a Grain?

All grain kernels have three parts. See 18-2. The parts are bran, endosperm, and germ.

18-2 All grains have three parts.

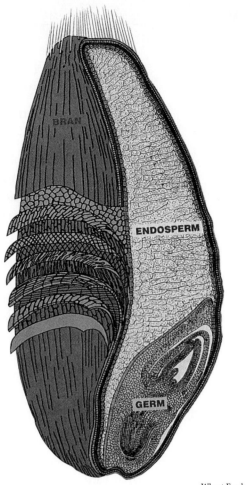

Wheat Foods Council

Bran

Bran is the seed's tough outer coat. It protects the inner parts of the seed. Bran contains most of the kernel's fiber.

Endosperm

The *endosperm* is the largest part of the seed. It contains many tiny pieces of starch called *granules* (GRAN-yools). The starch supplies energy. If the seed sprouts, the new plant gets the energy. If you eat the seed before it sprouts, you get the energy. The endosperm also provides some protein. It is low in vitamins, minerals, and fiber.

Germ

The ***germ*** is the smallest part of the seed. A new plant sprouts from the germ. The germ contains most of the seed's nutrients. It is rich in protein, minerals, vitamins, and fat.

Cereal foods that include all three parts of the kernel provide the most nutrients. They are called ***whole grain foods***.

White bread, pastries, and many other foods only use the endosperm. Most nutrients are lost when the bran and germ are removed. Foods made with just the endosperm are mainly starch. They have less fiber and lack many of the nutrients found in whole grain foods.

Many foods made with only the endosperm are ***enriched***. That means some of the nutrients lost during processing when the bran and germ were removed are added back to them. Cereal foods have thiamin, riboflavin, niacin, folate, and iron added to them. Enriched cereals are better for you than cereals made with just the endosperm and no added nutrients. Your best bet, though, is whole grain foods. They have all the nutrients added to enriched cereals and more!

Types of Grains

There are many types of grains. The most popular are wheat, corn, rice, oats, barley, and rye.

Wheat

Wheat is one of the most important crops grown worldwide. It is grown mainly in the United States, Canada, Europe, and Russia.

Almost all wheat kernels are ground into a fine powder called *flour*. There are two main types of wheat flour: whole wheat flour and white flour. *Whole wheat flour* is made by grinding the entire wheat kernel. This flour contains the bran, endosperm, and germ. It provides all the nutrients in the kernel. *White flour* is made by grinding only the endosperm. The bran and germ are removed. White flour is mainly starch and has almost no fiber, vitamins, and minerals. Most white flour is enriched. Even though it is enriched, it still lacks many of the nutrients found in whole wheat flour.

Wheat flour is an ingredient in many foods. For instance, it is used to make biscuits, bread, cookies, noodles, pizza crust, and waffles. It is also used to make crackers, muffins, pancakes, pastries, and rolls. The foods shown in 18-3 were all made with wheat flour. Which of the foods shown have you eaten?

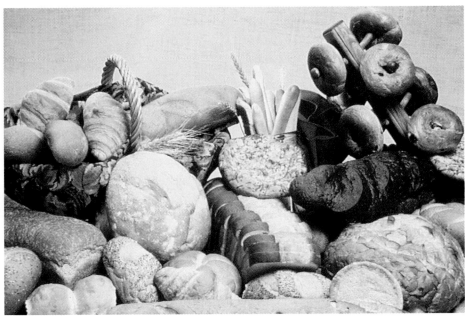

Wheat Foods Council

18-3 These foods were all made with wheat flour. How many have you tried?

Other foods are made from wheat, too. Have you tried any of these foods?

- *Wheat germ* is the germ of the kernel. It has a nutty flavor and is rich in vitamins and minerals. Often, it is toasted and served as a breakfast cereal. It makes a tasty topping for salads, vegetables, and soups.
- *Wheat bran* has a mild taste. Bran is high in fiber. It is added to some breakfast cereals, breads, and grain salads.
- *Farina* is a coarsely ground flour. Most of the bran and germ are removed. It is cooked and served as a hot breakfast cereal.

Corn

Have you tried breakfast cereals made with corn such as corn flakes and corn puffs? How about corn chips? Corn has been a major food in Mexico and Central America for centuries. Native Americans introduced this grain to the first New World settlers.

Like other grains, corn kernels contain an endosperm, germ, and bran. The endosperm is used to make hominy, grits, corn syrup, and cornstarch. Other products come from the germ or the whole corn kernel.

- *Hominy* is large, dried pieces of endosperm. It is boiled and served as a side dish.
- *Grits* are made by coarsely grinding hominy. Grits are served as a hot breakfast cereal.
- *Corn syrup* is very sweet. It sweetens many candies and desserts. It is made by changing the endosperm's starch into sugar.
- *Cornstarch* is a fine, white powder. It is the starch from the endosperm. Cornstarch is used to thicken puddings, pie fillings, sauces, and gravies.
- *Corn oil* comes from the germ. Squeezing the germ causes the oil to run out. Corn oil is used in cooking and to make margarine.
- *Cornmeal* is made by grinding the whole kernel or just the endosperm. Cornmeal made with whole kernels has more nutrients than cornmeal made with only the endosperm. Cornmeal made with just the endosperm often is enriched. Cornmeal is used to make corn bread, tortillas, and to coat fried foods.
- *Popcorn* is a special type of corn. There is a tiny drop of water inside each kernel. When popcorn is heated, the water turns into steam. The pressure of the steam causes the kernel to explode, 18-4.

Rice

Rice is the main food of over half the people on earth. More than two billion people eat rice at every meal. Most of the rice supply of the world grows in the hot, humid regions of Asia.

There are more than 7,000 kinds of rice. All can be grouped according to the length of the rice grains: short, medium, or long. *Long grain rice* is light and fluffy when it is cooked. *Short* and *medium grain rice* stick together when cooked.

18-4 Popcorn explodes when the tiny drop of water inside the kernel gets hot enough to become steam.

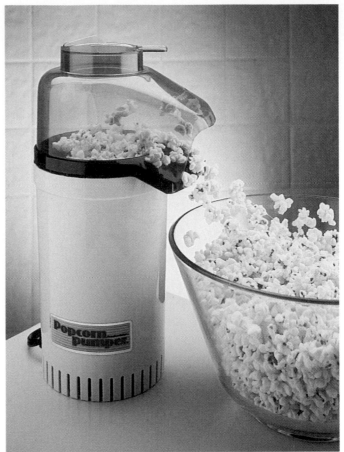

Hamilton Beach/Proctor-Silex

Three main types of rice are sold in supermarkets: brown, polished, and converted.

- *Brown rice* is the whole rice kernel. It contains more nutrients and fiber than other types of rice.
- *Polished rice* is just the endosperm. It has less than half as many nutrients as brown rice. Enriched polished rice has more nutrients than polished rice.
- *Converted rice* is made by steaming whole rice kernels. Steaming draws some of the nutrients from the bran and germ into the endosperm where they are trapped. After the kernels dry, the bran and germ are removed. Converted rice has more nutrients than polished rice. Converted rice is another name for parboiled rice.

Focus on Nutrition

The Clue of the Shaky Chickens

Scientists are like detectives. They look for clues and track down killers. The baffling puzzle of the shaking chickens took years to unravel.

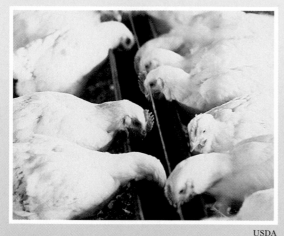

USDA

When investigating the cause of beriberi, Dr. Eijkman found that chickens fed white rice got beriberi. The chickens fed brown rice didn't get beriberi.

In the late 1800s, a brutal killer was loose in Asia. The work of this killer was well known for many years. Suddenly, the killer went on a rampage. It claimed thousands of victims. People called the killer "Beriberi."

Beriberi means "I can't, I can't." This killer causes muscles to waste away. The victims become paralyzed. When they are asked to walk, victims say "I can't." When their hearts become paralyzed, they die. Beriberi is a disease. Many people suffered from it. Yet, no one knew how they got it.

A doctor named Dr. Eijkman was working in Asia. He began studying this killer. He thought beriberi was caused by a germ. He looked for a germ, but couldn't find one. The disease was getting worse. It had spread to chickens. The chickens shook. They wobbled when they tried to walk. Many of them died. What was causing this terrible disease?

One day, Dr. Eijkman walked by a local chicken farm. He found a valuable clue. He noticed that the chickens didn't shake and wobble anymore. He questioned the farmer. He wanted to know how the chickens were cured.

The farmer said, "The price of white rice has gotten too high so, I stopped feeding my chickens white rice. Now I feed them brown rice."

The price of white rice had gone up after a new method for processing rice was developed. This method removed the bran and germ. Only the white endosperm was left. People wanted the pretty white rice. They didn't want "dirty looking" brown rice anymore. They ate white rice at every meal.

Dr. Eijkman thought about his clue. "Is there something in brown rice that prevents beriberi?" he wondered. He set up an experiment to find out.

He fed one group of chickens brown rice. He fed a second group white rice. The chickens fed brown rice didn't get beriberi. Those fed white rice got beriberi. When he fed the chickens with beriberi brown rice, they got better. When he fed people with beriberi brown rice, they also got better quickly.

Dr. Eijkman was right! There is something in brown rice that prevents and cures beriberi. What is it? About 30 years later, a scientist working in London found the answer. It is a vitamin. The vitamin is called thiamin. Thiamin is in the germ of grains. The white rice lacked thiamin. That is because white rice is only the endosperm. When the germ is removed, so are the vitamins and minerals.

Beriberi became a big problem in Asia when the people switched from brown to white rice. Amazing as it may seem, this killer is still at work. Many people in the Philippines die from this disease every year! They could be saved if they ate brown rice or enriched rice.

Another type of rice you may find in stores is wild rice. *Wild rice* is not rice at all. It is not even a grain. Wild rice is the seeds of a water plant. It has a dark brown color and nutty flavor.

Rice is used in many foods, 18-5. It may be served alone, ground into flour, or used in:

- breakfast cereals (puffed rice)
- soups (chicken rice soup, tomato rice soup)
- salads (ham and rice salad)
- desserts (rice pudding)
- main dishes (sausage and rice)
- side dishes (rice pilaf, rice cakes)

18-5 Rice is an ingredient in many main dishes.

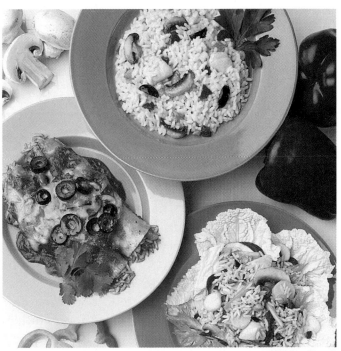

USA Rice Council

Oats

Oats are native to Europe where they are added to many foods. In the United States, oats are served most often as oatmeal. Oats may be an ingredient in muffins, crackers, cookies, and breads. This grain is sometimes used as a topping on fruit desserts.

How many of these foods made with oats have you tried?

- Apple crisp
- Breakfast cereals
- Granola
- Oat bran muffins
- Oatmeal cookies

Barley

Barley is eaten more often in Europe than in the United States. This grain may be added to soups, breakfast cereals, and baby foods.

When barley sprouts, it produces a sticky, sugary substance called *malt.* Malt is an ingredient in malted milk drinks and candies.

Rye

Rye is an important grain crop in Europe and Russia. Most rye is ground into flour. The flour is used to make pumpernickel bread, rye bread, and crackers. Rye is seldom served as a breakfast cereal.

Buying Cereals

Cereals are available year-round. They can be stored easily for long periods. This helps keep their prices low.

There are many cereal food choices. For example, some cereal foods contain whole grains, while others contain just the endosperm. Some cereal foods have added nutrients, but some don't. Cereal foods may be plain or have added ingredients such as sugar, nuts, and spices. Some cereal foods can be eaten right out of the package. Other cereal foods only need to be heated or cooked. The many cereal food choices include breakfast cereals, rice, pasta, and noodles.

Breakfast Cereals

Breakfast cereals can be made with any part of the grain. Most cereals use just the endosperm. Some use whole kernels. Others include only the bran or germ. Breakfast cereals make a good meal or snack. They also can be crushed into crumbs and used to coat meat, poultry, and fish. Sometimes they are added to cookies, breads, and desserts.

There are more than 100 types of breakfast cereals sold in United States supermarkets, 18-6. When buying breakfast cereal, you'll need to make several decisions. Do you want one with no, some, or a large amount of added sugar? (Compare labels. Some breakfast cereals contain more sugar per serving than some cookies!) Do you want a breakfast cereal made with whole grain cereals or one made with just the endosperm? Do you prefer a plain breakfast cereal or one with added ingredients, such as dried fruit? Do you want one with added nutrients? It is important to read the cereal's label to be sure you get what you need.

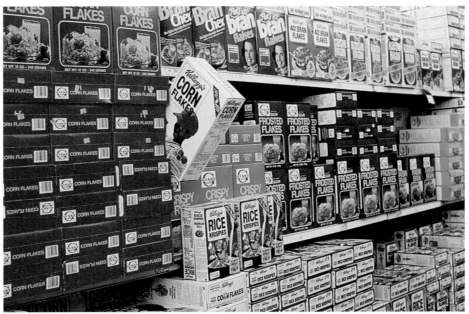

USDA

18-6 There are many choices of breakfast cereals.

Your choice also depends on your budget. The price you pay for a breakfast cereal is based on the package size, ease of preparation, and ingredients used.

It's a good idea to buy breakfast cereal by the weight of the package, not the size. This is because boxes are only partly filled. Also, the package's size might be misleading. For example, puffed corn takes up more space than corn flakes. A small box of corn flakes may weigh more and have more servings than a large box of corn puffs.

Unit pricing on the supermarket shelf gives you the price per unit of a breakfast cereal. Often, large packages are a better buy than small ones. Single serving boxes are the most costly.

The easier the breakfast cereal is to prepare, the more it will likely cost. If it can be eaten right from the package, it will probably cost more than a cereal that needs to be cooked. Oatmeal and farina are cooked cereals. Instant, individual packets of cooked cereals are the most costly type of cooked cereals.

Some cereals have extra ingredients added. Presweetened breakfast cereals have sugar added. Some cereals have nuts and dried fruits added. All extra ingredients increase the price of a cereal. You can save money by buying plain cereals and adding the sugar and extra ingredients yourself.

Rice

Dried, canned, and frozen rice is sold in supermarkets. The most common and least costly form is dried.

Rice is found in many convenience forms. For example, instant or precooked dried rice has been cooked, rinsed, and dried before you buy it. This type of dried rice cooks faster than other types of dried rice, but costs a little more. Dried rice mixes and canned or frozen rice dishes are quick and easy to prepare. They cost much more than the same dishes made from scratch.

You also can buy rice that's ready to eat. Cooked rice sold in delicatessens and as take-out food costs much more than making rice at home. You pay a higher price so you don't have to cook it yourself.

Pasta and Noodles

Pasta and *noodles* are made with wheat flour and water. These ingredients are mixed to make a thick paste. The paste is formed into hundreds of shapes, 18-7. Noodles are made by adding egg to the pasta dough. There are five basic shapes of pasta: tubes, rods, ribbons, special shapes, and pillows (pasta filled with meat or cheese).

Most pasta and noodles are pale yellow. Sometimes other ingredients are used to add color to the pasta. For example, green pasta has spinach added. Tomatoes give pasta a pink color. The colors and shapes help make meals more appealing.

18-7 All pasta products are made from the same ingredients: flour and water. Pasta comes in many shapes, sizes, and colors.

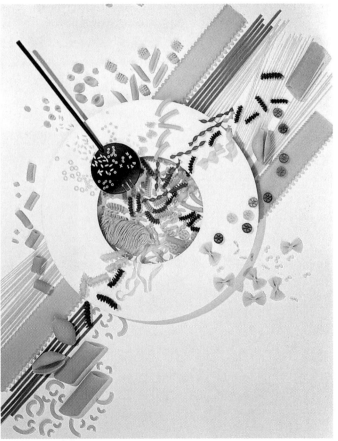

National Pasta Association

Pasta and noodles are sold in dried, fresh, canned, frozen, and ready-to-eat forms. Dried is the most common and least costly form. It is made by removing the water from fresh pasta or noodles. Fresh pasta contains more water and cooks faster than dried pasta. It is more costly than dried pasta. Canned and frozen pasta and noodles cost more than dried and fresh pastas. That is because much of the preparation already has been done when you buy them. Canned macaroni and cheese and frozen ravioli are examples.

You can buy take-out pasta and noodle dishes that are ready to eat, too. They can save you time, but they are more costly than pasta and noodle dishes made at home.

Flour

Flour is usually made from wheat, but it can be made from other grains as well, 18-8. Flour is the main ingredient in baked goods such as breads, cakes, and muffins. It also is used to thicken sauces, gravies, puddings, and pie fillings.

18-8 Flour comes in a variety of colors and textures.

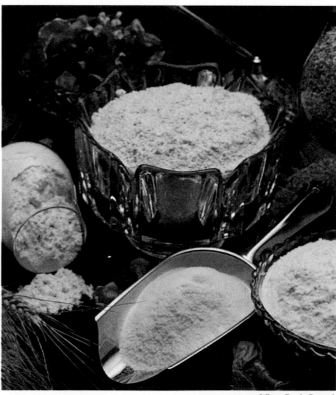

Wheat Foods Council

Whole wheat flour and several types of white flour are sold in supermarkets. There are five types of white flour. *All-purpose flour* is the most common type. It can be used in nearly all recipes. *Self-rising flour* is all-purpose flour that has salt and baking powder added to it. This flour can be used to make many breads including biscuits, muffins, and waffles. *Instant flour* is a special form of all-purpose flour. It is processed in a way that allows it to mix easily in cold liquids. It is good for making gravies and sauces. *Cake flour* feels smooth and silky. It is used to make cakes that have a light and delicate texture. *Bread flour* is used to make hearty, firm breads. It feels coarse.

All-purpose flour is usually the best buy, and it has the most uses. Whole wheat flour and other types of white flour cost a few cents more per pound. This is because they are for special purposes.

Storing Cereal Products

Properly stored dried cereal products remain fresh for a long time. Scientists have found grains stored in pyramids by ancient Egyptians, 18-9. These grains are still edible today, after 3,000 years!

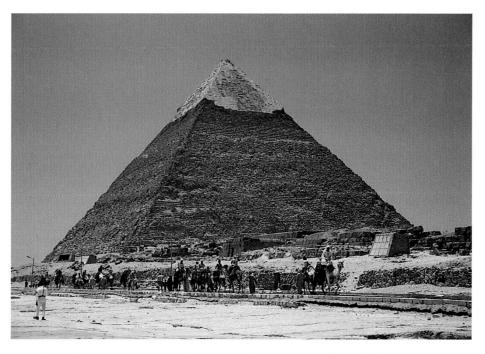

18-9 Dry, desert air preserved the grains that were stored inside the pyramids many years ago by ancient Egyptians.

Most dried cereal foods should be stored in a cool, dry place. The storage container you use should keep out pests, air, and moisture. You can keep dried cereal foods in the boxes and packages they were sold in or transfer them to airtight containers.

You can store dried rice, pasta, noodles, and white flour for a year or more. Whole grain cereal foods and breakfast cereals stay fresh for three months or longer.

Whole grain cereal foods, such as brown rice and whole wheat flour, need special care. It is best to put them in airtight containers and store them in the refrigerator. They will stay fresh longer when you store them this way. That's because oxygen in the air causes the oil in the germ to spoil. It spoils more quickly at room temperature than in the refrigerator.

After dried cereal products are cooked, put them in covered containers. Store them in the refrigerator and use them within a few days. Fresh pasta should be stored the same way. If you freeze these foods, they will retain their quality for six months.

Store unopened canned cereal foods in a cool, dry place. They will maintain their quality for a year. Place frozen cereal foods in the coldest part of your freezer. Use frozen cereal foods within three to six months.

Preparing Cereals

Cereal foods can be served at every meal. For breakfast, you could have oatmeal, toast, waffles, or muffins. At lunch, you might have cornbread, noodle soup, or a sandwich. For dinner, you may serve rice, biscuits, stuffing, or tortillas. Cereal foods, such as rye crackers and rice cakes, make good snacks.

All cereal grains must be cooked before they can be eaten. This is because the kernels are very hard. During cooking they become softer and easier to chew. Think about how hard a rice kernel is. Now think about how easy it is to chew after it is cooked. Also think about popcorn kernels before and after they are popped.

Proper cooking also improves the flavor of grains. If grains are undercooked, they are bland, crunchy, and hard to digest. Undercooked noodles and pasta are gummy and sticky. If rice, noodles, and pasta are cooked too long, they get mushy and bland.

Cooking waffles, cornbread, and other breads too long causes them to burn and become too dry.

Cereal foods provide many nutrients. Following a few tips will help you preserve their nutrients during cooking.

- Cook only until the food is done. Long cooking times destroy nutrients.
- Use the right amount of water for cereals cooked in water. Too little water causes the cereal to burn or not cook completely. Burning destroys many nutrients. If the food is not completely cooked, you probably won't eat it. That means you will miss out on the nutrients it contains. Too much water causes many nutrients to leak out of the grain into the water. When you pour off the excess water, many nutrients go down the drain.
- Don't rinse cereal foods cooked in water. Rinsing noodles, pasta, rice, and other cereals cooked in water washes away nutrients.

Hot Breakfast Cereals

Hot breakfast cereals taste great on cold mornings. The most appealing hot cereals are smooth and creamy. They don't have any hard, dry lumps.

Cooking causes the cereal's starch granules to absorb liquid. The liquid causes the granules to swell and soften. Hot breakfast cereals will be smooth if all the starch granules swell to the same size. Lumps form when the cereal sticks together during cooking. The lumps trap some granules and keep them from swelling.

To make smooth, lump-free hot cereal

1. Measure the amount of water and cereal indicated on the cereal package.
2. Bring the water to a rapid boil.
3. Stir the dry cereal slowly into boiling water. The stirring and bubbles keep the starch granules from sticking together and forming lumps.
4. After all the cereal is added and it begins to boil again, turn the heat to low.

5. Cover the pot until the cereal is done. No water should be left when the cereal is cooked. Cooking times vary, so follow the directions on the package.

Instant hot breakfast cereals are even easier to prepare. Just add boiling water to the cereal. Stir it and eat.

Rice

The best rice is tender and moist. It becomes mushy if it is cooked too long in too much water. Undercooked rice has a hard center.

Short and medium grain rice cling together when cooked. These types of rice are popular in China and Japan because they are easy to eat with chopsticks. After cooking, short and medium grain rice can be shaped by pressing it into molds. See Figure 18-10.

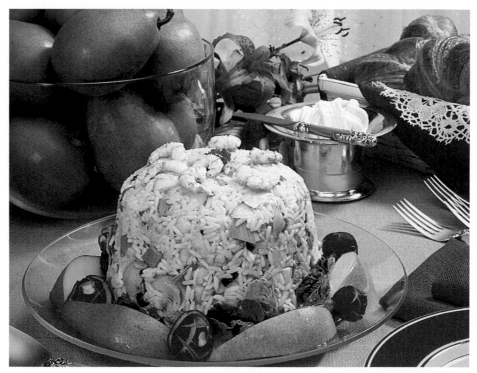

Oregon Washington California Pear Bureau

18-10 Short and medium grain rice kernels stick together when cooked. These types of rice can be used to make rice rings or molded salads.

Cooked long grain rice is light and fluffy. The grains do not stick together. This rice is used in salads, stews, and main dishes.

To cook dried rice

1. Measure the amount of water and rice indicated on the package.
2. Place the rice and water in a pot.
3. Bring the water to a boil and stir it.
4. Cover the pot and lower the heat. Simmer until done. Test doneness by tasting a cooled piece. No water should be left when the rice is cooked. Cooking times vary, so follow the directions on the package.
5. When the rice is done, fluff it gently with a fork. Serve right away.

Pasta and Noodles

When dry or fresh pasta and noodles are cooked, they absorb water and become softer. The starch in them swells and causes them to double in size.

The best pasta and noodles do not stick together, 18-11. They are cooked until they are ***al dente*** (all-DEN-tay). Al dente means that they are firm and chewy. They are not crunchy, mushy, or gummy. They are done as soon as they are not white in the center.

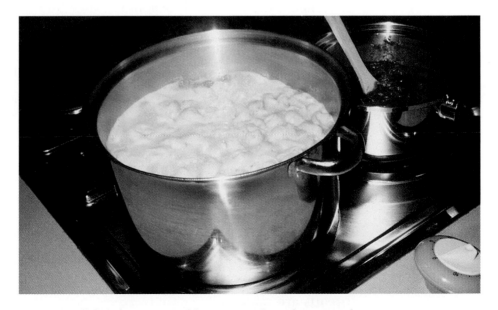

18-11 Pasta absorbs water and becomes softer when it cooks.

To cook dried pasta and noodles

1. Measure the amount of water and pasta or noodles indicated on the package.
2. Bring the water to a rapid boil.
3. Add the pasta or noodles slowly so the water doesn't stop boiling. If the water stops boiling, the pasta or noodles may stick together. Adding a teaspoon of vegetable oil to the water helps keep them from sticking together.
4. Stir once or twice gently. Rough stirring will break the pasta or noodles. If they stick together, lift the pan and carefully swirl it to shake them apart.
5. Cook only until al dente. Cooking time ranges from 1 minute to over 10 minutes. Check the package for cooking times. Test doneness by tasting a cooled piece.
6. When cooked, drain in a colander. Serve right away.

Using Flour or Cornstarch to Thicken Liquids

Flour is used to thicken gravies, sauces, puddings, and pie fillings. Cornstarch can be used to thicken liquids. When flour and cornstarch are heated in liquid, their starch granules absorb water. The water causes them to swell. They take up more space and crowd together. This causes the liquid to become thicker. This process is called *gelatinization.* The more flour or cornstarch used, the thicker the liquid will become.

The best gravies, sauces, puddings, and pie fillings are smooth and creamy. They don't have any lumps. They are smooth when all the starch granules in the flour or cornstarch swell evenly.

Lumps form when the starch granules stick together during cooking. This happens when flour or cornstarch is added to a hot liquid. To avoid lumps

1. Mix the flour or cornstarch with a small amount of sugar, fat, or cold liquid. Your recipe will tell you which to use.
2. Add the flour or cornstarch mixture to the other ingredients.
3. The mixture is cooked for a minute or more. If the mixture is cooked on the range, stir until it is thick and bubbly.

Flours from various grains are also used to make many different types of breads. In the next chapter, you'll find out how breads are made.

Cultures of the World

Italy: Your Pasta Passport

Italy is a long and narrow country. It is shaped like a boot. Most of it juts into the Mediterranean Sea. There are many well-known cities in Italy, like Rome, Genoa, and Venice. Venice is unique because instead of having streets, Venice has canals. People travel around town in boats called gondolas (gohn-DOE-lahs) instead of cars and buses.

Grains, fruits, and vegetables thrive in Italy's sunny weather and fertile soil. Rice and corn dishes are common in northern Italy. Rice is used to make a dish called *risotto* (rih-ZOE-toe). A pudding called *polenta* (poh-LEN-tah) is made with cornmeal. Wheat is used to make bread and pasta. Many bakeries in Italy bake bread twice a day. Shoppers can buy warm, fresh bread for breakfast and for dinner. Pasta is popular all over Italy. Many people eat it for lunch and dinner. There are over 500 types of pasta and a wide range of sauces for it.

Olives and tomatoes are grown in Italy. Olive oil is used in cooking and for salad dressing. Tomatoes are one of the most liked vegetables in Italy. They may be eaten fresh or cooked to make a tomato sauce for pasta. *Pasta Bolognese* (boh-loh-NAYS) is a popular pasta dish made with tomato sauce.

Many sheep, goats, and cattle are raised in northern Italy. These animals provide meat, milk, butter, and cheese.

Italy is famous for its cheeses. *Parmesan* (PAR-mih-zhahn) and *Romano* (roe-MAHN-oh) cheeses are sprinkled on pasta dishes. Creamy *ricotta* (rih-COT-ah) cheese is added to lasagna and ravioli. Pizza is topped with *mozzarella* (motz-ah-RELL-ah) cheese. In Italy, mozzarella often is made with buffalo milk.

Milk may be used to make ice cream. Italians call this cool, tasty food *gelati* (jeh-LAH-tee). It was invented by the Italian cafe owner *Tortoni* (tore-TOE-nee) in the 1700s. Since he invented gelati, ice cream has become popular worldwide.

Italians value very fresh food. Some visit three or more food stores each day. They may buy pasta in one store and cheese in another. Sausages such as salami, pepperoni, and mortadella may be sold in yet another store. The next time you go to the supermarket, consider putting foods from Italy on your shopping list.

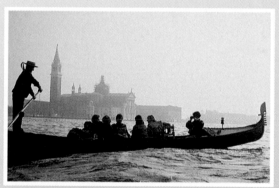

Abercrombie & Kent International

The canals of Venice make it one of Italy's most unique cities.

In a Nutshell

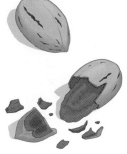

- Many people all over the world rely on cereals for most of their nutrients and calories.
- Grain kernels have three parts: bran, endosperm, and germ.
- The most nutritious cereal foods include all three parts of the grain kernel.
- Foods made with only the endosperm often are enriched with thiamin, riboflavin, niacin, folate, and iron.
- Wheat, corn, rice, oats, barley, and rye are types of grains.
- Cereals can be stored easily for long periods.
- Cereal buying decisions depend on your time schedule, your tastes, and your budget.
- All cereal grains must be cooked to make them easier to eat and digest.
- Cooking causes the starch granules in cereals to absorb liquid, swell, and soften.

In the Know

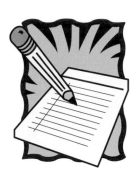

1. Draw and label the three parts of a grain kernel. List the nutrients each contains.
2. White flour is made from the _____ portion of the kernel.
3. List six types of grains. Name an example of one food made from each type.
4. Which cereal is likely to cost the least?
   A. Sugar-coated wheat flakes.
   B. Puffed rice.
   C. Oatmeal raisin cereal.
   D. Corn flakes with nuts and berries.
5. True or false? Fresh pasta should be stored in a cool, dry place.
6. How can you prevent lumps in a sauce thickened with flour?
   A. Mix the flour with cold water.
   B. Mix the flour with sugar.
   C. Mix the flour with fat.
   D. All of the above.
7. True or false? Pasta that is gummy and sticky was cooked in too much water.
8. Explain how flour thickens liquids.

What Would You Do?

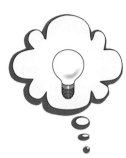

Pretend that your family eats three or four boxes of cereal each week. Their favorite cereals have added nuts, dried fruits, and sugar. These cereals are quite costly. When your mother quit work to go to college, everyone agreed to help cut costs. How can your family save money on breakfast cereals?

Expanding Your Knowledge

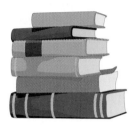

1. Design a mobile that shows foods made with grains. You could limit your mobile to food made with just one grain such as corn. Collect or draw pictures of cereal foods and glue them to pieces of poster board. Punch a hole in the top of each drawing or picture. Thread a string through the hole and tie one end to the picture. Tie the other end to a coat hanger. Repeat until all the pictures are tied to the hanger. Display the mobile in the school cafeteria.

2. Set up a taste panel to compare the flavors, smells, textures, and colors of breakfast cereals made from different grains. For example, you could sample corn flakes, oatmeal, puffed rice, shredded wheat, and farina.

3. Test the effects of cooking time on pasta. Prepare one cup of dried pasta by placing it in two cups of boiling water. Remove a few pieces of pasta after 30 seconds, 1, 2, 3, 5, 10, and 15 minutes. Compare the taste, color, and texture of the seven samples.

4. Write and produce a radio or television commercial to sell a cereal food. Include facts about its nutrients and how to prepare it. Test your advertisement by asking yourself, "Does the ad make me want to eat this grain food?" Tape record or videotape the advertisements to play for classmates or younger children.

5. Show how gelatinization works. Prepare a flour paste that could be used to thicken a sauce. Compare the texture of the two samples.
   Variation A:
   Mix 3 tablespoons of flour in ½ cup of cold water. Slowly add to ½ cup of boiling water. Boil one minute, stirring constantly.
   Variation B:
   Bring 1 cup of water to a boil. Add 3 tablespoons of flour. Boil one minute, stirring constantly.

6. Visit a supermarket. Make a list of all the foods made from grains that you see. How are grain foods packaged? Do you think the packaging protects the grain foods and keeps them fresh? Why or why not?

7. Grains are good sources of fiber. Do some research to find out more about fiber. You could research its sources and functions. Also find out why scientists think fiber could help prevent heart disease and certain cancers. Report your findings to the class.

8. Prepare instant, quick-cooking, and regular oatmeal. Compare the flavor, texture, and appeal of each. Also compare the cost and preparation time. Which do you prefer? Why?

9. Discover how proper storage affects popcorn. Count out two batches of 100 popcorn kernels each. Place one batch in an airtight container and store in a cool, dry place. Place the other batch in an open container and store in a warm, dry place (maybe over an oven). After two weeks, pop one batch. Count the number of unpopped kernels. Lay 15 popped kernels side by side. Use a ruler to measure their length. Repeat this procedure for the second batch. How do the batches compare? Which batch had the most unpopped kernels? Which batch produced the largest popped kernels? Why do you think these differences occurred? (HINT: Heat and uncovered storage cause water to evaporate.) How can you use this information? (To shorten the time needed for this activity, place the batch of popcorn kernels to be stored in an open container in a warm location in a cake pan. Heat them for 90 minutes in a 200°F (90°C) oven. This procedure simulates two weeks of improper storage.)

Chapter 19
Bountiful Breads

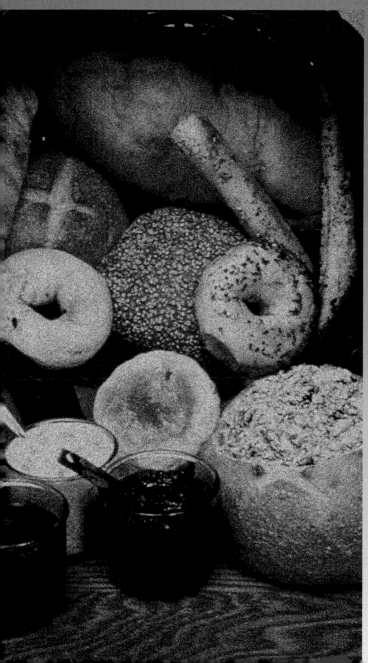

Objectives

After reading this chapter, you will be able to
- ❏ describe the types of breads available.
- ❏ store breads to maintain freshness.
- ❏ explain the function of each ingredient in breads.
- ❏ explain how to blend bread ingredients.

New Terms

leavening agent: ingredient added to baked goods that produces gas bubbles which cause the baked goods to rise.

gluten: a sticky, elastic protein that forms when flour is mixed with liquid.

batter: a mixture consisting of flour and liquid that can be poured.

dough: a mixture consisting of flour and liquid that is thick and stiff enough to be handled or kneaded.

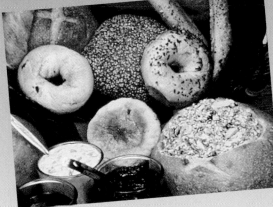

Wheat Foods Council

437

Breads are popular in every corner of the world. Bakers in the United States have borrowed many bread recipes from other countries. That means your taste buds can travel the globe without going any further than your kitchen.

When your menu includes pancakes, you are serving a bread from Sweden. Your breakfast waffles are a creation from Belgium. The tortilla holding your tasty taco comes from sunny Mexico. Soda bread is a treat from Ireland. There is pita bread from the Middle East and pumpernickel from Russia. The variety is almost endless.

Bread baking is one of the oldest industries in the world. Records show that there were bakeries over 4,000 years ago. Bread has always been a vital food. It has provided nutrients and calories to humans for thousands of years, 19-1.

All breads are good sources of carbohydrate and protein. The other nutrients in bread depend on the ingredients used. For example, bread made with milk will contain calcium. Nuts and seeds supply fat and fiber. Fruits add vitamins and minerals.

19-1 People in every nation eat breads. These low-cost, nutritious foods are popular in the United States, too. Millions of loaves are baked in the United States every day.

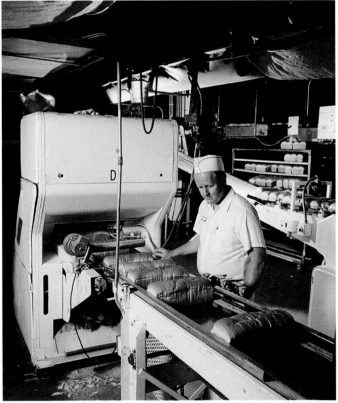

©Eastman Chemical Company, 1994

Types of Bread

There are so many bread choices, you could eat a different bread every day of the year! You might choose bite-size muffins or a long, crusty loaf of French bread. Chewy bagels, crumbly cornbread, and hot rolls are other options. Sweet raisin bread and dark rye bread are tasty choices, too.

All breads can be placed in one of two groups: leavened and unleavened. Leavened breads are puffy and light. That's because they contain a ***leavening agent***. This is an ingredient that produces gas bubbles in breads and other baked goods. The gas bubbles cause baked goods to expand and rise, 19-2. Unleavened breads do not contain leavening agents. These breads are flat, dense, and heavy.

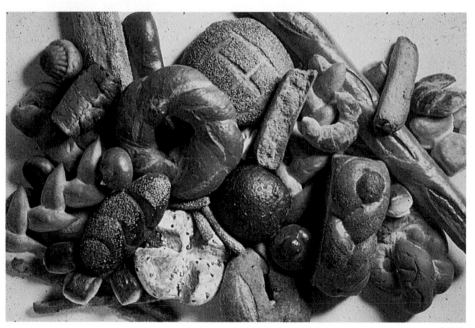

USDA

19-2 Leavened breads are puffy. They expand when they are cooked.

Unleavened Breads

Unleavened breads are also called flat breads, 19-3. These breads rise very little during cooking. They are much flatter than leavened breads.

19-3 Unleavened breads are flat. They rise little when cooked because they lack a leavening agent.

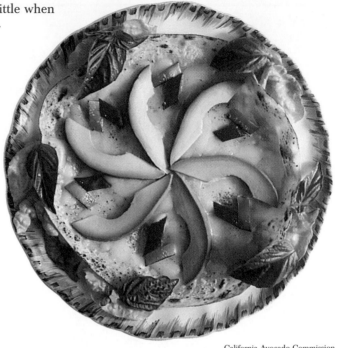

California Avocado Commission

People began making flat breads over 12,000 years ago. The first breads did not rise because no one knew about leavening agents. Tortillas and crepes are examples of flat breads. Leavening agents were discovered about 5,000 years ago. Since that time, people could choose flat breads or leavened breads.

Leavened Breads

Leavened breads contain baking soda, baking powder, or yeast. These leavening agents produce a gas called carbon dioxide (CAR-bun DIE-ox-eyed). The gas causes the bread to rise during baking. Sometimes eggs are used as a leavening agent to add another gas—air—into breads. Leavened breads increase in size and become light and fluffy.

Leavened breads can be either quick breads or yeast breads. The leavening agents in quick breads arc baking soda, baking powder, or both. These leavening agents produce gas quickly. This is why these breads are called "quick" breads. Biscuits, waffles, and muffins are quick breads. Sometimes eggs are also used as a leavening agent in quick breads.

Cultures of the World

The Breads of India

India is a large country on the north coast of the Indian Ocean. Its landscape includes rugged mountains, deserts, and rainforests. The Taj Mahal is one of this country's most famous buildings. It is made of white marble.

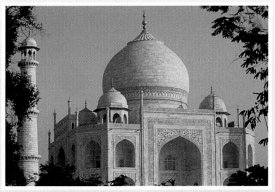

Abercrombie & Kent International

The Taj Mahal is just one of the many interesting places to see in India.

Farming is very important in India. Three out of four people work to grow crops. Rice, wheat, corn, peas, and beans are the major food crops.

In India, wheat is a major part of the diet. Most families eat wheat bread at every meal. Many breads, such as chapatis, purees, and parathas, are unleavened. *Chapatis* (cha-PAH-tees) are baked on the cooktop. *Purees* (POOH-rees) are deep-fried bread. *Paratha* (pah-RAH-tah) is a bread stuffed with meat or vegetables. *Naan* (NANH) is a leavened bread that is baked in a clay oven called a *tandoor* (tan-DOOER).

Chapatis are the best known bread from India. Many rural families grind their wheat to make chapatis every day. In cities, people make chapatis at home or buy them at food stores. Some people work as chapati makers. Each day, they go house to house making chapatis.

Spices give Indian food its unique taste. Common Indian spices include saffron, fenugreek, cumin, coriander, turmeric, and fennel. Foods made with these spices are called *curry* (KUR-ee). The flavor of curried foods differs in each region of India. The taste depends on the amount of each spice used.

Buttermilk, fruit juice, water, coffee, and tea are common drinks in India. Coconut milk is a popular beverage in towns along the coast. Water buffalo are the main source of milk. Milk is used to make yogurt, buttermilk, butter, and sweets.

Sweets are made by simmering milk until it is thick. Then sugar, nuts, cinnamon, fruits, rice, or wheat are added. *Halva* (HAHL-vah) is a thick pudding made with milk, wheat, and dried fruit or nuts. The sweet *basundi* (bah-SOON-dee) is made with the spice saffron, which gives it a bright yellow color.

In rural areas, the main meal is served at midday. In cities, dinner is usually the main meal. The meal may include chapatis, a vegetable stew, rice, and perhaps chutney. If the family is not vegetarian, meat or fish may be served. For a real treat, look for opportunities to try foods from India.

Yeast, a tiny plant, is the leavening agent used in yeast breads. Yeast breads take longer to rise than quick breads because yeast slowly produces gas. Italian bread, bagels, and rolls are yeast breads.

Buying and Storing Breads

Supermarkets sell many convenience forms of bread. You can buy bread mixes, refrigerated and frozen breads, and ready-to-eat breads. Of course, you also can buy the ingredients needed to make bread from scratch.

The cost of bread depends on the amount of convenience it offers. Ready-to-eat breads often cost more than those that require some preparation. Breads made from scratch usually cost less than convenience forms. You may find that convenience forms are worth the extra cost if your time is too limited to make breads from scratch.

Bread Mixes

Bread mixes need more preparation than other convenience forms. The ingredients in the mix are already measured and mixed together. You will need to blend in one or more ingredients and cook the bread. Supermarkets carry mixes for waffles, pancakes, biscuits, muffins, cornbread, and fruit breads. You can buy yeast bread mixes for use in bread machines, too.

Bread mixes can be stored in their package or in an airtight container. Keep mixes in a cool, dry location. Carefully stored mixes stay fresh for six months or more.

Refrigerated and Frozen Batters and Doughs

Refrigerated and frozen batters and doughs are a blend of all the ingredients needed to make bread. These batters and doughs are ready to cook. No other preparation is needed. These products often cost more than mixes and less than ready-to-eat bread.

Refrigerated batters and doughs include croissants, biscuits, and rolls. Keep them in the refrigerator until you are ready to cook them. They will stay fresh for a month or more.

Frozen batters and doughs include pancake batter, bread dough, and pizza crusts. They will stay fresh in the freezer for three months or more. Keep them frozen until you are ready to prepare them.

Frozen Breads

Frozen breads are already cooked. They are ready to serve once they are thawed. Many people prefer to heat them before serving. Frozen waffles, pancakes, and muffins are types of frozen breads. Ready-to-eat breads cost more than frozen breads.

Keep frozen breads frozen until you are ready to eat them. If they are kept frozen, they will stay fresh for three months or more.

Ready-to-Eat Bread Products

Ready-to-eat bread products, such as muffins, biscuits, rolls, and breads, are sold in bakeries. These items need no preparation. They are made fresh daily, and they are the most costly form of bread, 19-4.

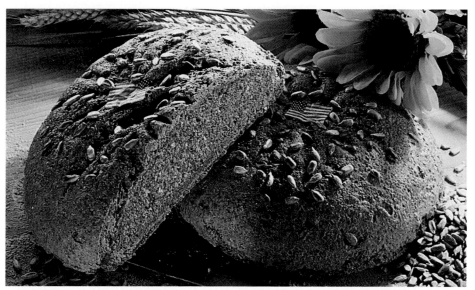

National Sunflower Association

19-4 Bakery breads usually cost more than other types of breads.

Ready-to-eat breads sold in supermarkets often cost less than bakery items. These breads are made at large commercial bakeries. Then they are wrapped and shipped to many supermarkets.

The cost of supermarket shelf bread depends on the size of the loaf, ingredients used, and brand. Large loaves usually cost less per serving than small loaves. Special ingredients, such as cheese, fruit, and nuts, increase the price. Store brands usually cost less than name brands.

Most supermarket shelf breads are cooked completely. You can eat them right out of the package. However, brown-and-serve breads are partially baked. They are very pale and look uncooked. These breads need to be browned in the oven before serving.

Ready-to-eat breads lose their freshness rapidly. They become stale and dry out fast. After bread mixes, refrigerated and frozen batters and doughs, and frozen breads are prepared, they can become stale quickly, too. To preserve the quality of breads, store them in a tightly closed container in a cool, dry place. They will stay fresh for about one week.

In hot, humid weather, mold forms quickly on breads. This is why breads should be stored in the refrigerator. They may become stale faster in the refrigerator, but the bread will stay mold-free longer.

Ready-to-eat breads and breads prepared from mixes, batters, and doughs can be frozen. Wrapped tightly, they will stay fresh in the freezer for two to four months. When you are ready to serve the frozen bread, thaw it at room temperature. To serve it warm, wrap the bread in aluminum foil and heat it in the oven. Loosely wrap it in a cloth or paper towel if you plan to heat it in a microwave oven.

Preparing Breads

Freshly baked bread is difficult to resist. It smells delicious and tastes great. Quick breads are fast and easy to make, 19-5. Yeast breads require a little more time to prepare.

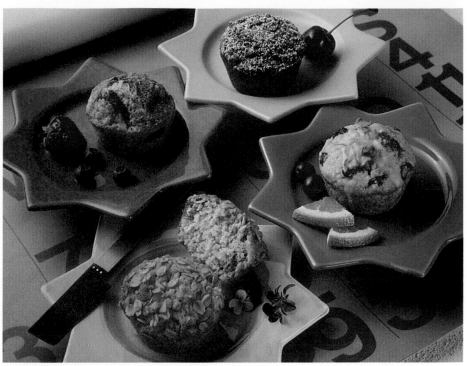

19-5 Home-baked breads make a delicious addition to any meal.

Basic Ingredients

Hundreds of different breads can be created by varying the amounts of six basic ingredients. These ingredients are flour, liquid, eggs, sugar, fat, and leavening agents.

Flour

Flour gives bread its structure. The structure is created by *gluten* (GLOO-ten). Gluten is a protein found in wheat that forms when flour is mixed with liquid. Gluten makes the flour and liquid mixture sticky and elastic.

Under a microscope, gluten looks like threads. The gluten threads are elastic. They can stretch and contract. Gluten lets the flour mixture stretch and trap bubbles. It works just like bubble gum, 19-6.

19-6 Leavening agents produce gas and cause bread to puff up. The same thing happens when you blow a gum bubble. You blow gas from your lungs (such as carbon dioxide) into the gum. The gum traps the gas and expands.

Thousands of tiny gas bubbles form when a leavening agent is added to the mixture. As the bread cooks, the tiny gas bubbles expand. The gluten stretches like a balloon to trap the expanding gas bubbles. The trapped gas makes the bread rise.

During cooking, the gluten becomes stiff. Once cooking is finished, the bread will be firm. It will keep its new shape. When you look at a slice of bread, it is easy to see where the tiny bubbles were.

Most breads use all-purpose flour. Whole wheat flour or cornmeal can be used, too. Recipes always tell you when a special flour is needed.

Leavening Agents

Leavening agents produce the gas bubbles that cause bread and other baked goods to expand and rise. As the bread rises, it becomes light and porous. The three leavening gases are air, steam, and carbon dioxide. In some breads, like cream puffs, one leavening gas produces most of the gas. In others, such as banana bread, all three gases work together to cause the bread to rise.

Air becomes incorporated in breads when you sift flour, beat eggs, cream fat and sugar together, and beat or knead ingredients. All breads use some air as a leavening gas.

Steam is produced when most breads are cooked. Hot cooking temperatures cause the liquids to boil and become steam. Liquids expand when they become steam. For instance, the steam produced by one cup of liquid water may fill two cups or more. This expansion causes breads to rise.

Carbon dioxide is produced by reactions between ingredients in bread. Three ingredients that may be used to produce carbon dioxide are baking soda, baking powder, and yeast.

Baking soda produces carbon dioxide when mixed with an acid. Acids are found in fruit, fruit juice, chocolate, buttermilk, sour cream, and yogurt. If no acid is added, baking soda cannot produce carbon dioxide gas.

Baking powder is a blend of baking soda and a dry acid powder. Baking powder releases carbon dioxide when mixed with a liquid and heated.

Yeast is a tiny plant. It grows and produces gas when mixed with warm, moist ingredients. Packages of yeast are stamped with a date. The yeast should be used before that date. After that date, the yeast won't produce as much gas and your bread will not rise as much as it should.

Liquid

Liquid ingredients moisten and blend the dry ingredients. They help flour to form gluten. When cooked, liquids also form steam that acts as a leavening agent.

Most recipes use milk, water, or juice. Some recipes call for yogurt or sour cream. Recipes list the type and amount of liquid needed.

Sugar

Sugar adds flavor and sweetness to bread. It also helps the bread form a brown, crisp crust, 19-7.

19-7 Through experimentation, food technologists have determined the effect of each ingredient used in breads.

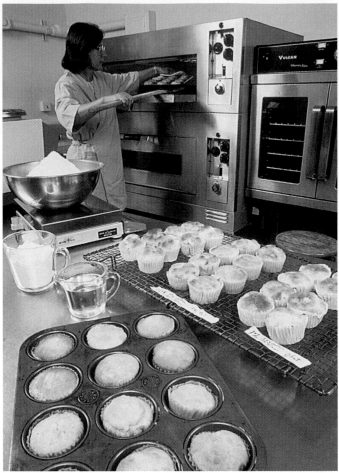

USDA

Sugar makes breads tender, too. It does this by preventing the gluten from becoming too elastic. The bread is chewy and tough when the gluten becomes too elastic.

Breads can be sweetened with many different ingredients. The recipe will tell you which to use. Sugar, brown sugar, honey, molasses, and syrup are commonly added to bread.

Eggs

Eggs add color and flavor to breads. Egg yolks are an emulsifier, so they help blend the ingredients.

Eggs also help bread to rise. When eggs are beaten, they form many tiny air bubbles. The air bubbles expand during cooking and cause the bread to rise.

Fat

Fat adds flavor to bread. It helps to make the bread tender by keeping the gluten threads from becoming too long. Long gluten threads make bread tough.

Recipes list the type and amount of fat needed. Some breads are made with solid fats. Margarine, butter, vegetable shortening, and lard are examples. Liquid fats, such as corn oil and sunflower oil, are used in other bread recipes.

Ingredient Mixtures in Breads

Breads are made of two types of mixtures: batters or doughs. The main difference between batters and doughs is the amount of liquid compared to the amount of flour used.

Batters have a large amount of liquid compared to the amount of flour. They are thinner than doughs. Batters have so much liquid that they can be poured or dropped from a spoon. Pancakes and muffins are made from batters.

Doughs are thick and stiff. They have a small amount of liquid compared to the amount of flour. Doughs are thick enough to be kneaded or rolled. Biscuits and rolls are made with dough.

Methods for Combining Ingredients

There are two methods for blending quick bread ingredients. Batters are mixed using the muffin method. Doughs are mixed using the biscuit method.

Muffin Method

The muffin method is used to mix batter for fruit bread, pancakes, waffles, cornbread, muffins, and brownies, 19-8. In the muffin method, the dry ingredients are sifted together in a bowl. Oil or melted fat is used and combined with the liquid ingredients in another bowl. The last step is to combine the liquid and dry ingredients into one bowl. The ingredients should be mixed only enough to moisten the dry ingredients. Some small lumps will remain in the batter. Overmixing will cause the bread to be tough and have tunnels running through it.

19-8 The ingredients for these breads were combined using the muffin method.

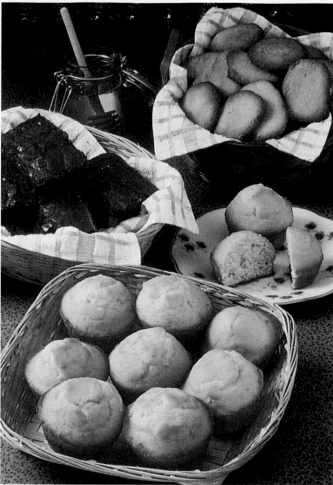

USDA

 Science in the Kitchen

Making Muffins

Each ingredient in bread plays an important role. Omitting an ingredient can change the muffin's color, flavor, and appeal. This experiment lets you examine the effect of each ingredient in muffins. To begin, gather the ingredients needed for each variation of this experiment.

Variation A:
1 cup sifted flour
½ cup milk
½ teaspoon salt

Variation B:
all ingredients in Variation A plus 1½ teaspoons baking powder

Variation C:
all ingredients in Variations A and B plus 1½ tablespoons oil

Variation D:
all ingredients in Variations A, B, and C plus 1½ tablespoons sugar

Variation E:
all ingredients in Variations A, B, C, and D plus 2 tablespoons beaten egg

For each variation, follow these steps.

1. Preheat an oven to 425°F (220°C) and grease a muffin pan.
2. Sift together the dry ingredients in a bowl.
3. Blend all liquid ingredients together in a second bowl.
4. Add the liquid ingredients to the dry ingredients. Stir only 15 times. The batter will be lumpy.
5. Place ¼ cup of batter in each greased muffin cup. Bake 20 minutes.
6. Remove from pan and cool.

Observe the color, shape, and visual appeal of each variation. Measure the height with a ruler. Cut each muffin variation in half and check its color and appearance. Taste it and note its tenderness and flavor. Ask yourself these questions.

1. How did the baking powder affect the muffins? Which muffin was flattest? Which was tallest?
2. What effect did the oil have on the muffins? Which muffin was toughest (needed the most chews)? Which was the most tender (needed the least chews)?
3. What effect did the sugar have on the muffins? Which muffin had the best color? Which had the best flavor? Which was the most crisp?
4. What effect did the egg have on the muffins?
5. How can you use this information?

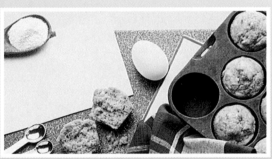

USDA

Each ingredient plays an important role in producing great tasting muffins.

Biscuit Method

The biscuit method is used to mix dough for dumplings, turnovers, biscuits, rolls, and pot pie crusts. Dough can be rolled out and cut or dropped by spoonfuls onto a baking sheet.

In the biscuit method, the dry ingredients are sifted together in one bowl. Solid fat is used with this method. This ingredient gives breads a flaky texture. The solid fat must be cut into the dry mixture with a pastry blender or two knives. The mixture should look like coarse crumbs. The liquid ingredients are combined in a second bowl and added to the dry ingredients. The ingredients are mixed with a fork until a dough ball forms around the fork. In 19-9, you can see how the blending of ingredients in the muffin and biscuit methods differ.

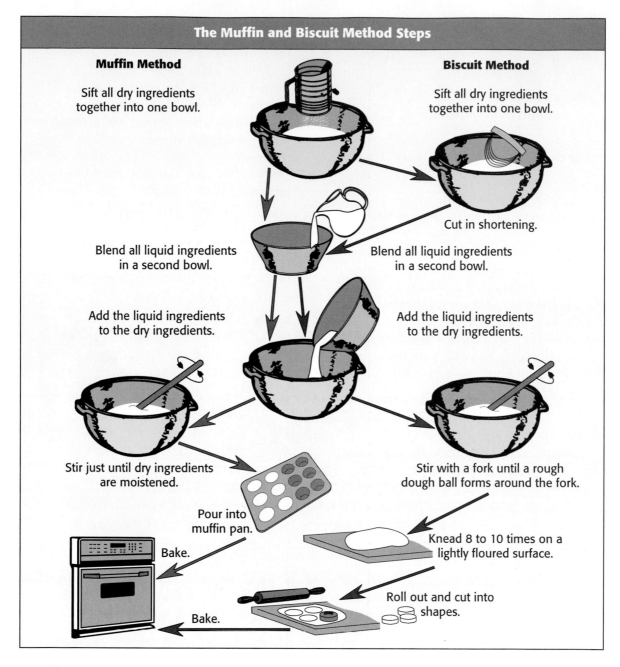

The Muffin and Biscuit Method Steps

Muffin Method

Sift all dry ingredients together into one bowl.

Blend all liquid ingredients in a second bowl.

Add the liquid ingredients to the dry ingredients.

Stir just until dry ingredients are moistened.

Pour into muffin pan.

Bake.

Biscuit Method

Sift all dry ingredients together into one bowl.

Cut in shortening.

Blend all liquid ingredients in a second bowl.

Add the liquid ingredients to the dry ingredients.

Stir with a fork until a rough dough ball forms around the fork.

Knead 8 to 10 times on a lightly floured surface.

Roll out and cut into shapes.

Bake.

19-9 This diagram compares and contrasts the muffin and biscuit methods of making breads.

Once ingredients blended using the biscuit method form a dough ball, the dough ball needs to be placed on a lightly floured surface. After it is quickly and gently kneaded 8 to 10 times, it is ready to roll out, cut into shapes, and bake.

Baking and Cooking Breads _____

After the ingredients are mixed together, they are cooked. Most breads are baked. Some are cooked in a skillet, griddle, or waffle iron. Doughnuts may be deep-fried.

The breads you make will be tasty and appealing if you follow the recipe carefully. You can ensure success by asking yourself these questions each time you make breads. You can find most of the answers in the recipe!

- How do I blend the ingredients? The recipe will tell you what method to use.
- What size pan do I need? Many recipes list the size pan needed. The right size pan is important. If the pan is too big, the batter or dough will spread out too far. The bread will be thin and dry. If the pan is too small, the bread will overflow.
- Do I need to grease the pan? Some breads are baked in a greased pan, others are not. Check the recipe to see if you need to grease the pan. Some batters stick if the pan is not greased. If the batter sticks, your bread will tear when you try to remove it from the pan.
- How hot should the oven be? Most breads are baked in a preheated oven. The recipe will tell you what the oven temperature should be. The oven temperature determines how fast your bread will bake. If the temperature is too high, the crust will bake too fast. The crust gets hard and cracks when the bread tries to rise. High temperatures also make the crust too brown. If the oven temperature is too low, the bread cooks too slowly. The mixture doesn't become firm fast enough, and the leavening gas escapes. The bread will be flat and dry.
- Where should I place the pans in the oven? Be sure to keep pans from touching the sides, top, bottom, or door of the oven. Also, don't let pans touch each other. The part of the pan that touches the oven or another pan gets too hot. Parts that are too hot will become very brown and dry. If you have one pan, center it on the middle shelf of the oven. This allows the air to move around it. If you have more than one pan, arrange them as shown in the diagram, 19-10.

One Pan

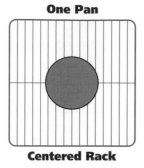

Centered Rack

Two Pans

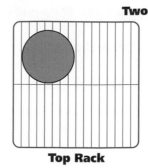

Top Rack

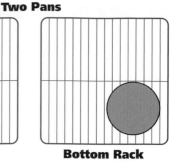

Bottom Rack

19-10 It is important to arrange pans on oven racks so air can move around the pans. If you are placing two pans in the oven, place them as shown here.

Focus on Food

Hungry People

More than half the people in the world do not get enough to eat. Most of world's hungry people live in Asia, Africa, and Latin America. Their hunger is so severe that they are often sick. They are so weak that they cannot work hard or concentrate in school. Children and teens do not grow normally.

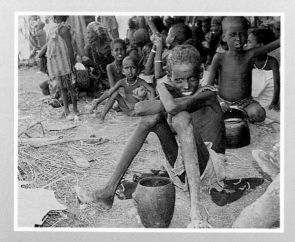

Many people in the world do not have enough to eat. There are ways you can help to solve this problem.

The world's farmers grow enough food to feed every person on earth. Why, then, do some go hungry? The main reason is that they are very poor. They have too little money to buy the food they need. Over half of the people on earth earn less than $5 per week. They spend almost all of it on food. Even then, it's not enough money to buy all the food they need.

Poor, hungry people are likely to remain poor and hungry throughout their lives. In many parts of the world, parents must pay for children to go to school. Poor families often cannot afford to send their children to school. People who never learn to read or write can only get low-paying jobs.

Most of the poor, hungry people live in rural areas. It is hard to deliver food to these areas because many poor countries have few roads and lack delivery trucks and planes. It is difficult for these people to grow enough food to feed their families. This is because they lack the money needed to buy seeds, tools, and fertilizer.

Their land is often too rocky, dry, or mountainous to farm. Large companies usually own the best farmland. They use it to grow foods that can be sold to richer countries. Local people may be hired to work for the large companies. However, the pay is so low that workers often cannot afford to buy the crops they tend.

Some of the food that poor people are able to grow or buy rots or is eaten by pests. This is because they lack places to store their food to keep it safe.

The governments of poor countries often cannot offer much help to hungry people. This may be because they are forced to spend their money to defend the country from invading groups. They may have to spend it to rebuild hospitals damaged by floods or earthquakes. They may not be aware that people are going hungry.

People all over the world are working to end hunger. Through the following steps, you can help, too.

1. Learn more about hunger. Read the newspaper. Do research on the Internet. Check your local library for books on hunger. Then, teach others what you have learned. You could give presentations in your neighborhood. You could write a letter for the school newspaper. Ask your friends to help.

2. Become involved with local groups who are working to end hunger. If you can't find a group, think about starting one.

3. Write letters to government officials. Let them know your concerns about hunger. Ask them what they are doing to end hunger. You may want to write your governor, senators, and representatives. You could even write to the President of the United States.

- Can I cook bread in a microwave oven? Breads can be cooked or thawed in a microwave oven. To keep them from looking pale and uncooked, you can use a special browning dish. You also can brown the bread in a conventional or convection oven after it's cooked. Also, you can top breads cooked in a microwave oven with brown sugar to disguise their paleness.
- How do I know when the bread is done? Recipes state the amount of cooking time needed. Breads are done when they are golden brown and firm. They should spring back when you touch them lightly. The *toothpick test* is another way to see if quick bread is done. To perform this test, insert a toothpick in the thickest part of the bread. Remove the toothpick and examine it. If batter coats the toothpick, the bread needs to cook longer. The bread is done when the toothpick comes out clean.
- When should I remove bread from the pan? Some breads are removed as soon as they are taken out of the oven. Others need to cool a few minutes before removing them. Some cool completely in the pan. Check the recipe to find out when the bread

should be removed. When it's time to remove a bread, run a spatula around the edge of the pan. Place a rack over the top of the bread. Carefully turn the pan and the rack over together. Gently shake the pan to loosen the bread. If you followed the recipe carefully, you should find a delicious, golden brown bread when you lift off the pan.

In a Nutshell

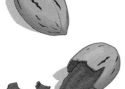

- Breads are eaten in every country.
- Breads are good sources of carbohydrate and protein.
- Unleavened breads rise very little during cooking because they do not contain a leavening agent.
- Leavened breads contain a leavening agent that causes the bread to rise during cooking.
- Supermarkets sell many convenience forms of bread.
- Flour, liquid, eggs, sugar, fat, and leavening agents are the basic ingredients used to make breads.
- Bread ingredients are blended using either the muffin method or biscuit method.

In the Know

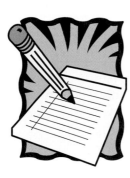

1. Describe two main differences between unleavened and leavened breads.
2. True or false? Once bread mixes are prepared, they should be stored like ready-to-eat breads.
3. Describe the roles of each of the six basic ingredients in breads.
4. Name two leavening agents used in quick breads.
5. Explain how leavening agents cause bread to rise.
6. Mixtures of bread ingredients are called either batters or doughs. Describe how these differ.
7. Bread ingredients blended using the _____ method are kneaded on a lightly floured surface.
8. The oven temperature is too high if the crust _____.
   A. cooks too fast
   B. becomes hard and cracks
   C. is too brown
   D. All of the above.
9. Make a diagram of how you would arrange two pans in the oven.

What Would You Do?

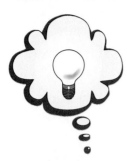

Your family enjoys toasted white bread for breakfast. Sliced Italian bread or rolls are served at lunch and dinner. Your dad heard that most people do not get enough fiber. He wonders if your family should make some changes in the breads served. What advice would you give him? What breads would you recommend? What can you do to help your family try new breads?

Expanding Your Knowledge

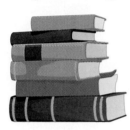

1. Design a bulletin board that uses a map to show where breads originated. For example, you could place a picture of a crepe near France or a chapati near India. Use string and tacks to connect the picture of the bread with its origin.
2. Visit a bakery and watch bakery products being prepared. What types of ingredients are used? How are the ingredients measured? How are they mixed and cooked? Ask the baker how he or she prepared to become a baker.
3. Examine bread recipes in cookbooks. Which recipes blend the ingredients using the muffin method? Which use the biscuit method? Select a recipe using the muffin method and another using the biscuit method. Prepare the breads and compare them.
4. Select a basic muffin recipe. Prepare the same recipe using different flours. You could use these flours: white, bread, cake, rye, whole wheat, and soy. Observe the color, texture, and appeal of muffins made with different types of flour. Set up a taste panel to sample the muffins.
5. Visit a supermarket and record the cost of a bread mix, refrigerated bread dough, frozen bread, and ready-to-eat bread from the bakery and supermarket. Find a bread recipe in a cookbook and determine the cost of its ingredients. Which form of bread is the best buy? How much time does it take to prepare each form?
6. Make biscuits from scratch, refrigerated dough, and a mix. Compare the taste and appeal of each. Which do you prefer? Why?

Chapter **20**
Dairy Delights

Objectives

After reading this chapter, you will be able to

- ❏ describe the types of dairy products on the market.
- ❏ select dairy products in the supermarket.
- ❏ store dairy products to preserve nutrients, appeal, and safety.
- ❏ explain how to heat milk and cheese.

New Terms

homogenized: milk or cream in which the fat has been broken into tiny pieces by a special process. This process keeps the fat and watery liquid in milk or cream from separating.

pasteurized: milk or cream that has been heated to a high temperature for a few seconds to kill harmful bacteria.

cultured milk products: dairy products produced by adding certain helpful bacteria to milk.

curds: the solid pieces in milk that can stick together to form lumps.

whey: the liquid portion of milk that is left after curds form.

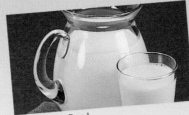

National Dairy Board

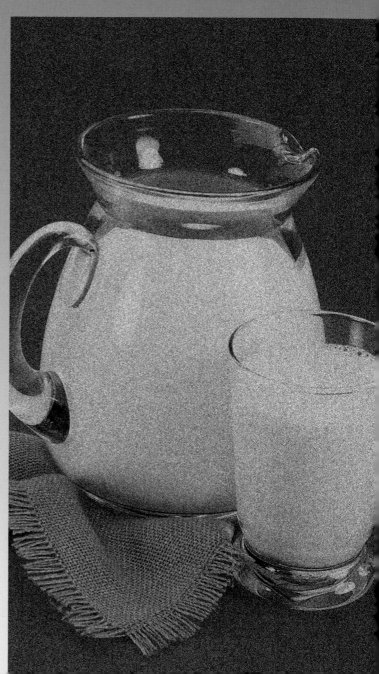

People all over the world eat dairy products. In fact, milk is the first food almost every baby eats. Milk isn't just for babies, though. Everyone, at all ages, needs dairy products in their diet each day.

Dairy products provide valuable nutrients. They are rich in protein, calcium, vitamin A, and riboflavin. Dairies fortify most dairy products with vitamin D.

All dairy products start out as milk. Milk can come from a cow, goat, or even a camel, 20-1. Dairy products are much more than just a glass of milk!

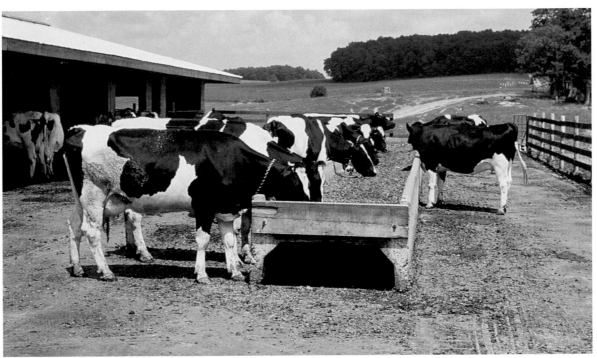

USDA

20-1 Most dairy products sold in the United States are made with milk from cows.

Types of Dairy Products

Hundreds of foods are made with dairy products. Scalloped potatoes and puddings are made with milk. Salads and pizza can be topped with cheese. Sour cream or plain yogurt adds a tasty touch to baked potatoes. With so many choices, it's easy to include dairy products at every meal.

Supermarkets sell many types of dairy products. Most are found in the refrigerated section of the store. Some, such as canned and dry milk, do not need to be refrigerated. They can be found on supermarket shelves.

Dairy products are grouped by the way the milk is processed. The types of dairy products are milk and cream, cultured products, frozen dairy desserts, cheese, and butter.

Milk and Cream

Milk and cream are mostly a watery liquid and fat. The fat floats on top unless the milk or cream is **homogenized**. The fat in homogenized milk has been broken into tiny pieces. These pieces will stay mixed with the milk or cream. They won't float to the top.

Only pasteurized milk and cream are sold in the United States. **Pasteurized** foods are heated to a high temperature for a few seconds. The heat kills harmful bacteria. Pasteurization makes milk and cream safe to drink. It doesn't affect their taste or destroy nutrients.

Fresh Milk

The fresh milk you drink is grouped by the amount of fat it contains. *Whole milk* contains the most fat. If all the fat is skimmed off before the milk is homogenized, you get *fat free milk*. (Fat free milk is sometimes called skim milk.) If only some of the fat is skimmed off, you get *lowfat milk*.

Skimming off fat lowers the calories in milk. For example, a cup of fat free milk has about half as many calories as a cup of whole milk. See 20-2.

Lowfat and fat free milk have all the nutrients found in whole milk except for vitamin A. This is because vitamin A is dissolved in the fat in the milk. Vitamin A is removed when the fat is skimmed off. Dairies fortify lowfat and fat free milk to replace the lost vitamin A.

Some fresh milk has added flavorings such as chocolate. Flavored milks are tasty, but they often have added sugar and more calories than plain milk.

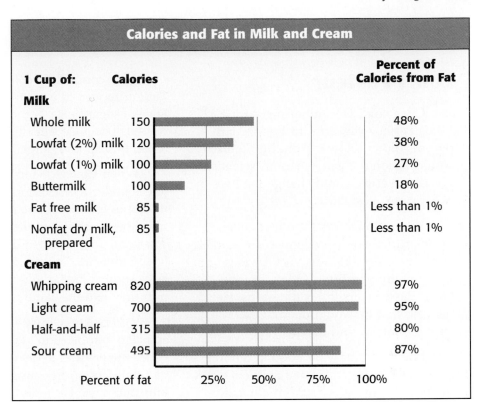

Calories and Fat in Milk and Cream

1 Cup of:	Calories		Percent of Calories from Fat
Milk			
Whole milk	150		48%
Lowfat (2%) milk	120		38%
Lowfat (1%) milk	100		27%
Buttermilk	100		18%
Fat free milk	85		Less than 1%
Nonfat dry milk, prepared	85		Less than 1%
Cream			
Whipping cream	820		97%
Light cream	700		95%
Half-and-half	315		80%
Sour cream	495		87%

Percent of fat   25%   50%   75%   100%

20-2 The main difference in these dairy foods is calories and fat. Cut calories and fat by choosing lowfat and fat free milk products.

Canned Milk

Evaporated milk and sweetened condensed milk are canned milks. *Evaporated milk* is made by removing half the water from fresh milk and canning it. Many recipes for sauces, soups, and desserts include evaporated milk. It can be used full strength in place of cream. You also can mix it with an equal amount of water and drink it like fresh milk. *Sweetened condensed milk* is made by adding a very large amount of sugar to evaporated milk and canning it. This sweet, thick milk is used in dessert recipes. It is very high in calories. To save calories, choose lowfat or fat free canned milks.

Dry Milk

Nonfat dry milk is made by removing all the fat and water from whole milk. All of the other nutrients remain except vitamin A. This is why dry milk is fortified with vitamin A. Nonfat dry milk mixed with water is the same as fat free fresh milk.

Science in the Kitchen

Louis Pasteur

On a cold, December night in 1822, Louis Pasteur was born in France. His parents didn't know it then, but Louis would become a world-famous scientist. His discoveries would change the lives of every person on earth.

When Louis was a teenager, he decided to become a chemist. He worked hard in college. He was very curious and asked many questions. Often, no one knew the answers to his questions. He realized that he would need to do experiments to find the answers.

Louis became very good at doing experiments. He found the answers to many of his questions and made many discoveries.

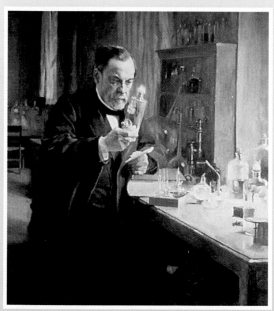

Institute Pasteur, Edefelt

Louis Pasteur discovered the process that makes milk safe to drink. The process, named in honor of him, is called pasteurization.

After completing college, Professor Pasteur moved to a town that processed the juice of sugar beets. Some vats of beet juice soured. The juice was ruined. Pasteur was asked to help find out why this happened.

When Louis looked at the spoiled juices under a microscope, he saw many microbes (germs) shaped like rods. These microbes were not in the unspoiled juice. These microbes turned the sugar in the juice into acid. The microbes made the juice spoil. Vinegar and wine makers told him they had the same problem.

Pasteur knew microbes caused the spoilage, but he didn't know how to get rid of them. After years of experimenting, he finally found the answer. Heat! Heat kills microbes. He found that if he heated the juice, the microbes died. The liquid wouldn't spoil.

Another liquid Pasteur studied was milk. People knew that milk was rich in nutrients. They also knew that it could cause deadly disease. Pasteur tried heating the milk. The heat killed the microbes that caused deadly disease. Pasteur had found a simple way to make milk safe to drink. This heat process was named in honor of Louis. It is called *pasteurization*. This process is used all over the world. In the United States, all milk must be pasteurized.

Pasteurization made Pasteur a hero, but his work didn't end there. He went on to prove that many diseases are caused by microbes. Before his discovery, no one believed that something you couldn't see (microbes) could kill people. This is one of the most important scientific findings in history!

UHT Milk

A newer form of milk is called *UHT milk*, 20-3. UHT stands for Ultra High Temperature. This milk was given this name because it is pasteurized at a higher temperature than the temperature normally used. The milk is placed in a sterilized container. The higher temperature and sterilized container preserves the milk. UHT milk stays fresh for several months when stored in a cool, dry place. It doesn't need to be refrigerated until you open the carton.

20-3 UHT milk is processed for long-term storage.

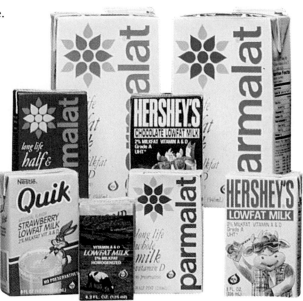

Aseptic Packaging Council

Frozen Milk Concentrate

Frozen milk concentrate is becoming available in more and more food stores. Frozen milk concentrate is made by removing most of the water and fat from milk. Then, the milk is frozen. When you're ready to serve frozen milk concentrate, add three cans of water and stir. Adding water makes it like fresh milk.

Fresh Cream

Fresh cream is like milk, but it contains much more fat. See 20-2. Whipping cream contains the most fat. It is thick, and can be whipped into a dessert topping.

Light cream has less fat than whipping cream. Light cream also is known as coffee cream. It may be whipped, used in dessert recipes, or added to coffee.

Half-and-half is a mixture of milk and cream. It has the least fat of all creams. Half-and-half may be added to coffee. It also may be used to make rich milk drinks such as egg nog. You can use it to make desserts such as puddings and custards, too.

Cultured Milk Products

Buttermilk, yogurt, and sour cream are ***cultured milk products.*** These products are made by adding certain helpful bacteria to milk. The bacteria grow and increase in number. When they do this, they form what is called a bacteria culture. This is why these foods are called cultured milk products.

The bacteria cause the milk to develop a tangy flavor. They also cause the milk to become thick and smooth.

Buttermilk

Buttermilk is available in whole, lowfat, and fat free varieties. It has very little butter in it. It's called buttermilk because it was originally made with the milk that was left after cream was churned into butter. Buttermilk is used in baking and can be served as a beverage.

Yogurt

Yogurt is made by adding bacteria to fat free, lowfat, or whole milk. Yogurt is a tasty snack. See 20-4. It often is used in dips and salad dressings. It is sold plain or with added fruit and sugar. The fruit added to most yogurt is really jam. Plain yogurt is low in calories. Adding jam to plain yogurt greatly increases the calories. The jam adds a large amount of sugar, too.

Sour Cream

Sour cream is made by adding bacteria to light cream. It is high in fat and calories. Sour cream is smooth and thick like yogurt. It is used in dips and to top baked potatoes and vegetables. In many recipes, plain yogurt can be used instead of sour cream. This is an easy way to cut fat and calories.

20-4 Yogurt is a delicious way to boost your calcium intake.

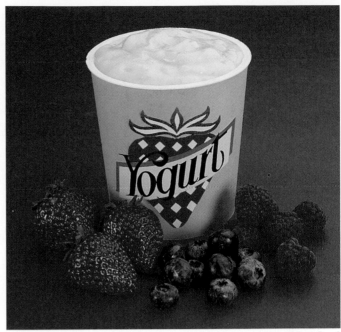

National Dairy Board

Frozen Dairy Desserts

Dairy desserts are tasty, 20-5. Ice cream, frozen yogurt, and sherbet are frozen dairy desserts.

Ice cream is made by freezing cream or milk, sugar, and flavorings. Frozen yogurt is a mixture of yogurt and milk. Sherbet is made with milk, fruit juice, water, sugar, and flavorings. It contains more surgar and less milk, vitamins, and minerals than other frozen dairy desserts.

Cheese

Most cheeses are made with the milk from cows, goats, and sheep. Some cheeses are made with milk from buffalo, yaks, reindeer, and camels. Even horse milk can be used!

The first step in making cheese is to separate the tiny solid pieces in milk from the watery portion. The solid pieces include protein, fat, vitamins, and minerals. When the solids stick together, they form lumps called *curds*. The liquid around the curds is called *whey*. (Remember Miss Muffet?) Cheese is made from the curds.

20-5 Frozen dairy desserts taste great on a hot day. They provide protein and calcium, too.

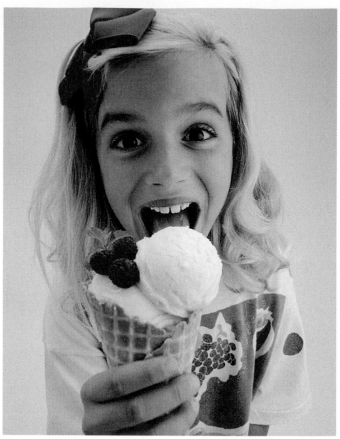

©Eastman Chemical Company

 Cultures of the World

The Middle East

The Middle East is the crossroads of the world. It is located where Africa, Europe, and Asia meet. The landscape is vast with deserts and rugged mountains. The Middle East is one of the driest areas on earth. Some villages only get rain every 10 years!

Farming in this hot, dusty region is hard, but vital. Most farming is done along the fertile river banks, sea coasts, and in mountain valleys. Fruits, vegetables,

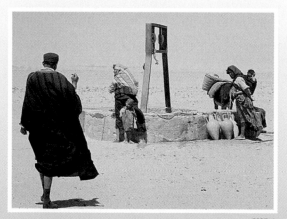

USDA
In the deserts of the Middle East, water is scarce.

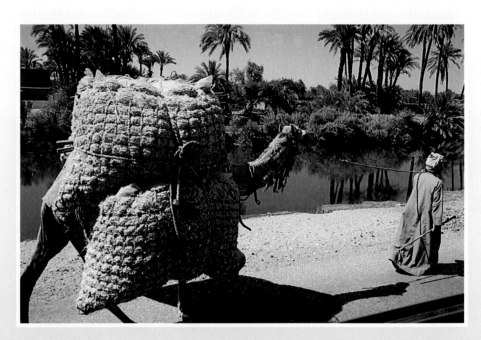

Camels are often used to transport goods back and forth to the market.

grains, and legumes thrive in the fertile areas. Lamb, sheep, goats, and camels graze on the sparse grass near the edge of the desert. These animals provide milk, meat, and hides. Camels also provide transportation. In the desert, they are used like cars.

The cuisine of the Middle East is very old. Early "cookbooks" in the Middle East were written on stone tablets 4,000 years ago!

Yogurt, wheat, legumes, lamb, and eggplant are common foods. Wheat bread is eaten at almost every meal. Chickpeas are a favorite legume. Middle Easterners like to boil, toast, or fry them. Street vendors sell them as a fried patty called *falafel* (fah-LAW-full). It is served in pita bread. Falafel is the fast food of the Middle East. Lamb is popular all over the Middle East. It may be cubed and grilled on a skewer. This style of cooking is called *shish kebab*. It was created in the Middle East.

Desert nomads have used milk to make yogurt, cheese, and butter for centuries. In fact, scholars believe that cheese and yogurt were made first in this parched land.

Yogurt is the preferred form of milk throughout the Middle East. Many families make a big bowlful of creamy yogurt every day. They serve it as a side dish or snack. They add it to soup and dessert recipes. They also make yogurt sauces for many meat and vegetable dishes. They even make a cool drink called *ayran* with it. Yogurt is a staple food in the Middle East. Middle Eastern foods are flavorful and delicious. Give them a try sometime soon!

There are hundreds of types of cheeses, 20-6. The differences in cheeses depend on the kind of milk used and how the curds are processed. The five groups of cheeses are fresh, aged, pasteurized process, pasteurized process cheese food, and cold pack.

20-6 Each cheese has its own special flavor, texture, and color. Cheeses may be salty or sweet. Some are sharp, others mild. Cheeses can be firm or soft. They may be white, creamy yellow, dark yellow, or even green. How many have you tried?

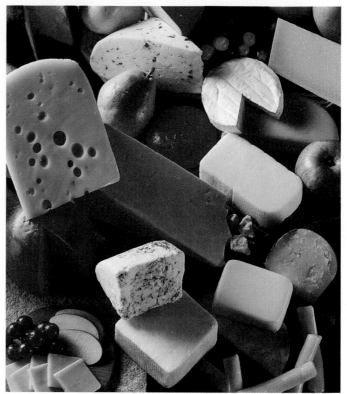

National Dairy Board

Fresh Cheese

Fresh cheese is ready to eat as soon as it is made. Fresh cheeses are usually soft and smooth. Most have a mild flavor. Cottage cheese, cream cheese, farmer's cheese, ricotta, and Neufchatel are fresh cheeses.

Aged Cheese

Aged cheese is stored by the cheese maker for a time before it is sold. The storage time may be a few weeks up to two years. This storage time is called *aging*. Aged cheeses are stored in areas with carefully controlled temperature and humidity. Sometimes caves are used.

Aging adds interesting flavors and textures. Cheddar and Parmesan are aged cheeses. Some cheeses have mold or bacteria added during aging. For instance, blue cheese has mold added. The mold grows and leaves blue veins in the cheese. The bacteria added to Swiss cheese produce gas bubbles, which form the holes in the cheese.

Pasteurized Process Cheeses

Pasteurized process cheeses are a blend of two or more cheeses. After blending, these cheeses are pasteurized. Heating them prevents further aging.

Pasteurized process cheeses are soft. They are often used in baked dishes and grilled cheese sandwiches. These cheeses melt quickly and smoothly when heated. They mix easily with other foods.

Pasteurized Process Cheese Food

Pasteurized process cheese food is often sold in jars or pressurized cans. It is similar to pasteurized process cheese, but it has a milder flavor. It also has less cheese and fat and more water than pasteurized process cheese. Cheese food melts and spreads easily because it is very soft.

Cold Pack Cheese

Cold pack cheese is a blend of cheeses. Cold pack cheeses are similar to pasteurized process cheese, but they are not heated. Cold pack cheeses are softer than aged cheeses. Spices and other flavorings may be added to cold pack cheese.

Butter

Butter is the fat found in milk. It floats on milk that has not been homogenized. The fat is skimmed off, formed into sticks, and sold as butter. Often, yellow coloring and salt are added to butter. The coloring makes the butter look more appealing. The salt helps to preserve it. Sweet butter has no salt added.

Butter is almost pure fat. It lacks the protein and minerals found in other milk products. It is a good source of vitamin A.

Buying Dairy Products

The price of dairy products depends on the form. The price also depends on the container size. Larger containers often have a lower unit price than smaller containers. Try to buy only the amount you need. Money is wasted if food spoils before you can use it.

You can get an idea of how long a dairy product will stay fresh by checking the date on the package. Fresh dairy products will stay fresh and safe to eat for a week or more after the date passes.

Milk

The price of milk depends on whether it is fresh, UHT, canned, frozen, or dry. When choosing milk, think about when you plan to use it. Fresh milk spoils quickest. UHT, canned, and frozen milk are more costly than fresh milk, but they can be stored longer. Dry milk can be stored for long periods and costs the least.

✚ Health Alert

Food Sensitivities

People who are allergic to peanuts or have trouble drinking milk have food sensitivities. Food allergies are one type of food sensitivity. A food allergy occurs when a person reacts to a protein in a specific food. The allergy may cause minor symptoms like a rash or itching. Sometimes the allergy causes symptoms that can be deadly. For instance, the throat may swell so much the person cannot breathe. Eggs, peanuts, and milk are the foods to which people are most often allergic.

Another common type of food sensitivity is called lactose intolerance. Lactose is the sugar found in milk. A special chemical substance called lactase is made in the intestine to digest lactose. Most people make lactase when they are babies.

As they grow older, some people make less lactase. Others stop making it at all. People who do not make lactase feel ill after eating dairy products. They may have intestinal gas, cramps, and diarrhea. Fortunately, they often can enjoy dairy products if they eat them with meals in small amounts. They can buy low-lactose milk. They can also eat cheese and cultured dairy products like yogurt and buttermilk. These foods have very little lactose.

Anyone can have food allergies or lactose intolerance. Food allergies are more common in children than in adults. African American, Hispanic, Asian, and Southern European adults are more likely than others to have lactose intolerance. When serving food to friends, it's a good idea to ask if they have any food sensitivities.

Cheese

Cheese prices are affected by the following three factors:

- The type of cheese: Aged cheeses often are priced higher than fresh cheeses. The longer the cheese is aged, the more costly the cheese will be. Fresh cheeses and pasteurized process cheeses usually are cheaper than aged cheeses. Pasteurized process cheese foods have the lowest price, except when they are sold in pressurized cans.
- The origin of the cheese: Cheese made in the United States often costs less than cheese imported from other countries.
- The size of the pieces: Cheese is sold in blocks, slices, and shredded. Large, uncut blocks often cost the least per unit, 20-7. Shredded cheese tends to cost more. Individually wrapped slices are convenient, but cost more than unwrapped slices. You may be able to save money by shredding or slicing blocks of cheese yourself.

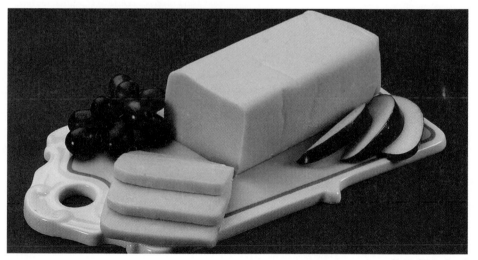

National Dairy Board

20-7 You can often save money by buying cheese in blocks and slicing it yourself.

Yogurt

Yogurt is one of the most costly forms of milk. It is priced higher than fresh milk and ice cream. Plain yogurt usually costs less than yogurt with added fruit and sugar. You can save money and calories by buying plain yogurt and adding fruit yourself.

Frozen Dairy Desserts

Many types and flavors of frozen diary desserts are sold in supermarkets. Ice creams are labeled as reduced fat, lowfat, light, or fat free. Products labeled ice cream have the most fat. Fat free ice cream has no fat. Ice creams often cost more than frozen yogurt and sherbet. Special ingredients, such as nuts and chocolate chips, add to the price. Ice cream bars and sandwiches cost more per unit than frozen diary desserts sold in cartons. Premium ice cream with special ingredients is the most costly frozen dairy dessert.

Storing Dairy Products

Fresh milk, cream, cultured dairy products, cheese, and butter spoil quickly. Protect these foods by storing them in tightly closed containers in the refrigerator. Dairy products will stay fresh longer when returned to the refrigerator as soon as you finish with them. For example, put the milk carton back in the refrigerator right after you pour a glass of milk.

Store fresh, aged, and cold pack cheese tightly wrapped in the refrigerator. Fresh cheese spoils quickly, so eat it within a week. Most aged and cold pack cheeses will keep a month or more. Cut off any mold that forms before serving aged cheese. The remaining cheese will still be safe to eat. Pasteurized process cheese foods can be stored in a cool, dry place until opened. Once they are opened, refrigerate them and use within a few weeks. Many aged and cold pack cheeses can be frozen. Be sure to thaw frozen cheese in the refrigerator and use it soon after thawing. Frozen and thawed cheeses taste best when they are cooked.

Yogurt, butter, and frozen dairy desserts can be stored in the freezer for about two months. Other dairy products don't freeze well. If you freeze butter or yogurt, be sure to thaw it in the refrigerator.

Unopened canned milk can be stored in a cool, dry place for a year. Canned milk doesn't need to be refrigerated until you open it. Once the can is opened, the milk will spoil quickly. When opened, store it like fresh milk.

Nonfat dry milk stays fresh in an airtight container for six months or more. Keep it in a cool, dry place. Frozen milk concentrate can be stored in the coldest part of the freezer for about six months. Once dry or frozen milk is mixed with water, it is like fresh milk. It will sour fast, so refrigerate it and use it within a few days.

Cooking with Dairy Products

Dairy products can be served as any part of the meal. They make nutrient-rich beverages. Piping hot cocoa or a frosty milk shake are good choices. Cheese wedges make a great snack or appetizer. Salads often include cheese. For example, a chef's salad has strips of cheese. Fruit salads can be served with a yogurt dressing. Cream soups, macaroni and cheese, and cheese fondue can be main dishes or side dishes. Ice cream sundaes, pudding, and cream pies are delicious dairy desserts.

Dairy products arc important ingredients in many recipes. See 20-8. They add nutrients, flavor, and texture to foods. They help baked products brown, too.

20-8 Milk is a key ingredient in many cream soup recipes.

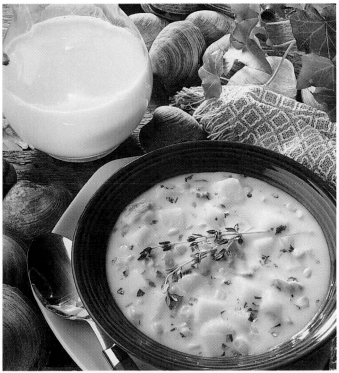

National Dairy Board

Dairy products are very sensitive to heat. They burn easily. You can keep them from burning by using a heavy pan and low cooking temperatures. Short cooking times help prevent burning. Frequently stirring milk and cream while it's cooking also helps prevent burning. Dairy products can be cooked in a microwave oven, too. Moderate or low microwave oven power settings help preserve the flavor and quality of dairy products.

Milk

When you heat milk to make hot chocolate or soup, a skin may form. The skin traps heat and may cause the milk to boil over. You can prevent the skin from forming by stirring the milk while you heat it. Covering the pot will also help. Another way to prevent the skin from forming is to whip the cold milk until it's foamy and then heat it. If a skin forms, remove it. If you leave it in the pan, it will make lumps in the milk.

 Focus on Food

Nondairy Products

Nondairy products do not contain any milk. Whipped topping, coffee whiteners, and margarine are nondairy products. These foods are used in place of dairy products. It's important to keep in mind that they do not supply the nutrients found in dairy products. Also, some are high in fat.

People who have trouble digesting milk may find these products useful. Others like the convenience of these foods. For example, coffee whiteners don't need to be refrigerated. Whipped toppings are ready to serve.

Margarine can be used in place of butter. Both are almost pure fat. Margarine is made from vegetable oils, such as corn oil. Margarine contains no animal fat or cholesterol. It costs less than butter.

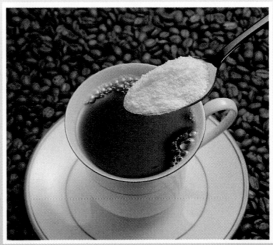

©Eastman Chemical Company

Nondairy products are often used in place of dairy products.

Cheese

Cheese gets tough and greasy if it cooks too long. Cheese only needs to melt. It doesn't need to cook. For the best results, add cheese in the last few minutes of cooking. For example, top pizza with cheese a few minutes before it is done. Heat grilled cheese sandwiches only long enough to brown the bread. Sprinkle cheese over food and broil just until the cheese melts and is bubbly.

When preparing dairy products, always remember to cook them gently. Gentle cooking will help preserve the appeal of dairy products and make your dairy dishes a delight to eat.

In a Nutshell

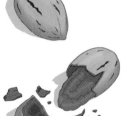

- Dairy products are rich sources of protein, calcium, vitamin A, and riboflavin.
- Most dairy products are fortified with vitamin D.
- The fat in homogenized milk does not separate from the watery portion of milk.
- Pasteurized foods are heated to a high temperature for a few seconds to kill harmful bacteria.
- Skimming fat off milk lowers the milk's calories.
- Cultured milk products are made by adding certain helpful bacteria to milk.
- Cheese is made from milk curds.
- Butter is the fat found in milk.
- Store fresh milk, cream, cultured dairy products, cheese, and butter in the refrigerator.
- Store frozen milk concentrate in the coldest part of the freezer.
- Unopened packages of dry milk, canned milk, and UHT milk can be stored in a cool, dry place.
- Dairy products burn easily. A heavy pan, low temperatures, short cooking times, and frequent stirring help prevent burning.

In the Know

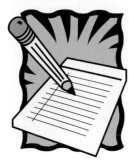

1. Fat floats to the top of milk that has not been _____.
   A. fortified
   B. pasteurized
   C. homogenized
   D. None of the above.
2. True or false? Pasteurized milk spoils more quickly and is not as safe to drink as unpasteurized milk.
3. If you want to decrease your fat intake, which would be the better choice?
   A. Fat free milk.
   B. Lowfat milk.
   C. Whole milk.
   D. Evaporated milk.
4. Name two cultured dairy products. Describe their flavor and texture.
5. True or false? Fresh cheese is stored by the cheese maker for up to two years before it is sold.
6. _____ is a dairy product that is almost pure fat.
7. Which dairy product must be refrigerated even if its package has not been opened?
   A. UHT milk.
   B. Evaporated milk.
   C. Sour cream.
   D. Sweetened condensed milk.
8. Explain how to keep a skin from forming when you heat milk.

What Would You Do?

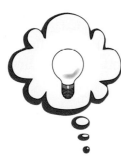

Your dad noticed the date stamped on the milk was yesterday. Only half the milk was used. This happened last week, too. He is concerned that your family is wasting money on milk. He also wonders if he should pour out the milk. What advice would you give him?

Expanding Your Knowledge

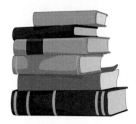

1. Visit a dairy farm. Watch how the cows are milked. Ask the dairy farmer to describe what will happen to the milk before it gets to the supermarket.

2. Set up a taste test of frozen dairy desserts. You could compare the flavor and texture of premium ice cream, ice cream, lowfat ice cream, and frozen yogurt. Be sure to use the same flavor of each. Drink a sip of water between each taste. Which had the best flavor? Which had the best texture? Which did you prefer? Why? Which was the best buy?

3. Visit a supermarket. Record the cost and volume of containers of whole milk, lowfat milk, fat free milk, evaporated milk, and nonfat dry milk. Calculate which type of milk has the lowest unit price. Also check the dates stamped on the containers. Has the date stamped on any of them passed?

4. Prepare homemade yogurt. Preheat an oven set to the lowest setting for 5 minutes. Turn off the oven but leave the oven light on. On the range, heat 2 cups of milk and 3 tablespoons of non-fat dry milk powder in a saucepan until it reaches 120°F (48°C). Remove the milk from the heat. Stir in ¼ cup of supermarket yogurt that contains live bacteria cultures. (Some brands of supermarket yogurt contain live cultures, others don't. Read the yogurt label to find one that does.) If the temperature is higher than 120°F (48°C), the bacteria will die. Cover the saucepan with aluminum foil and place it in the oven for 8 to 24 hours. Chill the yogurt. Save 2 tablespoons to start your next batch. Set up a taste panel to compare the homemade yogurt with yogurt from the supermarket. Your homemade yogurt will stay fresh for about five days if you keep it refrigerated.

5. See how cottage cheese is made. Place 3 tablespoons of vinegar and 3 cups of fat free milk in a double boiler. Heat until the milk reaches 140°F (60°C). Stir constantly. Strain the liquid by pouring it into a colander lined with cheesecloth. Let it drain for 10 minutes. Mix in a pinch of salt and 1 tablespoon of heavy cream. Chill and serve.

6. Do some research to find out why cheeses are sometimes aged in caves. Write up your findings and share them with the class.

7. Have a cheese-tasting party. Select five cheeses you have never tasted. Ask everyone tasting the cheese to describe the flavor, color, and texture of each. Before the party, collect some information on each cheese. You could make an information card for each cheese that states the type of milk used, where the cheese originated, and how long it was aged.

8. See how heat affects cheese. Make a quick pizza by splitting an English muffin. Spread one tablespoon of pizza sauce on each half. Top one pizza with 2 teaspoons of grated mozzarella cheese. Bake both for 5 minutes at 450°F (230°C). Top the second pizza with 2 teaspoons of mozzarella cheese. Bake both pizzas 2 minutes more. Which pizza had the best tasting cheese? Which cheese was tough? Which was greasy?

9. Make butter. Pour 1 cup of whipping cream in a jar. Tighten the lid. Shake the jar vigorously until a lump of butter forms. Pour off the milk and save it for later. Spread the butter on crackers and taste it. Describe its taste. How does it compare with butter purchased at the supermarket?

Chapter 21

Meat, Fish, and Poultry

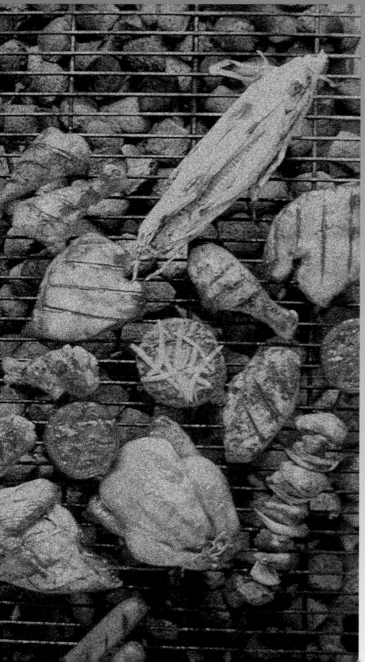

Objectives

After reading this chapter, you will be able to
- ❏ describe the different kinds of meat, fish, and poultry.
- ❏ explain how to select meat, fish, and poultry in the supermarket.
- ❏ store and prepare meat, fish, and poultry to keep them safe and appealing.

New Terms

marbling: streaks of fat running through lean meat.

connective tissue: long, thin tissue that holds muscles together.

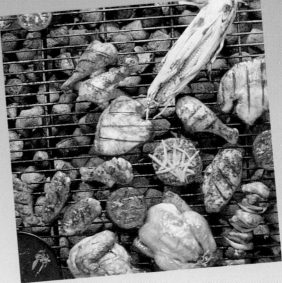

Purdue Farms

479

For many years, meats have had the starring role in meals, 21-1. This role might go to a juicy steak or spicy barbecued pork. Grilled lamb chops, chicken nuggets, and fish sticks are other stars.

Meat often sets the stage for meals. Vegetables, fruits, breads, and dairy foods play vital supporting roles. They are chosen to complement the meat dish. For example, many families serve roasted turkey at Thanksgiving. The flavors of yams, squash, and bread stuffing blend with the turkey to create a mouth-watering feast.

Meat is a rich source of protein, iron, and zinc. It also is high in fat and cholesterol. Eating large amounts of fat and cholesterol may lead to heart disease and certain cancers. In recent years, health conscious people have started eating less meat. They include more fruits, vegetables, and breads in their meals.

21-1 Meat can be prepared in many different ways.

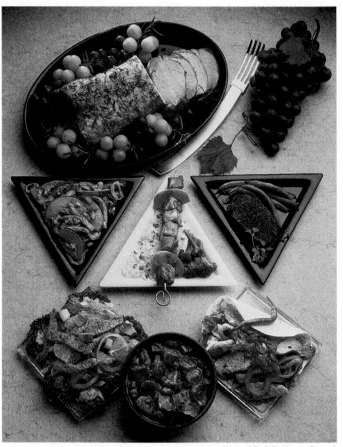

National Pork Producers Council

Nutrition experts agree that eating less meat is a good idea. They suggest putting meat in a supporting role instead of featuring it as the star. This means serving smaller portions of meat. An easy way to do this is to serve casseroles, soups, and stews more often. Beef stew and tuna casserole are examples.

Eating less meat not only is good for your health, it's good for your budget, too. Meat is one of the most costly foods in the supermarket.

What Is Meat?

Meat has three major parts: muscle, fat, and connective tissue. Most of the nutrients in meat are in the muscle. Muscle is rich in protein and minerals such as iron and zinc.

Fat is high in calories. Fat is found mostly along the sides of the muscle. By slicing off this fat, you can save many calories. Streaks of fat also run through the muscle of cows, calves, pigs, and lamb. These streaks are called *marbling*. See 21-2. The more marbling meat has, the more fat it contains. Lean beef, veal, lamb, and pork have little marbling. This makes them lower in fat.

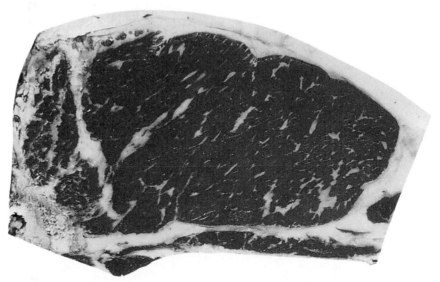

National Cattlemen's Beef Association

21-2 Well-marbled meat is tender and juicy.

The fat in poultry is mostly just below the skin. It keeps the poultry moist and tasty. You can save many calories by removing the skin and eating only the poultry muscle.

Fish have very little fat. Fish muscle that is white or very light in color has less fat than fish muscle that is dark.

Connective tissue is long and thin. It looks like threads. These threads hold the muscle together. Connective tissue is strong and can make meat tough.

Connective tissue in young animals is more tender than that in older animals. As animals get older, the connective tissue becomes stronger. Most beef and older poultry is tougher than meat from young animals. Lamb, pork, young poultry, and some parts of beef usually have tender connective tissue. Fish is tender because it has very little connective tissue.

Red Meat

Red meats include beef, veal, lamb, and pork. They are called red meat because the muscle has a red or pink color.

In the United States, all of these animals and their carcasses must be inspected. Red meats that pass the inspection are stamped "U.S. Inspected." See 21-3. This stamp tells you that the animal is safe to eat. It also tells you that the meat was processed in a clean area. You will find this stamp on fresh red meat and all foods containing red meat.

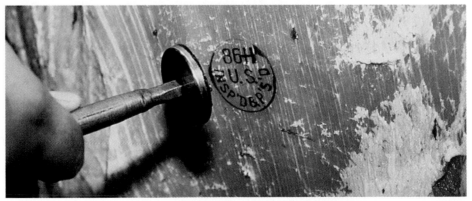

USDA

21-3 Meats passing federal inspection are stamped "U.S. Inspected." The stamp means that the animal is safe to eat.

Animal carcasses are cut into smaller portions called *cuts*. Some cuts are more tender than others. Cuts from well-exercised muscles, such as the legs, are tough. Well-exercised meat is tough because it has more connective tissue than less exercised muscle. Cuts from muscles that get little exercise, such as the back, are the most tender. For example, T-bone steak is a cut from the back. It is more tender than shank cuts that come from the well-exercised front legs.

Beef and Veal

Beef is the meat from cattle that is over a year old. The best beef has a bright red color. It is firm and has creamy white fat.

Veal is the meat from cattle that is a few weeks old. It has little fat. Veal has a mild flavor and light pink color.

Most beef is graded, but grading is not required, 21-4. The grades are set by the U.S. Department of Agriculture. *Grades* are based on the age of the animal, amount of marbling, and the color and texture of the muscle. The highest grades go to meat from young animals with a lot of marbling. That's because young animals are more tender than older ones. Also, marbling helps make the meat tender and juicy.

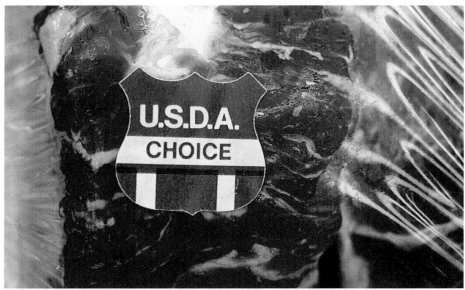

USDA

21-4 U.S. Choice is a common beef grade found in most supermarkets.

The grades try to predict how good the taste and texture of beef will be. Top grades are more tender and tasty than lower grades. Veal may be graded, too. *Prime* is the top grade of beef and veal. It is often sold to restaurants. Supermarkets often sell the next highest grades, *choice* and *select*. All grades have the same nutrients, except for fat. Lower grades are leaner. They have less fat and waste than higher grades.

Lamb

Lamb is the meat from a sheep that is less than one year old. The best lamb is deep red. Its fat is white. Lamb is tender and has a mild flavor. It may be graded, but often it is not. That's because lamb is usually tender and juicy.

Mutton is meat from an older sheep. It is not as tender as lamb and has a stronger flavor. Mutton is not eaten much in the United States. It is most popular in Middle Eastern countries and in Australia and New Zealand.

Pork

Pork is the meat from pigs. Most pork sold in the United States is from animals less than a year old. Pork is tender and juicy. High quality pork ranges in color from rosy pink to grayish pink. Some pork is graded, but most is not.

Many people think pork is high in fat. This was true years ago. Farmers have bred pigs to have less fat, 21-5. Today, pork has about the same amount of fat and protein as beef.

Variety Meats

Variety meats are the organs of an animal. Liver, kidney, heart, tongue, and brains are examples. These meats are very tender and rich in nutrients. However, most of them are high in cholesterol.

21-5 Today, pork has less fat than it did in the past.

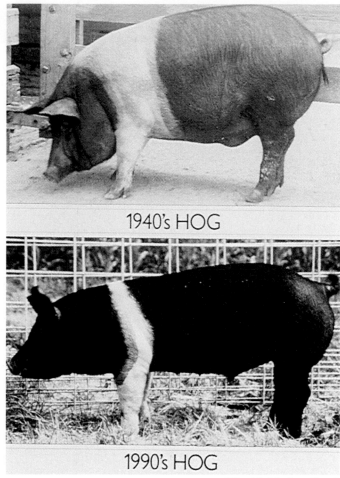

1940's HOG

1990's HOG

National Pork Producers Council

Fish

There are two groups of fish. They are finfish and shellfish.

Finfish have backbones and fins. Sardines, snapper, and sole are examples. There are more than 20,000 types of finfish. Each has a different flavor and color. Lean finfish have white, mild-flavored flesh. Cod and haddock are lean finfish. Finfish that have more fat have a darker color and stronger flavor. Salmon and tuna are examples. These fish often live in very cold water. For example, salmon are common in the waters around Alaska.

New Technology

Aquaculture

Did you ever hear of farmers who let their animals graze in ocean pastures? Everyone knows about cattle ranchers, but how about salmon or lobster ranchers?

You may be surprised to learn that fish are being raised on farms. These farms may be in freshwater or saltwater. Raising fish like crops is called *aquaculture.*

Aquaculture probably began in Asia. Fish have been raised in ponds there for thousands of years. Aquaculture is an important industry in many other areas of the world, too. For example, Ecuador is known for its shrimp farms. Israel and India get more than one-fourth of their fish from their fish farms.

Aquaculture is an important business in the United States, too. Catfish are raised in lakes and ponds in Mississippi, Alabama, and Arkansas. Fish farmers in Idaho raise freshwater trout. In Washington, farmers fence off part of the ocean. They put salmon in floating nylon pens and feed them many times each day. When the fish are large enough, ranchers "round them up" and sell them.

Farmers in the United States grow shellfish, too. Lobsters are raised in California. Shrimp are farmed in Texas. One of the world's largest oyster farms is in New York. Crawfish are raised in southern states. These small, tasty shellfish look like tiny lobsters.

Aquaculture is a growing business. Fish farmers need much more information, though. They need to know more about breeding, feeding, and taking care of fish. Scientists and technologists are working with farmers to find out more about aquaculture. Knowing more can help farmers raise more fish. This can help to increase the world's food supply.

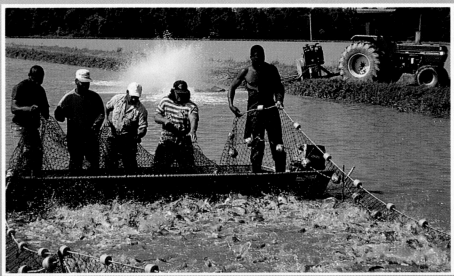

Catfish Institute

Catfish are being harvested at this catfish farm.

Fish do not have to be inspected or graded. Inspection may be required in the future. Some businesses ask the United States government to inspect and grade their fish. The highest grades are given to fresh, healthy fish with few cuts and bruises. The best canned fish have a federal inspection mark.

Shellfish have hard shells. Clams, oysters, scallops, crabs, lobsters, and shrimp are shellfish, 21-6. These fish don't have any bones or connective tissue. They are very tender and have a slightly sweet taste.

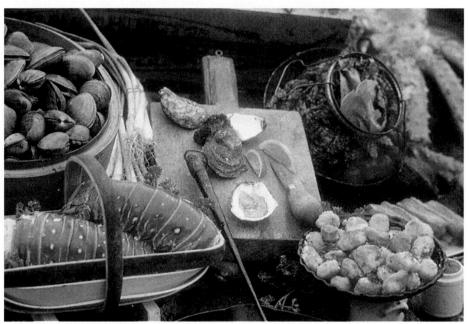

American Heart Association

21-6 There are many types of shellfish.

Poultry

Poultry is any bird raised for meat. Chickens, ducks, geese, and turkeys are poultry. Rock Cornish game hens, guinea hens, and squab (pigeon) are other types of poultry.

Poultry is inspected by the United States government, 21-7. The inspection stamp is found on all fresh poultry and any processed food containing poultry.

21-7 Poultry inspected by the United States government has this inspection seal. Poultry doesn't have to be graded. If it is, it has this grade shield.

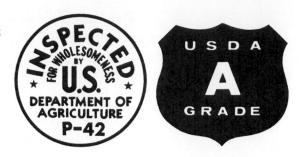

Poultry can be graded, but grading is not required. Grading tries to predict flavor and tenderness. The highest grade poultry is labeled U.S. Grade A.

High-quality poultry is young. Chickens labeled broiler, fryer, roaster, or capon are young and tender. As birds get older, they get tougher. Stewing hens are older birds.

Processed Meat

Fresh meat spoils quickly. Thousands of years ago, people discovered they could preserve meat by curing, drying, or smoking it. These meats are called *processed meat.* Processed meats include any meats that have been prepared in some way other than cutting or grinding. Cured meats, sausages, luncheon meats, dried meats, and canned meats are the most common types of processed meats.

Today, it's not necessary to process meat because refrigerators are available. However, people like the flavor and variety processed meats add to meals.

Cured Meats

Cured meat is made by rubbing fresh meat with salt or soaking it in saltwater. The salt draws the moisture out of the fresh meat. It also keeps harmful bacteria from growing. Some cured meats are flavored with sugar and spices.

An ingredient called *sodium nitrite* is added to cured meats. It gives them a pink color and helps preserve them. It also prevents the foodborne illness botulism.

Ham and bacon are cured pork. Corned beef is cured beef. Most cured meats should be stored in the refrigerator.

Sausages and Luncheon Meats

There are hundreds of types of sausages and luncheon meats. Kielbasa, bologna, and hot dogs are examples. The difference in these depends on the ingredients used and whether they are uncooked, smoked, or cooked.

Both sausages and luncheon meats are made from a variety of cuts of beef, pork, and poultry. The meat is ground and mixed with spices. Often, this mixture is stuffed into a mold or casing. A *casing* is a thin skin shaped like a tube. The mixture is then cooked in the casing and the casing is usually removed. Fresh sausage may be stuffed into a casing or sold in bulk form. Fresh sausage must be cooked.

Luncheon meats, like olive loaf, don't need to be cooked. They are ready to eat. Smoked cooked sausages, like pepperoni and thuringer, are ready to serve.

Sausages and luncheon meats are tasty, but they are generally very high in fat, 21-8. For example, 80 percent of the calories in bologna come from fat! Salami gets 70 percent of its calories from fat. Some meat processors now offer reduced-fat products.

21-8 Sausages and luncheon meats often are high in fat.

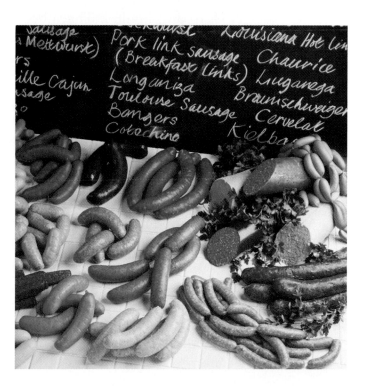

Dried Meats

Drying was one of the first ways humans preserved meat. Any meat can be dried. Native Americans made jerky by drying thinly sliced buffalo meat in the sun. Beef jerky is still sold today. Dried seafood is still very common in China. Dried meat is lightweight, and it doesn't require refrigeration. It is often used on camping trips.

Canned Meats

There are many choices of canned meats. You can buy tuna, sardines, deviled ham, and potted beef. You can even buy a whole boneless chicken.

Canned meats are quick and easy to prepare because they are cooked during the canning process. You can eat them right from the can. No cooking is needed. Most canned meats can be stored in a cool, dry place until the can is opened.

Buying Meat, Fish, and Poultry

Many families spend a large part of their food budget on meat, fish, and poultry. That's because these foods are among the most expensive in the supermarket. To find the best buy, compute the cost per serving before making comparisons. To learn more about cost per serving, see the *Math in the Kitchen* feature in this chapter.

The choices you make depend on your tastes and budget. The way you plan to use these foods also affects your choices. For example, if you plan to make beef stew, you can buy beef chunks. If you want to serve hamburgers, you will need to buy ground beef.

Prices are based on the type of meat. Lamb and veal often cost more than beef and pork. Variety meats cost less than muscle meats. Finfish tend to be priced lower than shellfish. Turkey and chicken often have lower unit prices than other types of poultry.

The grade and method of processing also affect price. Higher grades cost more than lower ones. Sausages and cured, dried, and ready-to-eat meats often cost more per unit than fresh, canned, and frozen meats. The higher price reflects the labor, time, and equipment needed to process the meat.

÷ Math in the Kitchen

Computing Cost Per Serving

The price of meat includes the parts you eat and those you don't eat. You pay for fat and bone even though you throw them away. Bone and fat raise the cost per serving of a cut of meat. The *cost per serving* is the price you pay to serve one person at one meal. A serving is about four ounces of lean meat.

When you compare prices at the supermarket, cuts with little fat and bone may seem costly. Cuts with a lot of fat or bone may appear to be bargains. They often have a lower price per pound than leaner, boneless cuts.

A lower price per pound doesn't always mean that it is the best buy. Meat with a low price that has a lot of bone and fat may have a high cost per serving. Lean, boneless cuts that cost more per pound may have a lower cost per serving.

To get the best buy of meat, you will need to compare costs per serving. Here's how to find the best buy:

1. Estimate how many people you can serve per pound. Each person should get about four ounces of lean meat.

For example, you can serve four people with a pound of lean, boneless meat. Some cuts have so much fat or bone that you can serve only one or two people with a pound.

2. Compute the cost per serving. To do this, locate the cost per pound on the meat label. Then, divide the cost per pound by the number of people you estimate you can serve per pound. The equation for computing the cost per serving looks this this:

$$\frac{\text{Cost}}{\text{per pound}} \div \frac{\text{Number of people who can be served per pound}} = \frac{\text{Cost per serving}}$$

The equation would look like this if the meat costs $3.00 per pound and you could serve two people per pound:

$$\frac{\$3.00}{\text{per pound}} \div \frac{2 \text{ people}}{\text{can be served per pound}} = \frac{\$1.50}{\text{per serving}}$$

Now that you know how to compute cost per serving, visit a supermarket. Find five cuts of meat you might buy. Compute their cost per serving. Which is the best buy? Find three recipes you could use to prepare the meat that is the best buy.

Canned and frozen foods containing meat are often costly. These foods can save you time, but they cost much more than making the food at home. For example, you can buy clam chowder, beef ravioli, and chicken chop suey. Keep in mind that many of these prepared dishes contain very little meat. This is why it's a good idea to read the ingredient label to find out where meat falls in the list. Remember, the ingredient label lists all the ingredients used to make the food in order of weight.

21-9 Save money by combining small amounts of poultry, meat, or fish with grains and vegetables.

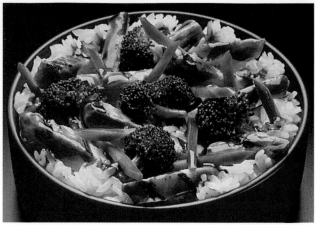

U.S.A. Rice Council

One way to spend less on meat, fish, and poultry is to serve recipes that use small amounts of these foods, 21-9. Chili con carne is an example. It is made by mixing a small amount of ground beef with a large amount of beans and tomatoes. Chicken a la king is a second example. It combines a small amount of chicken with other ingredients.

Red Meat

The price of red meat depends partly on the cut. Tender cuts are in demand, so their price is high. Other cuts are less in demand, so their price is lower.

The amount of fat and bone a cut has affects the price, too. You are charged for fat and bone even though you throw them away.

You can learn more about the meat you want to buy by checking the package label. Most meat labels list the type of meat, wholesale cut, retail cut, net weight, cost per pound, and total price. See 21-10.

21-10 The labels on meat often include this information.

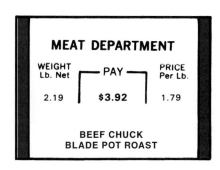

MEAT DEPARTMENT

WEIGHT Lb. Net	PAY	PRICE Per Lb.
2.19	$3.92	1.79

BEEF CHUCK
BLADE POT ROAST

Fish

The best quality fresh finfish have a mild smell. Their eyes are clear and bulging. They have bright, shiny skin with firmly attached scales. Their gills are red and their flesh is firm, 21-11. If a fish is soft or slimy, it isn't fresh. A fishy odor, dry skin, and cloudy, sunken eyes also tell you the fish is old.

The freshest shellfish have a mild scent. Mussels and clams have shells that are closed tightly. If open shells don't snap shut when you touch them, the animal is dead. They could be dangerous to eat. The best live lobsters and crabs are active.

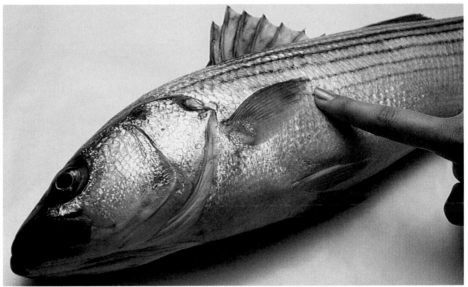

American Heart Association

21-11 Fresh fish have firm flesh.

You can buy whole, uncleaned fish, and cut pieces of fish. A *whole fish* is sold just as it was when it was caught. A *drawn fish* is a whole fish with only its inner organs removed. A *dressed fish* is a drawn fish with its scales, head, tail, and fins removed. *Fish steaks* are crosswise slices of a dressed fish. The slices are made from the back to the stomach. *Fish fillets* are the sides of a dressed fish. They are cut along the backbone from behind the head to the tail. Fillets have few bones. *Fish sticks* are wide strips cut from fillets. Most fish sticks are breaded and sold frozen.

The best frozen fish are tightly wrapped and frozen solid. There should be no odor or dark, discolored areas.

The price of fresh fish depends partly on the type of fish. Shellfish tend to cost more per unit than finfish. The demand for some fish is greater than for others. Fish in demand cost more than less popular fish.

The season also affects the cost of fish. Some fish are more available at certain times of the year than at other times. A fish is in season when it is plentiful. Its price is lowest when it is in season. Whole and drawn fish are priced lower than other cuts of fish. You can save money by cleaning and cutting whole or drawn fish yourself. Many cookbooks explain how to do this.

Poultry

The best poultry has a lot of meat on the bone. It looks plump and clean. The skin is thick, moist, and free of bruises and feathers.

The price of poultry depends on the type. Turkey costs the least per unit. Pheasant, quail, duck, goose, Rock Cornish game hens, guinea hens, and squab cost the most.

Price also depends on the size of the bird. Small birds are young and tender. They cost more per pound than larger birds.

To get the most servings per pound, look for plump birds. They are a better buy because they are meaty. They have more meat to eat and less bone to throw away.

Supermarkets sell poultry whole and in parts. Whole birds cost less per pound than parts. Parts cost more because you are paying someone else to cut up the bird for you. You can save money by buying a whole bird and cutting it up yourself. Many cookbooks show you how to do this.

Storing Meat, Fish, and Poultry

Fresh meat, poultry, and fish spoil very quickly. Preserve their freshness by keeping them in the refrigerator or freezer. See 21-12. Processed meat can be stored for a longer time than fresh meat.

21-12 A label like this is placed on fresh meat and poultry packages. The label reminds consumers how to safely store and prepare fresh meat and poultry.

Safe Handling Instructions

This product was inspected for your safety. Some animal products may contain bacteria that could cause illness if the product is mishandled or cooked improperly. For your protection, follow these safe handling instructions.

Keep refrigerated or frozen.
Thaw in refrigerator or microwave.

Keep raw [meats or poultry] separate from other foods. Wash working surfaces (including cutting boards), utensils, and hands after touching raw [meat or poultry].

Cook thoroughly.

Refrigerate leftovers within 2 hours.

USDA

After buying fresh meat and poultry, store it in the coldest part of the refrigerator. Meat that is prepackaged can be stored in its original wrapper. Meat that was packaged by the butcher should be rewrapped in plastic wrap or aluminum foil. Wash and dry fresh poultry. Put the poultry on a plate and cover it loosely. Use fresh meat and poultry within a few days.

Keep fresh finfish and shellfish tightly wrapped in the refrigerator. If you bought whole fish, clean it before storing it. Use fish within a day of purchase.

If you want to freeze fresh meat, poultry, or fish, remove the supermarket package. Wrap it first in plastic wrap then in aluminum foil or freezer paper. If it was frozen when you bought it, you can freeze it in the supermarket package.

It is important to wrap frozen foods tightly. If the wrap is loose or torn, the food may become freezer burned. Foods with *freezer burn* have pale, dry, tough patches. Freezing a food too long also can cause freezer burn.

Refrigerate leftover meat, fish, and poultry. Also refrigerate canned meats once they are opened. Store them in an airtight container and use them within three days. Leftovers and canned meats can be frozen, too.

Preparing Meat, Fish, and Poultry

Meat, fish, and poultry can be served in many ways. They can be boiled with water and strained to make bouillon. This meat-flavored liquid can be served as a warm beverage or soup. Meat, fish, and poultry can be served in salads. Tuna salad, chef's salad, and chicken salad are examples. Most often, meat, fish, and poultry are served as the main dish. Beef tacos, grilled salmon steaks, and fried chicken are well-known main dishes. Meat, fish, and poultry are almost never used in desserts. Older recipes for mince meat pie contain meat. Can you think of any other desserts that include meat, fish, or poultry?

Before cooking frozen meats, thaw them in the refrigerator or microwave oven. If thawed meat is refrozen, it will be mushy when cooked. Check the label on prepared frozen foods before thawing them. Most don't need to be thawed before cooking.

Cooking Methods

Cooking makes meat, fish, and poultry tender, tasty, and appealing. During cooking, the connective tissue softens and becomes tender. The fat melts and makes the meat juicy. The protein becomes firm and develops an appealing texture.

The best way to cook meat depends on how tender it is. Fish, lamb, pork, and young poultry are tender. Rib, short loin, and sirloin beef cuts are tender, too. Tender meats can be cooked with dry heat, such as broiling, roasting, or frying. They can be cooked by moist heat methods, too.

Less tender cuts of meat need to be tenderized during cooking. There are three ways to tenderize meat:

- Cook meat in liquid. Cooking in liquid softens the connective tissue in less tender cuts of beef and older poultry. Meats are more tender and juicy when cooked with a moist heat method such as braising or stewing.
- Grind, pound, or cut meat. These methods break the connective tissue.
- Marinate the meat in an acid, such as lemon juice or vinegar. The acid helps dissolve the connective tissue.

Cultures of the World

On the Pampas in Argentina

Argentina is in South America. Most of Argentina is covered by the large grassy plains called the *pampas* (PAHM-pahs). This flat, fertile land is an ideal place to grow crops. Cattle and sheep thrive on the lush grass in the pampas.

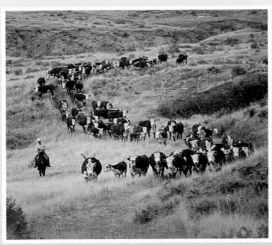

USDA

Gauchos herd cattle on the pampas of Argentina.

The pampas are the heart of Argentina's farmland. In fact, the pampas makes Argentina a world leader in beef and wheat production. Argentine farm produce is exported all over the world.

The native foods of Argentina include potatoes, tomatoes, pineapples, bananas, squash, and hot chili peppers. Early settlers from Spain and Italy brought cows, sheep, rice, wheat, garlic, onions, and coffee. Argentina's cuisine has become a blend of native foods and foods from the settlers' homelands.

In Argentina, beef is a major part of the diet. It is plentiful and low cost. Some families serve it with wheat bread at every meal.

Most people like their beef roasted. This is called beef *asado* (ah-SAH-doe). They prefer to roast it outdoors on a grill called a *parrilla* (pah-REE-yah). At mealtime, you can smell meat roasting all over Argentina. This smell is so common that some say it is the "national scent" of Argentina!

Argentine cowboys are called *gauchos* (GOW-chohz). They like to top roasted meat with a peppery sauce called *chimichurri* (chihm-ee-CHUHR-ee). Argentines have many other recipes for beef. *Metambre* (meh-TAHM-bray) is a tasty beef appetizer. It is made by rolling vegetables up in steak and roasting it. Slices of metambre look like colorful spirals. *Carbonada criolla* (car-boh-NAH-dah cree-OH-yah) is a rich beef vegetable stew that is served in a hollowed out pumpkin shell. The *empanada* (ehm-pah-NAH-dah) is another well-known food. It is a turnover filled with chopped meat, olives, raisins, and onions. When you get the chance, give Argentine foods a try!

Meat, fish, and poultry can be cooked in a microwave oven. Moderate or low power settings are needed to keep meat from becoming tough during cooking. Tender meats and meats tenderized by grinding, pounding, cutting, or marinating are the best choices for microwave cooking. Large roasts and turkeys should not be cooked in a microwave oven. They are too large to cook evenly. Some parts may get overdone, while others remain undercooked.

Cooking Temperature

The look and taste of cooked meats depend on the cooking temperature used. Meats should be cooked slowly at low temperatures. At low temperatures, meat is more tender, juicy, and tasty than when cooked at high temperatures. Slow cooking gives the connective tissue enough time to soften.

At high temperatures, fat burns and juices evaporate. Cooking is so fast that there isn't enough time for the connective tissue to soften. Meat cooked at high temperatures is tough and dry.

Cooking Time

Total cooking time depends on the grade, cut, and type of meat. Higher grades and tender cuts need the shortest cooking time. Thick, large cuts take longer to cook than thin, small ones. Most fish cooks more quickly than red meat and poultry.

The length of cooking time also depends on how well done you want your meat. Beef can be cooked rare to well done. Many food scientists believe it's a good idea to cook beef at least until only a little pink remains. Harmful bacteria may survive in rare beef.

All poultry and pork should be cooked until they are well done. Cooking kills harmful bacteria found in chicken. It also kills the parasite that is found in the muscles of some pigs that causes trichinosis.

Fish and shellfish should be completely cooked. Raw fish may contain harmful bacteria. If you are eating dishes made with raw fish, be certain that the fish came from unpolluted water. Sushi (SOO-shee) is a popular Japanese dish made with raw fish. Reputable sushi restaurants use only fish from clean water.

Uncooked fish is translucent. It has a more solid, milky color when it is cooked properly. Finfish is finished cooking when it is firm and flakes easily. See 21-13.

21-13 Fish is done when it flakes.

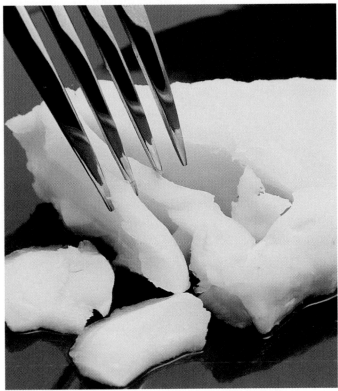

Sharp Electronics Corporation

Whole and drawn fish must be cleaned before cooking. Dressed fish, steaks, fillets, and sticks are ready to cook. No cleaning is needed.

Clams and mussels are done when their shells open. Fresh lobster is blue green. It turns bright red when it is cooked. Shrimp become pink when they are cooked.

Meat, fish, and poultry are versatile, protein-rich foods. In the next chapter, you'll learn about eggs and legumes, which are other protein-rich foods with many uses.

In a Nutshell

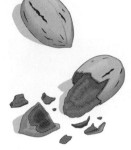

- Meat is a rich source of protein, iron, and zinc. It also contains fat and cholesterol.
- All beef, pork, veal, lamb, and poultry animals and their carcasses must be inspected. Inspection of fish is voluntary.
- Red meat and poultry grades try to predict how good the taste and texture will be.
- Finfish have backbones and fins.
- Shellfish have hard shells. They don't have any bones or connective tissue.
- Poultry is any bird raised for meat.
- Meat, fish, and poultry often are the most costly foods in the supermarket.
- Fresh meat, poultry, and fish should be stored in the refrigerator or freezer.
- Cooking makes meat, fish, and poultry tender, tasty, and appealing.
- Meat, fish, and poultry cooked at low temperatures are more tender, juicy, and tasty than when they are cooked at high temperatures.

In the Know

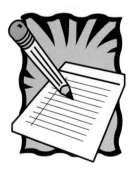

1. The three major parts of meat are _____, _____, and _____.
2. True or false? In the United States, all beef, pork, lamb, and veal carcasses must be graded.
3. Explain why meat cuts from the back of a cow are more tender than meat cuts from the legs of a cow.
4. The best quality fresh finfish have _____.
   A. a fishy smell
   B. bulging eyes
   C. shiny skin with firmly attached scales
   D. soft, slimy flesh
5. Explain why meat is cured.
6. Draw and label the parts of a meat label.
7. A _____ fish is sold just as it was when it was caught.
   A. drawn
   B. whole
   C. dressed
   D. fillet

8. Which is NOT true about the price of poultry?
   A. Whole birds cost less than parts.
   B. Small birds cost more per pound than larger birds.
   C. Duck costs more per pound than turkey.
   D. Older birds cost more per pound than younger birds.
9. Describe three ways to soften connective tissue.
10. Explain how to prepare fresh poultry for storage in the refrigerator.

What Would You Do?

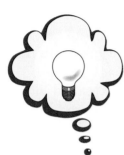

Your mom asks you to go to the supermarket with her. At the seafood counter, you notice that some fish are reduced to half price. Your mom thinks they are a good buy, but wonders if the fish are fresh. How can you tell if they are fresh? How can you tell if they are a good buy?

Expanding Your Knowledge

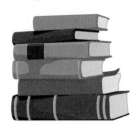

1. Visit a fish market or supermarket. Make a list of the types of fresh fish you see. Write a description of each fish. Include its colors, shape, and size. Also look for signs that the fish are fresh.
2. Interview a butcher. Ask the butcher to describe his or her job. Also ask: How is the meat department in a supermarket organized? How is meat inspected? How is it graded? Where is the meat produced? How is it shipped to the store? What training is needed to become a butcher?
3. Design a bulletin board on poultry. You could include pictures of the many types of poultry. You could also give tips for buying and storing poultry.
4. Start a file of meat, fish, and poultry recipes. Use these recipes to plan meals for three days.
5. Prepare two pieces of chicken. One piece should be from an older bird such as a stewing chicken. The other should be from a younger bird such as one labeled broiler, roaster, or fryer. Cut the two pieces in half. Cook one piece from each bird using dry heat. Cook the other two pieces using moist heat. Compare their taste, texture, and appeal.

6. Prepare three pieces of a less tender cut of beef (½ inch thick) as follows:
   A. Pound one piece with a meat mallet for two minutes on each side. Place on a broiling pan.
   B. Marinate the second piece in a mixture of ½ cup vinegar and ½ cup water for two hours. Place on a broiling pan.
   C. Place the third piece on a broiling pan.
   Broil each piece. Compare the taste, color, and texture of the three pieces.

7. Set up a taste panel to compare the flavor, smell, texture, and color of different forms of the same shellfish. For example, you could compare clams (canned, fresh, and frozen) or shrimp (dried, canned, fresh, and frozen).

8. Do some research to find out how sausages are made. Report your findings to the class.

9. Find out more about the Japanese seafood dish called sushi. Create a poster to display the information you gathered.

Chapter 22

Incredible Eggs and Legumes

Objectives

After reading this chapter, you will be able to
- ❑ explain how eggs are graded.
- ❑ select eggs in the supermarket.
- ❑ prepare and store eggs to maintain quality and safety.
- ❑ identify the functions of eggs as ingredients.
- ❑ describe how to buy, store, and prepare legumes.

New Terms

chalazae: two white stringlike structures that hold the yolk in the middle of an egg.

candling: shining a very bright light on eggs in order to judge their quality.

legumes: high-protein seeds, such as dry peas, dry beans, lentils, and peanuts, that grow in a pod.

vegetarian: person who does not eat meat, fish, or poultry.

tofu: a soft, custardlike food made from soybeans.

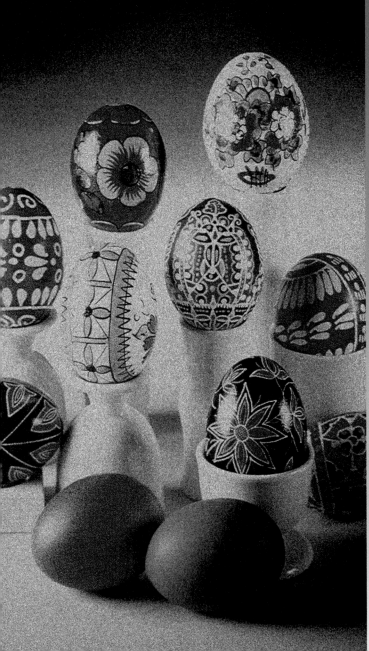

American Egg Board

Eggs and legumes are protein-rich foods. These nutrient-packed foods can be prepared in a variety of ways. They are often served in place of meat in meals. This chapter will allow you to explore the nutritious possibilities of eggs and legumes.

Eggs

Are eggs all they are cracked up to be? Yes! Eggs are tasty and good for you. They can come from a chicken, quail, ostrich, or any other bird.

Science in the Kitchen

Did You Know...

... some chickens lay green eggs?
The food some chickens eat makes the shells of the eggs they lay pale green. In fact, the shells could be any color. The shell color doesn't affect the flavor or nutrient content of the egg.

... a hard-cooked egg will spin like a top?
This makes it easy to tell a hard-cooked egg from an uncooked one without cracking them. Twirl an egg on its small end. If it spins, it's hard-cooked. If it falls over, it uncooked. Try it out!

... if you cook a whole egg in a microwave oven it will explode?
During cooking, steam forms inside the shell. The pressure from the steam builds up and causes the shell to explode. Before cooking an egg in a microwave oven, remove it from the shell and put it in a dish. Pierce the yolk with a fork. Cover the dish loosely with plastic wrap and cook on medium heat for about 40 seconds.

... one ostrich egg equals 20 hen eggs?
You could make a huge omelet with just one ostrich egg!

... if you grew as fast as a chicken, you would weight 350 pounds by the time you were two months old?

... hens lay about 240 eggs a year?

... there are more chickens than people in the world?

... you can put a whole egg in a bottle without breaking the shell?
Here's how! First, hard-cook an egg.– Don't remove its shell. Now, place the egg in a jar and cover it with vinegar. Place the lid on the jar and let set for five days. The egg will feel rubbery. You can easily put it into a bottle!
Here's why! Calcium makes the shell hard. (Calcium also makes bones and teeth hard.) Vinegar is a mild acid. Vinegar causes the calcium to leave the shell and enter the vinegar. Once the calcium is out of the shell, the shell is soft and rubbery.

Inside an eggshell is a food packed with nutrients. Eggs are a great source of protein. They also provide small amounts of many vitamins and minerals. Chicken eggs are low in calories, too. Each one has only about 80 calories.

You may already know that egg yolks are high in fat and cholesterol. Diets high in these may lead to heart disease. For this reason, health experts suggest eating no more than four egg yolks per week.

Most people think of eggs as a breakfast food. This low-cost food is great for lunch and dinner, too. In fact, people in France seldom eat eggs for breakfast. They like to make egg dishes part of a light supper.

What's in Eggs?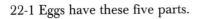

Eggs have five major parts. They are the yolk, chalazae (CHAH-lay-zah), white, membrane, and shell. See 22-1.

The *egg yolk* is where most of the nutrients are found. All the fat and cholesterol are the yolk, too. When freshly laid eggs are cracked onto a plate, the yolk stands high. As eggs age, the yolk flattens out.

Chalazae are part of the egg white. They look like two white strings. Their job is to hold the yolk in the middle of the egg. As eggs become older, the chalazae weaken. They aren't able to hold the yolk in place.

22-1 Eggs have these five parts.

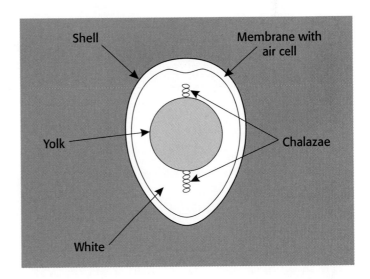

Cultures of the World

Vive la France!

France is located in the western part of Europe. The Eiffel Tower is in France. This famous structure is located in the capital city, Paris. Many people believe French cuisine is the finest in the world. The French view cooking as a fine art. Chefs try to release the flavor of each food. They combine food shapes, colors, and flavors to create appealing, tasty meals.

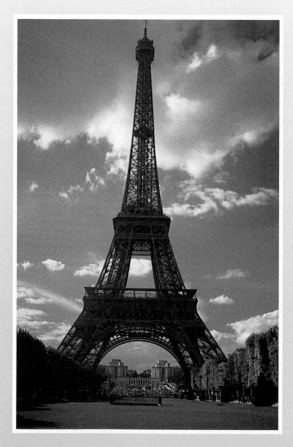

The Eiffel Tower is a popular sight in France. French cuisine is enjoyed throughout the world.

France is famous for its grapes, cheeses, breads, and egg dishes. Tons of grapes are harvested from French vineyards each year. More types of cheese are made in France than anywhere else in the world. *Camembert* (kam-ehm-BEAR), *Roquefort* (ROHK-fort), and *Brie* (BREE) are three popular cheeses from France.

Bread is served at every meal in France. Families buy it freshly baked twice a day. A favorite type of bread is long, thin, crisp loaves called *baguettes* (bah-GET).

French chefs have hundreds of ways of cooking eggs. Eggs are used to make French toast, crepes (KREPZ), and sauces. *French toast* is made by frying slices of bread that were dipped in egg. Crepes are thin pancakes that have meat, fish, vegetables, or fruit rolled up inside. Eggs are an ingredient in many sauces, such as *Hollandaise* (HAWL-ahn-dayz).

Egg dishes such as soufflés, quiche, and omelets are often part of a light lunch or dinner. Eggs are rarely eaten for breakfast. A *soufflé* is a light, airy egg dish made with whipped eggs. Other ingredients such as cheese or vegetables may be added. *Quiche* is a milk and egg mixture baked in a pastry crust. Quiche Lorraine has cheese and bacon in it, too. It is named for an area in the northeastern part of France. *Omelets* are prepared by beating eggs and cooking them on the range. Most omelets are filled with meat, cheese, vegetables, or fruit. The next time you have a quiche or omelet, imagine you're in a Paris cafe. After all, these foods are from France!

The *egg white* is almost pure protein. It is fat-free. One egg white has only 15 calories. In freshly laid eggs, the egg white is very thick and firm. Older eggs have thin whites.

A membrane is found between the shell and egg. This thin skin helps to protect the yolk and white. At the large end of the egg is an air cell. The air cell is between the membrane and the shell. Freshly laid eggs have a very small air cell. The air cell becomes larger as eggs age.

Eggshells may be thin, but they are very strong. They protect the food inside. Most eggshells are white or brown. The color depends on the breed of the hen. Shell color has no effect on the flavor of the egg or its nutrient content.

Eggshells have tiny pores. Bacteria, air, and odors can enter through the pores. As eggs age, air comes in through the pores. This causes the air cell to become larger and the yolk and white to become drier. Eggs stored in an open container can absorb odors from other foods in the refrigerator.

Buying Eggs

Before being sold, eggs often are graded and sized. Most supermarkets sell fresh eggs. You may be able to find frozen, dried, or even pickled eggs. Egg substitutes also are sold in many food stores.

Grading

Egg grades are set by the United States and state governments. Most fresh eggs are graded, but they don't have to be. The grade eggs receive is printed on their cartons, 22-2. The date the eggs were packed is stamped on the carton, too.

22-2 The grade given eggs at the time they were inspected is printed on egg cartons.

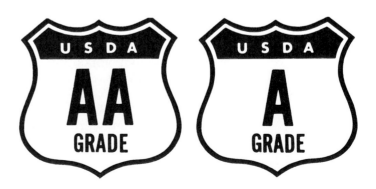

Inspectors grade eggs by shining a very bright light on them. The light lets the inspectors see through the shells and judge the quality of eggs. This process is called *candling.* See 22-3.

22-3 Candling is used to judge the quality of eggs.

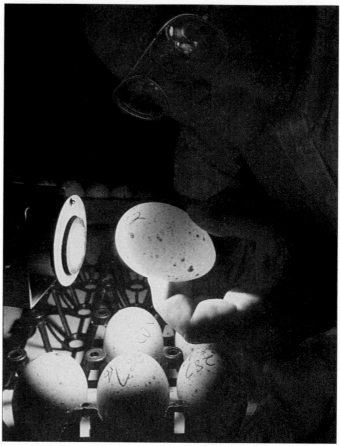

USDA

The best quality eggs are Grade AA. Grade AA eggs have smooth, clean shells and firm, clear egg whites. They have a small air cell. When cracked onto a plate, their yolks stand high.

Grade A and Grade B eggs have larger air cells. Their whites are runny. Their yolks flatten out. Lower grades don't look as nice as higher grades, but the nutrient content of all grades is the same.

Refrigerated eggs will maintain their grade for about five weeks after the date they were packed. Eggs stored outside the refrigerator drop to a lower grade in just a few days.

Egg Sizes

Eggs come in several sizes. The smallest eggs are called *peewees*. They weigh a little more than an ounce each. *Jumbo* eggs are the largest. They weigh about 2½ ounces each. There are four other sizes: *small, medium, large,* and *extra large*. The size is printed on the egg carton.

The United States government sets the standards for egg sizes. Size is based on the weight of a dozen eggs. For example, a dozen eggs of similar size that weigh 15 ounces are called peewees. A dozen eggs that weigh 30 ounces are called jumbos. See 22-4.

Most recipes are based on large eggs. Extra large or medium eggs can be used instead. You will need to adjust the recipe if you use jumbo or small eggs. Peewee eggs are rarely sold to consumers.

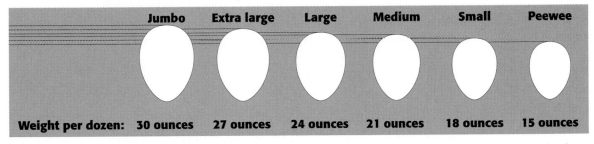

	Jumbo	Extra large	Large	Medium	Small	Peewee
Weight per dozen:	30 ounces	27 ounces	24 ounces	21 ounces	18 ounces	15 ounces

22-4 Egg size is based on the weight of a dozen eggs. Not every egg in the carton will be exactly the same size.

Fresh Eggs

When shopping for fresh eggs, buy those stored in refrigerated cases. Eggs lose freshness fast if they are not refrigerated. Open the carton to see that eggs are clean and not cracked. It's a good idea to lift each egg to be sure it isn't stuck to the carton. See 22-5.

The price of eggs depends on grade and size. Higher grades cost more than lower grades. Larger eggs often cost more than smaller eggs. The unit price will help you locate the best buy.

Frozen and Dried Eggs

You can buy frozen whole eggs, egg whites, and egg yolks. They can replace fresh eggs in recipes. Some supermarkets sell frozen heat-and-eat egg dishes such as omelets.

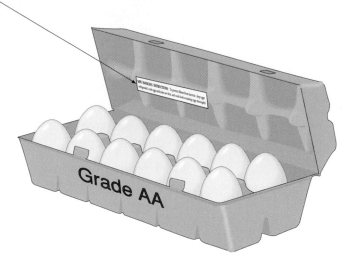

SAFE HANDLING INSTRUCTIONS: To prevent illness from bacteria: keep eggs refrigerated, cook eggs until yokes are firm, and cook foods containing eggs thoroughly.

Grade AA

22-5 To help keep consumers healthy, the Food and Drug Administration now requires this statement on cartons of fresh eggs that have not been commercially pasteurized.

Dried eggs are made by removing the water from whole eggs. They can be stored for months in a cool, dry place. Dried eggs are popular for camping and in places where refrigeration is not available. Add water to prepare dried eggs for cooking.

Egg Substitutes

Egg substitutes are made mostly from real egg whites. Most don't include any egg yolk. Other ingredients are added to fulfill the role of yolks. These ingredients usually are nonfat dry milk and vegetable oil.

People wanting to lower the cholesterol and fat in their diets often choose egg substitutes. This is because egg substitutes made with no egg yolks are cholesterol-free. Also, egg substitutes have much less fat than fresh eggs.

Most egg substitutes are frozen. You should thaw them in the refrigerator, in hot water, or in a microwave oven before using them. It is not safe to thaw them at room temperature. Store foods made with egg substitutes the same way you store foods made with fresh eggs.

The flavor and color of egg substitutes is similar to fresh eggs. Egg substitutes work well in many recipes calling for beaten eggs.

Storing Eggs

The best way to store eggs is in a covered container in the refrigerator. Covered containers prevent eggs from absorbing the odors of other foods. They also keep eggs from losing moisture through the pores. The best storage container for eggs is the carton. It protects them and helps maintain their quality.

Eggs should be stored with the large end pointing up. This keeps the yolk centered and slows the loss of quality.

Eggs can be frozen for long-term storage. Remove them from the shell and freeze them in an airtight container. If you freeze an egg in its shell, it will expand and break the shell. When you are ready to use the frozen eggs, thaw them in the refrigerator. They should be used as soon as they are thawed.

Moist foods that contain eggs should be stored in a covered container in the refrigerator. This includes dishes such as egg salad, omelets, and sauces. Most dry foods that contain eggs don't need to be refrigerated. For example, most cakes, cookies, and breads can be stored in a cool, dry place.

Preparing Eggs

Eggs can be served for any part of the meal. Eggnog is a beverage made with eggs. Deviled eggs are a tasty appetizer. Salads can include eggs, too. Egg salad and chef's salad are examples. Spinach omelets and quiche (KEESH) are main dishes made with eggs. Most desserts are made with eggs. The main ingredient in custard is eggs. Many cakes and cookies contain eggs, too.

When eggs are cooked, they become firmer. The egg white goes from clear to milky white. The yolk becomes more opaque. Cooking also kills harmful bacteria.

Salmonella bacteria hide on eggshells. Food scientists report this harmful bacteria also hides inside some raw eggs. Heat kills this bacteria. To avoid the risk of foodborne illness from salmonella, be sure to eat only cooked eggs. Eggs should be cooked at least until the whites are milky white and the yolk begins to harden. Avoid eating foods made with uncooked eggs that have not been commercially pasteurized. Commercial pasteurization kills bacteria.

The best egg dishes are tender. Eggs are most tender when cooked at low temperatures only until they are done. High temperatures and long cooking times make eggs tough, lumpy, and discolored. For instance, a hard-cooked egg that was simmered has a yellow yolk and a tender texture. A hard-cooked egg that was boiled has a greenish egg yolk and a rubbery and tough texture. Although is it safe to eat, it's not very appealing.

Science in the Kitchen

Cooking Up Some Eggs!

The best egg dishes look appealing and have a tender texture. Both appearance and texture are affected by cooking temperature and cooking time. To see how cooking temperature and time affect eggs, prepare a hard-cooked egg in the following ways. You will need two saucepans and two whole, raw eggs in their shells.

1. Place an egg in each pan and cover with enough cool water to come at least 1 inch above the egg. Cover the pan.

   Variable A:
   Bring to a boil. Let boil for 15 minutes.

   Variable B:
   As soon as the water boils, remove the pan from the heat. Let the egg stand in the water for 15 minutes.

2. Cool both eggs by putting them in cold water.

3. When the eggs feel cool, peel them.

4. Place each egg on a separate plate. Cut each in half.

How do the eggs differ in appearance? How are they alike? Taste each of the eggs. Which egg is the most tender? Which egg has a rubbery texture? Why do these differences exist? How can you use these observations?

There are many ways to prepare eggs. See 22-6. Some cookbooks contain nothing but egg recipes! Eggs can be simmered in their shell. They also can be fried, scrambled, baked, or poached. You can whip up an omelet in a minute or two. You can even cook eggs in a microwave oven. Just remember to crack eggs into a dish and pierce the egg yolk before cooking them in a microwave oven. Also, be sure to use a low power setting.

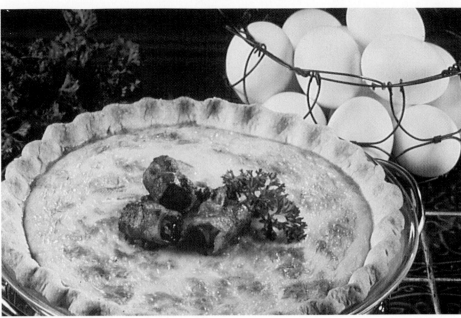

American Egg Board

22-6 Eggs are the main ingredient in many different dishes. Have you ever tried quiche?

When appearance is important, use higher grade eggs. For instance, Grade AA eggs are best for poaching, cooking in the shell, and frying. Lower grade eggs spread out. They don't look as appealing as higher grade eggs. Lower grade eggs are best used as ingredients in recipes or for scrambling.

Using Eggs as an Ingredient

Eggs perform many roles in foods. They add color, flavor, and nutrients to foods. For instance, eggs add color and flavor to breads, cakes, puddings, and ice cream. They help breads and cakes to have a brown crust. Eggs give puddings and ice cream a creamy yellow color and rich taste. Brushing a beaten egg on breads and pastries makes the crust shiny.

Whipping egg whites causes them to become foamy and stiff, 22-7. They increase three or four times in volume. Whipped egg whites are used to make meringues, puffy omelets, and soufflés. A meringue is a topping for a pie. It is a mixture of whipped egg whites and sugar. A puffy omelet is made by folding beaten egg

22-7 Beaten egg whites are foamy. They are used to make meringues, puffy omelets, and soufflés.

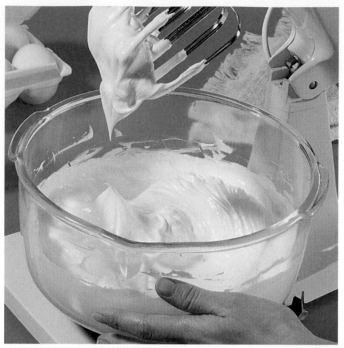

American Egg Board

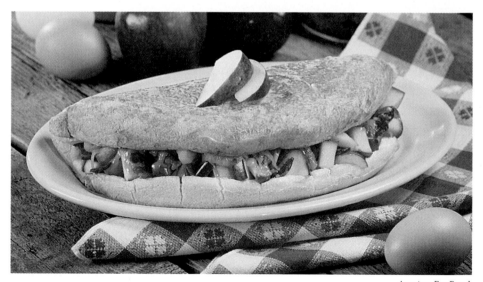

American Egg Board

22-8 The fillings in puffy omelets add many important nutrients.

yolks into whipped egg whites, 22-8. After cooking, puffy omelets may be filled with fruit or cheese. A soufflé (soo-FLAY) is similar to a puffy omelet. It has a sauce added to the eggs. Soufflés are baked in the oven. See 22-9.

22-9 Soufflés are made by folding beaten egg yolks into foamy egg whites.

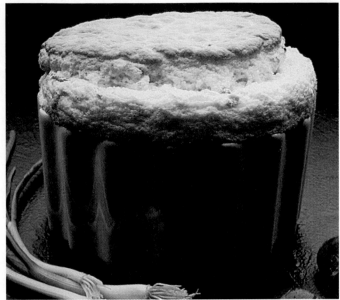

American Egg Board

Eggs also perform the following four other functions:

- *Binding ingredients together.* In the role of binding agent, eggs help to "glue" ingredients together. For example, eggs hold the ingredients in meatloaf together. Many fried foods are dipped in egg, then rolled in flour or bread crumbs. Eggs bind these coatings to foods. Eggs also help keep fried foods from absorbing too much fat.
- *Thickening foods.* Heat makes the protein in eggs thicken. This means that eggs can be used to make liquid foods thicker. Eggs may be a thickening agent in pie fillings, soups, ice cream, and sauces.
- *Emulsifying ingredients.* Egg yolks are an emulsifying agent. They help to blend ingredients that don't mix together, such as oil and water. Egg yolks mix with oil. They also mix with water. Water and oil can mix if an egg yolk is added. Egg yolks are used to emulsify the ingredients in mayonnaise and some sauces.
- *Leavening baked goods.* When eggs are beaten, they form many tiny air bubbles. Beaten eggs can be used to add air to foods. This makes foods light and fluffy. The air in beaten eggs may be a leavening agent in breads and cakes.

Eggs serve as binding, thickening, emulsifying, and leavening agents in many baked desserts. In the next chapter, you'll learn about baked desserts like pies, cakes, and cookies.

Legumes

Legumes are high-protein seeds that grow in a pod. They are produced by a certain plant family. This family includes many dry peas and dry beans. It also includes lentils and peanuts.

Legumes have been an important food for thousands of years. People all over the world eat this flavorful, nutritious, low-cost food. In the United States, legumes have always been popular among vegetarians. *Vegetarians* are people who do not eat meat, fish, or poultry. Today, more and more people are discovering how healthful and versatile legumes can be.

 ## Focus on Nutrition

Going Vegetarian

There are four main types of vegetarians. Most vegetarians eat any food from plant sources. This includes fruits, vegetables, grains, nuts, seeds, and dry peas and beans. *Vegans* eat only foods from plant sources. *Lacto-vegetarians* eat plant foods plus foods from the milk group. *Ovo-vegetarians* eat plant foods plus eggs. *Lacto-ovo-vegetarians* eat plant foods, eggs, and foods from the milk group.

Nutrients in a Vegetarian Diet

With careful planning, vegetarians can get all the nutrients they need. However, they need to pay special attention to protein, vitamin B_{12}, and iron. That's because the richest sources of these nutrients are from the meat and beans group. Vegetarians eat only dry beans and perhaps, eggs, from the meat and beans group. Vegetarians who do not eat foods from the milk group also need to pay special attention to calcium and vitamin D.

Protein

Vegetarians who eat eggs or foods from the milk group easily meet their protein needs. However, vegans will need to combine plant proteins to get all the needed amino acids.

Combining plant proteins is like putting a puzzle together. You must have the right pieces for them to fit. Grains, nuts, and seeds are one part of the puzzle. They lack some amino acids, but contain plenty of others. Dry peas and beans are another part of the puzzle. They are low in other amino acids, but have a lot of the amino acids that grains, nuts, and seeds lack. By combining dry peas and beans with grains, nuts, or seeds, a vegan can get all the amino acids needed.

Here are some examples of how these two pieces of the puzzle fit together. These plant protein combinations contain all the amino acids you need:

- Boston baked beans and brown bread
- Pasta fagiole (beans and pasta)
- Hoppin' John (black eyed peas and rice)

- Tofu and rice
- Refried beans and corn chips
- Lima beans and cornbread
- Peanut butter sandwich
- Hummus (chickpeas and sesame seeds)

Vitamins

Vegetarians who include eggs and foods from the milk group in their diets can get all the vitamins they need. Vegans may need to take vitamin B_{12} and vitamin D supplements or eat foods that have these vitamins added to them. Many ready-to-eat breakfast cereals have these vitamins added. Also, people who spend time in the sunshine can get all the vitamin D they need.

Minerals

All types of vegetarians need to make an extra effort to eat foods that contain iron. That is because meats are the best source of iron. Dark green vegetables and foods in the grains group can supply some iron. All types of vegetarians may need an iron supplement.

Ovo-vegetarians and vegans don't eat foods from the milk group. Therefore, they will need to depend on other sources of calcium. Dark green vegetables, almonds, sunflower seeds, and dry beans provide some calcium. Calcium supplements may be needed.

Menu Planning

Vegetarian diets can be very nutritious and easy to plan. With just a few changes to the Food Guide Pyramid, vegetarians can use it just like everyone else. The changes vegetarians should make to the Pyramid are shown here.

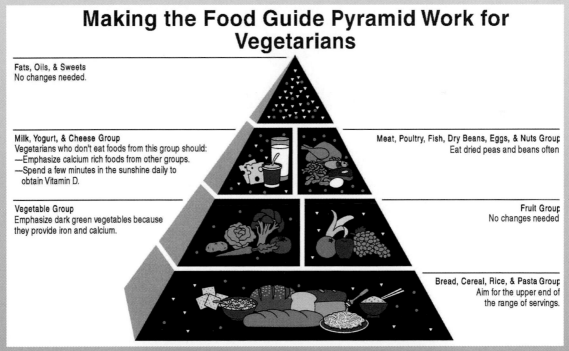

Making the Food Guide Pyramid Work for Vegetarians

Fats, Oils, & Sweets
No changes needed.

Milk, Yogurt, & Cheese Group
Vegetarians who don't eat foods from this group should:
—Emphasize calcium rich foods from other groups.
—Spend a few minutes in the sunshine daily to obtain Vitamin D.

Meat, Poultry, Fish, Dry Beans, Eggs, & Nuts Group
Eat dried peas and beans often

Vegetable Group
Emphasize dark green vegetables because they provide iron and calcium.

Fruit Group
No changes needed

Bread, Cereal, Rice, & Pasta Group
Aim for the upper end of the range of servings.

USDA

Vegetarians can use the Food Guide Pyramid by following these guidelines.

Legumes come in every color of the rainbow, 22-10. There are yellow peas and green lentils. Beans may be red, white, pink, black, or tan. Some are even spotted! Some peas have black eyes! No matter what color they are, legumes are a rich source of protein. In fact, legumes are considered to be part of the same group of the Food Guide Pyramid as meat. Legumes also are a good source of fiber, calcium, and iron. They are low in fat. Legumes not only add nutrients to your diet, they also add flavor, color, and texture.

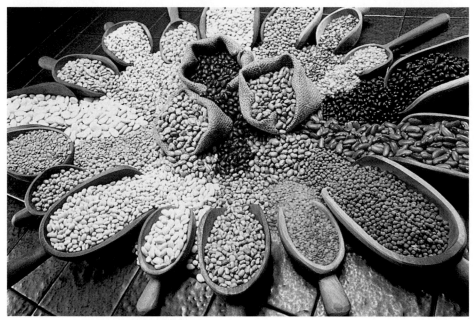

American Heart Association

22-10 How many of these legumes have you seen or tried?

Buying and Storing Legumes

Legumes are a very low-cost source of protein. They are much less expensive than meat, fish, and poultry. Legumes are a good way to save money on protein foods.

Supermarkets sell two main forms of legumes: dried and canned. Dry peas, beans, and lentils are usually sold in plastic bags. Some food stores have large bins of legumes. You can scoop out the amount you want to buy. Canned legumes may be plain or have added seasonings or sauces.

You can save money by buying dry peas, beans, and lentils. This is because they cost much less than those that are canned. However, dry peas, beans, and lentils take longer to prepare than canned ones.

When buying dry peas, beans, and lentils, choose those that have a bright color. A pale color tells you the legumes are old. Old legumes will take longer to cook and may not be as tasty as fresher ones. Also, choose legumes that are similar in size. They will not cook evenly if their sizes differ. The small ones will get done before the large ones. The best dry legumes are not wrinkled or cracked. They also are free of insect holes and nonfood materials like small twigs and stones.

Select canned legumes as you would any canned food. That is, buy cans that are not dented, rusted, or swollen.

Store dry peas, beans, and lentils in airtight containers placed in a cool, dry, dark location. This storage method will protect the quality of these legumes. Unopened cans of legumes will maintain their quality for a year or more if you store them in a cool, dry place.

Many food stores also sell a legume product known as tofu. *Tofu* is a soft, custardlike food made from soybeans. It has a very mild flavor. It is a rich source of protein and is low in calories and fat. Tofu can be eaten plain. Many people like to add it to stir-fried foods and casseroles. Buy tofu that is creamy white and firm, but not hard. Keep it refrigerated and use it within a week of purchase.

Preparing Legumes

Legumes can be used in many ways, 22-11. They may be used to make a bean burrito. They are often an ingredient in soups and stews like black bean soup and chili. They can be added to salads or casseroles. They also can be served as a side dish. For example, baked beans are a popular legume side dish. You can mash them to make a bean dip.

Canned legumes don't need any preparation. All you need to do is open the can. They are ready to eat or add to a recipe.

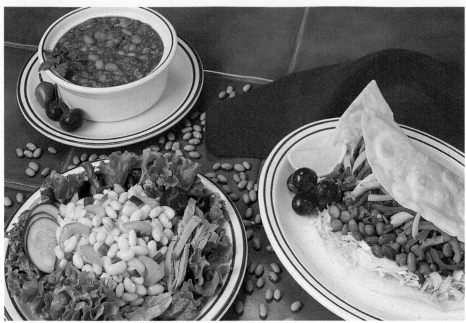

Idaho Bean Commission

22-11 There are thousands of recipes that call for legumes.

Dry legumes, especially dry peas and beans, take considerably more time to prepare. To prepare them, follow these steps:

1. Place the legumes in a colander and wash them thoroughly. Then remove any wrinkled, broken, or discolored peas or beans. Also remove any foreign objects, like tiny stones, that you find.

2. Soften the dry peas or beans. You can do this by placing them in a large pot. For every cup of peas or beans you place in the pot, add 5 cups of water. Cover the pot. Cook on high and bring to a boil. Boil for three minutes and then allow them to set for 2 hours before cooking. You can also allow the peas or beans to soak overnight in a covered pot. Soaking is very important. If the peas or beans are not soaked, they will not get soft when you cook them. Briefly boiling, then soaking also helps keep beans from causing gas in your digestive system.

3. Drain the peas or beans and rinse them well. Then, put them back in the pot and add fresh water.

4. Gently simmer them on the cooktop in a covered pan. Check the package to determine how much water to add and how long to cook them. Cooking time usually ranges from one to three hours.

Properly cooked peas and beans have a firm texture. If they are mushy, they were overcooked. If they are hard, they were under-cooked. Once the legumes are cooked, they are ready to eat. You could serve them plain. You can also use them as an ingredient in a recipe, 22-12. Many cookbooks include recipes that call for legumes.

22-12 Legumes add many nutrients to meals.

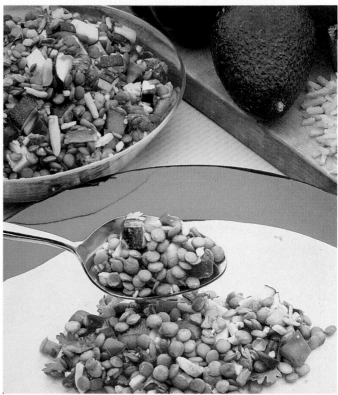

Since it takes a while for dry peas and beans to cook, it's important to plan ahead. You may want to make a large batch so that you have enough for more than one meal. Leftover cooked peas and beans need to be refrigerated or frozen. Be sure to use refrigerated cooked peas and beans within a week. Frozen legumes will maintain their quality for six months or so.

The next time you are planning a meal, think about having a legume dish. Remember, legumes are a low-cost and low-fat alternative to meat, fish, and poultry. They can help you to conserve your food dollars and protect your health.

In a Nutshell

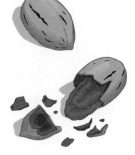

- Eggs are a rich source of protein.
- The five parts of an egg are yolk, chalazae, white, membrane, and shell.
- Inspectors grade eggs by judging their quality using a process called candling.
- Eggs maintain their quality longest if they are kept refrigerated.
- The United States government sets the standards for egg grades and sizes.
- The carton is the best container for eggs.
- The most tender and appealing eggs are cooked at low temperatures.
- Eggs are binding, thickening, emulsifying, and leavening agents.
- Legumes are rich sources of protein, fiber, calcium, and iron.
- Dry peas and beans are prepared by rinsing, soaking, and simmering them.

In the Know

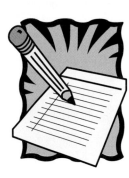

1. Draw and label the parts of an egg.
2. Which part of the egg is almost pure protein?
   A. Yolk.
   B. White.
   C. Chalazae.
   D. None of the above.
3. True or false? Brown eggs are more nutritious than white eggs.
4. Explain how candling works.
5. Which are the most nutritious?
   A. Grade AA eggs
   B. Grade A eggs
   C. Grade B eggs
   D. All of the above are equally nutritious.
6. Describe how to store fresh eggs.
7. A _____ is a topping for a pie made with whipped egg whites and sugar.
   A. meringue
   B. soufflé
   C. omelet
   D. chalazae
8. True or false? Raw eggs are safe to eat.

9. Explain how you can avoid getting salmonella food poisoning from eggs.
10. True or false? Eggs can be used to make liquid foods thicker.
11. List the characteristics of high-quality dry peas and beans.
12. True or false? Legumes are high in fat.

What Would You Do?

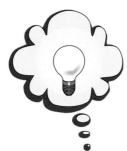

Your mom just found her grandmother's eggnog recipe. The recipe calls for raw eggs. She is thinking about serving it at a family party next week. What advice would you give her?

Expanding Your Knowledge

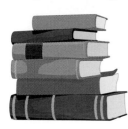

1. Select an omelet recipe. Prepare it in these two ways listed below. Then compare the flavor, texture, and appeal of the two products.
   - Use fresh whole eggs.
   - Use an egg substitute. NOTE: One fresh whole egg is equal to ¼ cup of egg substitute.
2. Test the effect of food odors on eggs. Place a chopped onion and a whole raw egg in its shell in a bowl. Cover tightly and refrigerate for one week. Place the egg in a saucepan. Cover with enough cool water to come at least 1 inch above the egg. Cover the pan and heat. As soon as the water boils, remove the pan from the heat. Let the egg stand in the water for 15 minutes. Run cool water over the egg to cool it completely. Taste the egg. How can you use this information?
3. Visit an egg farm. Make a list of questions to ask the farmer. You might ask: What are chickens fed? How many eggs does a hen lay each day? How are the eggs collected? Where are they candled? What happens to the eggs before they reach the supermarket?
4. Find out more about salmonella bacteria. Why is this bacteria commonly found on eggshells? How does it get inside some eggshells?

5. Look through cookbooks to find recipes that include eggs. Make a list of recipes that use eggs as leavening agents. Also make lists of recipes that use eggs as thickening, emulsifying, or binding agents.
6. Create a poster that shows many different ways legumes can be prepared. Use magazine pictures or drawings to illustrate the poster.
7. Interview a vegetarian. You could ask these questions. What foods do you eat? What are your favorite legume recipes? What do you order when you go to a restaurant?

Chapter 23
Delicious Desserts

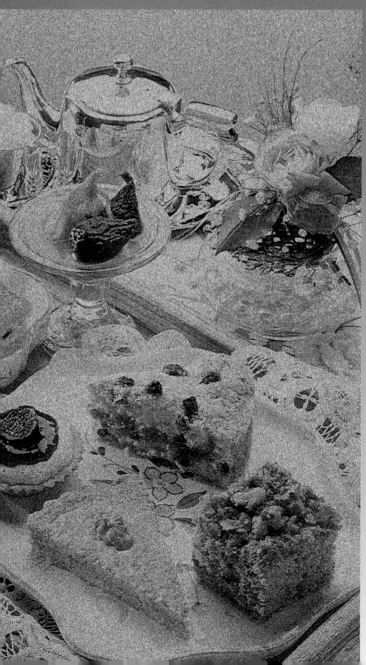

Objectives

After reading this chapter, you will be able to
- describe the types of cakes, cookies, and pies.
- explain how to blend ingredients for cakes, cookies, and pastry crusts.
- prepare cakes, cookies, and pies.
- store cakes, cookies, and pies to maintain freshness.

New Terms

shortened cakes: cakes that contain fat such as butter or shortening.

conventional method: mixing method used for shortened cakes in which fat and sugar are creamed together, the eggs added, and sifted dry ingredients are added alternately with the liquid ingredients.

quick-mix method: mixing method used for shortened cakes in which dry ingredients are sifted into a mixing bowl, the fat and liquid are added, then the eggs are added.

foam cakes: cakes that contain no fat; sometimes called unshortened cakes.

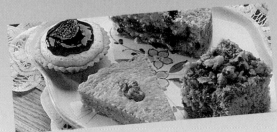

Sun-Diamond Growers

Greeks eat baklava. People in Iceland ask for vinarterta. Germans serve lebkuchen. New Zealanders serve Pavlova. Chinese people request pa-ssu-ping-kuo. In Kenya, people ask for chin-chin. What are all these foods? Desserts! People all over the world eat them.

Cultures of the World

Out of Africa

Ghana is located in the western part of Africa. This small country is hot, humid, and rainy most of the year. It is only dry in winter. During the winter, a hot dry wind from the Sahara desert blows across Ghana.

Most Ghanaians live on small farms. They raise cassava, yams, corn, and rice. Casava and yams are starchy root vegetables. They are ground into flour. They make up the largest part of the Ghanaian diet. Ghanaian farmers grow peanuts, peas, beans, and vegetables, too. Their land produces barely enough food.

Meat is eaten only for very special events. Ghanaians may eat the animals they raise or wild animals. Mice and insects, such as certain types of ants, caterpillars, and grasshoppers are eaten, too. These foods are rich in protein. In coastal areas, fish and shellfish are eaten.

Some farmers have enough land to grow cash crops like sugar cane and *cacao* (kuh-KOW) beans. These beans are used to make chocolate. Ghana is a leading producer of cacao beans. The chocolate candy bar you eat may be made with beans grown in Ghana. Ghana's biggest cacao bean customers are the United States, Holland, Germany, Great Britain, and Russia.

Most Africans eat one meal each day. This meal is served in the evening. When it's time to eat, families gather. They begin the meal by washing their hands and clapping. The main dish at dinner in Ghana is almost always *fufu* (foo-foo). Fufu is a thick paste of flour and water. It looks like oatmeal. A platter of fufu is placed in the middle of the table. Everyone eats with their fingers from the same platter. A small amount of stew, vegetables, or fruit may be served with the fufu. Desserts are usually fresh fruit. For special events, sugared fried pancakes, banana fritters, or cookies are served.

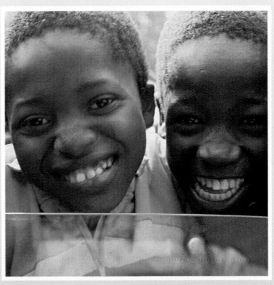

Doug Furtek, American Cocoa Research, Institute Molecular Biology Lab, Penn State

Desserts bring a smile from children. Children of Ghana often enjoy fresh fruit for dessert.

Desserts provide a sweet ending to meals. Desserts can be as simple as fresh berries or ice cream. They can be as fancy as a chocolate cake or coconut cream pie.

There are many dessert choices. All of them usually have one thing in common. They are sweet. Many are high in calories. Very sweet, creamy desserts have the most calories. Fresh fruit and low-fat milk desserts have the least calories.

Some desserts are good sources of vitamins and minerals. Of course, this depends on their ingredients. Fresh fruit desserts provide vitamins A and C. Milk desserts are rich in calcium. See 23-1. Most pies, cakes, and cookies provide small amounts of a few vitamins and minerals. They contain mostly carbohydrates.

23-1 This ricotta raspberry parfait dessert supplies both calcium and vitamins.

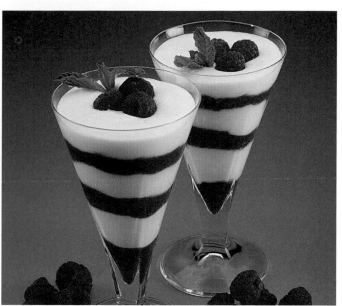

National Dairy Board

Cakes

There are many types of cakes! Some cookbooks contain only cake recipes. Cakes range from bite-size cupcakes to towering wedding cakes. Cakes may be served plain or decorated to look like a clown or cartoon character. Cakes can be almost any flavor. You could make a cherry, marble, or poppy seed cake. Carrot cake and pound cake are delicious treats, too. See 23-2.

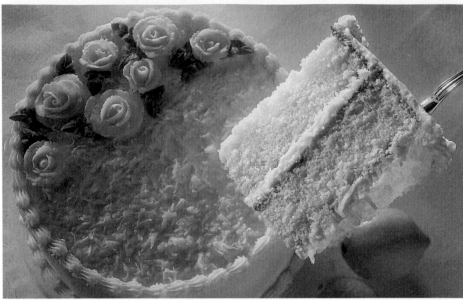

Eastman Chemical Company

23-2 Cakes make mealtimes special. A cake can be the centerpiece at a special event.

Cakes are made with many of the same ingredients used to make breads. Flour, sugar, eggs, liquid, and leavening agents are used. These ingredients function the same way in cakes as they do in breads. (See Chapter 19.)

Types of Cakes

Although there are many kinds of cakes, there are two basic types of cakes. All cakes are either shortened cakes or foam cakes.

Shortened Cakes

Shortened cakes contain fat such as butter or shortening. Chocolate, spice, and pineapple upside-down cakes are examples. Perfect shortened cakes are tender and light. They have a thin crust. The crust is smooth and rounded on top. The inside is silky and moist. Of course, they taste great, too. The cake in 23-2 is a shortened cake.

The ingredients in shortened cakes can be blended using either the conventional or quick-mix method. Your recipe will tell you which method to use.

The ***conventional method*** for mixing cakes takes three bowls. In the first bowl, cream the fat and sugar until light and fluffy. Beat in the eggs. In the second bowl, blend all the liquid ingredients. Sift the dry ingredients together in the third bowl. The second and fourth steps are to beat half the liquid ingredients into the creamed mixture. The third and fifth steps are to beat in half the dry ingredients. When all the ingredients are blended, it's time to bake the cake. See 23-3.

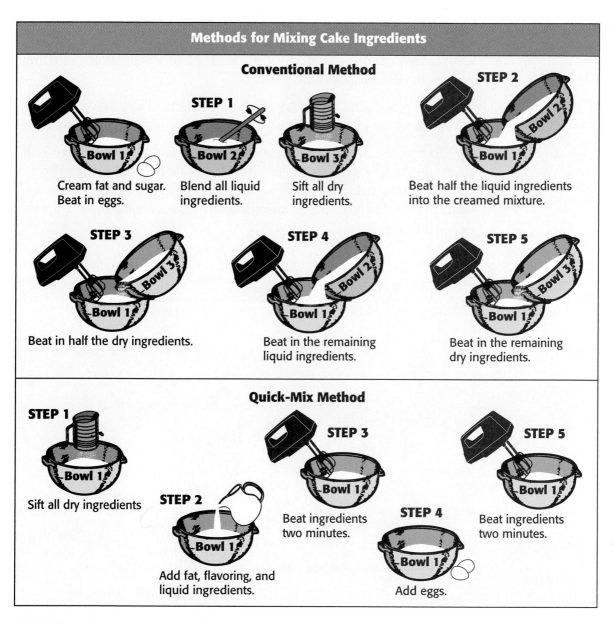

Methods for Mixing Cake Ingredients

Conventional Method

STEP 1

Cream fat and sugar. Beat in eggs. (Bowl 1)

Blend all liquid ingredients. (Bowl 2)

Sift all dry ingredients. (Bowl 3)

STEP 2

Beat half the liquid ingredients into the creamed mixture.

STEP 3

Beat in half the dry ingredients.

STEP 4

Beat in the remaining liquid ingredients.

STEP 5

Beat in the remaining dry ingredients.

Quick-Mix Method

STEP 1

Sift all dry ingredients

STEP 2

Add fat, flavoring, and liquid ingredients.

STEP 3

Beat ingredients two minutes.

STEP 4

Add eggs.

STEP 5

Beat ingredients two minutes.

23-3 Follow these steps for mixing shortened cakes.

The ***quick-mix method*** is also called the one-bowl method. To make a cake using this method, sift all the dry ingredients into a mixing bowl. Add the fat, flavoring, and liquid ingredients. Beat the ingredients for two minutes. The last step is to add the eggs and beat for two more minutes.

Foam Cakes

Foam cakes, sometimes called unshortened cakes, contain no fat. Angel food, sponge, and chiffon cakes are foam cakes. These cakes are leavened with air beaten into egg whites. Angel food cakes are fat-free. Sponge and chiffon cakes include egg yolks, so they have a small amount of fat.

The best foam cakes are fluffy and light. They have a tender crust. They are moist and not gummy. They are tasty, too. See 23-4.

To make a foam cake, beat the egg whites until they are stiff, shiny peaks. (See 22-7.) When you lift the beater, the peaks should stand up straight. Mix all the other ingredients together in a second bowl. Gently fold the ingredients in the second bowl into the egg whites.

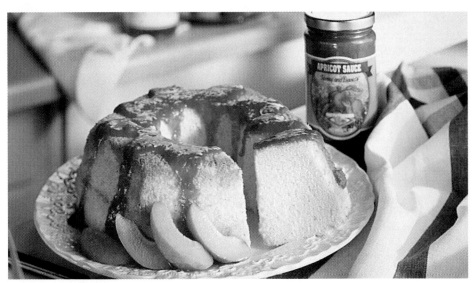

Harry and David

23-4 The best foam cakes are light, tender, and moist.

Baking Cakes

Cakes should be baked in a preheated oven. Be sure to set the oven to the right temperature. If the oven is too hot, the crust gets too brown and cracks. If it's too cool, the cake won't cook fast enough. The cake will be flat and dry. Try not to open the oven during baking. Every time the door opens, the oven temperature drops.

Cake pans come in many sizes and shapes. Check the recipe to see which size you need. If the pan is too big, the cake will spread out too far. It will be flat and dry. If the pan is too small, the cake batter will overflow. Cakes baked in light-colored pans will have light, tender crusts. Dark pans make the crust dark and tough. Grease the pan if you are making a shortened cake. Do not grease the pan if you are making a foam cake. Foam cakes are baked in a tube pan. The tube heats the center of the cake and allows the cake to bake evenly.

Bake cakes for the amount of time given in the recipe. A cake is done when it pulls away from the sides of the pan. It should spring back when you touch it lightly. Another way to test for doneness is to insert a toothpick in the center of the cake. The cake is done when the toothpick comes out clean. See 23-5.

23-5 You can test a cake for doneness by inserting a toothpick into the center of the cake. If the toothpick comes out clean, the cake is done.

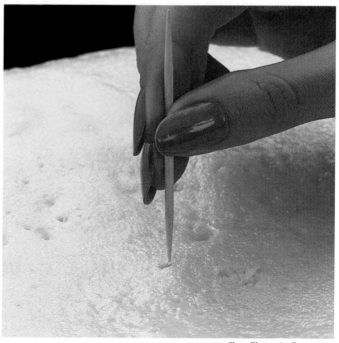

Sharp Electronics Corporation

Cool shortened cakes 5 to 10 minutes in the pan. Then, run a spatula around the edge of the pan to loosen the cake. Invert the cake onto a wire rack and remove the pan. Let the cake finish cooling on the wire rack. Leave baked foam cakes in the pan and turn and the pan upside down. Place the pan's tube on a funnel or bottle so the cake doesn't touch any surface. Leave the cake in the pan until it is cool.

Cake Toppings

Many people like to top cakes with frosting. Pudding and whipped cream are other tasty toppings. All of these add many calories to the cake.

You can save calories by topping cakes with fresh fruit. Another way to save calories is to sprinkle the cake lightly with powdered sugar. You can also drizzle on just a little frosting, 23-6. Cakes are great served plain, too.

Before you frost a cake, be sure it has cooled. A warm cake will cause the frosting to melt. Brush off all the loose crumbs. Then, place narrow strips of waxed paper between the edge of the cake and the serving plate. The waxed paper catches any frosting drips and helps keep the serving plate neat. Now, spread frosting on the top of the bottom layer. Stack the top layer on the bottom layer. Frost the sides. Then, frost the top. The last step is to remove the waxed paper strips.

23-6 Trim calories by using only a small amount of frosting.

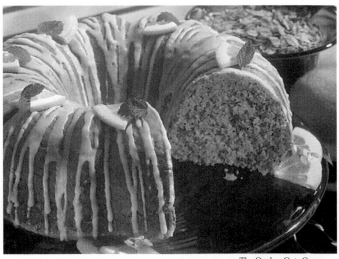

The Quaker Oats Company

Storing Cakes

It's hard to resist freshly baked cakes. They're best when eaten within a day or two. Wrap any leftovers tightly. Uncovered cakes dry out and become stale fast. Always store cakes made with pudding or whipped cream in the refrigerator.

You can make cakes up to three months ahead of time and freeze them. They can be frosted before freezing or after thawing. Before serving a frozen cake, thaw it at room temperature. If the cake is frosted, uncover it before thawing. This will keep the frosting from sticking to the covering.

Cookies

Making cookies is quick and easy. In less than an hour, you can be enjoying freshly baked cookies. The term *cookie* includes any small, sweet cake. Cookies are usually flat. Some are soft, others are crisp. Many are round, but cookies can be any shape.

Most cookies are made with sugar, fat, eggs, flour, and water. Some include special ingredients, such as chocolate chips, nuts, spices, or raisins.

Cookies can be put into six groups. These are drop, bar, molded, rolled, pressed, and refrigerator. The groups differ by the stiffness of the dough and how you handle the dough. Drop and bar cookies are made with soft dough. Molded, rolled, pressed, and refrigerator cookie doughs are stiff.

Drop cookies are made by dropping spoonfuls of dough onto a cookie sheet. Oatmeal and chocolate chip cookies are drop cookies. See 23-7.

Bar cookies are made by spreading the soft cookie dough in a pan. After baking, these cookies are cooled, cut, and served. Brownies and date bars are well-known bar cookies. See 23-8.

Molded cookies are shaped with the hands. Small balls and crescents are common shapes. Balls may be flattened with the bottom of a glass or a fork. Peanut butter cookies are molded cookies.

Rolled cookies are made by rolling out the dough and cutting it into shapes. You can use a knife or cookie cutters to cut the dough. Many people like to decorate rolled cookies with colorful sprinkles. Rolled cookies include sandwich cookies and sugar cookies.

23-7 Many drop cookies are soft and chewy.

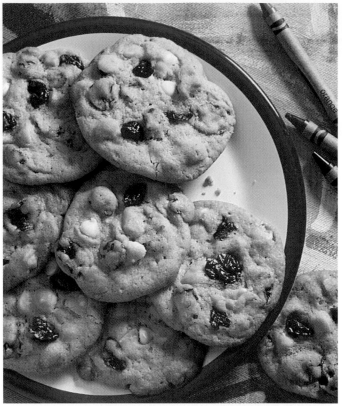

Cherry Marketing Institute, Inc.

23-8 Brownies are one of the most popular bar cookies.

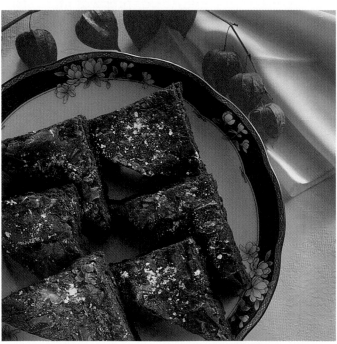

Eastman Chemical Company

Pressed cookies are made by pushing dough through a cookie press. Spritze and lemon crisps are two types of pressed cookies. See 23-9.

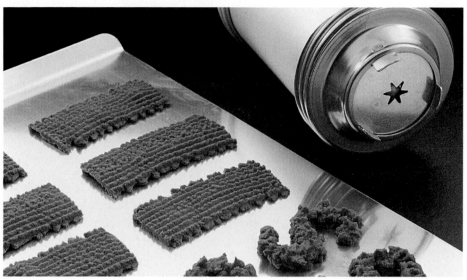

General Mills, Inc.

23-9 Pressed cookies come in fancy shapes.

Refrigerator cookies are formed when dough is shaped into a roll. It is then wrapped tightly and refrigerated. Once it is well chilled, the dough is cut with a knife into thin slices and baked. Pinwheel cookies are an example.

Preparing Cookies

The ingredients for most cookies are blended using the conventional method. All cookies are baked on a cookie sheet except bar cookies.

Cookie sheets don't have any sides. This makes it easy to remove cookies from the pan. Plus, it lets the cookies bake more evenly. If you don't have a cookie sheet, you can bake your cookies on the bottom of an inverted cake pan.

Place cookies on a cool pan. If it is hot, the cookies will melt and spread out. Light, shiny pans give cookies a tender crust. Dark pans cause the cookies to form a dark, heavy crust.

It's a good idea to make all your cookies the same size and shape. This way they will all get done at the same time. If the sizes vary, small cookies will burn before large ones get done.

Drop and refrigerator cookies spread out when they bake. They won't run together if you place them 2 inches apart. Rolled, molded, and pressed cookies spread less. They can be placed about 1 inch apart.

Bake cookies in a preheated oven. Cookies bake fast, so watch them closely. Refrigerator, pressed, rolled, and molded cookies are done when they are light brown and firm. Drop cookies are done if they spring back when you touch them lightly. Bar cookies pull away from the sides of the pan when they are done. If you touch them lightly, a slight dent remains.

The best cookies have a tender crust. Some cookies, such as peanut butter and chocolate chip, are soft and moist. Others, such as lemon wafers and gingersnaps, are crisp and dry. All cookies should taste great.

Storing Cookies

Keep cookies fresh by storing them in a container with a tight cover. If soft cookies become hard, put a slice of apple or bread in the container with them. Replace the slice every day or two. If crisp cookies become soggy, place them on a cookie sheet and put them in the oven at 300°F or 150°C for a few minutes. This will dry them out and make them crispy again.

Cookies can be frozen for long-term storage. When you want to serve frozen cookies, thaw them at room temperature. You can freeze cookie dough, too. Thaw cookie dough before baking.

Pies

Pies can be a sweet ending to any meal. You might be surprised to learn that some pies aren't sweet at all. The term "pie" refers to any food baked in a crust, 23-10. The crust can be filled with almost any food. Many dessert pies have a fruit or creamy filling. Main dish pies are filled with meat, eggs, or cheese. Chicken pot pie and quiche are popular main dish pies.

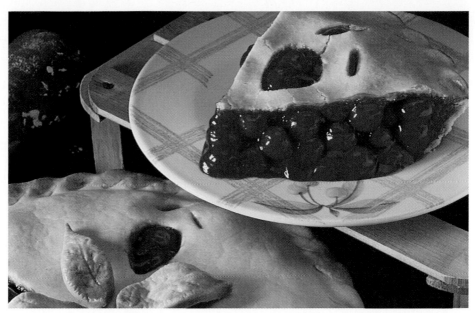

23-10 Pastry crusts are often used for desserts, like this cherry pie.

There are four types of dessert pies. *Fruit pies*, such as apple and peach pies, are a well-known type. Any fresh, frozen, or canned fruit can be used. The fruit is blended with sugar and cornstarch or flour. *Custard pies* are common, too. They contain eggs and milk. Pumpkin pie is an example. *Cream pies* begin with a baked crust. The crust is filled with pudding and topped with meringue or whipped cream. Lemon meringue and banana cream pies are examples. *Chiffon pies* are light and airy. They contain gelatin and beaten eggs. Some include whipped cream. Lime chiffon pie is an example.

Some pies are large enough to serve eight people. Others are so small they serve only one. Small pies are called *tarts*. Tarts are appealing because it's fun to have your own individual treat.

Most pies are baked in a pie pan. *Turnovers* are pies cooked on a baking sheet. They are pockets of pastry dough filled with any food used in a pie filling.

Preparing Pie Crusts

Some pies are made with crumb crusts. The crumbs are made by crushing crackers, cookies, or cereal. The crumbs are mixed with sugar and melted margarine or butter and pressed into a pie pan.

Most pie crusts are made with *pastry dough.* The best pastry crusts are golden brown. They are light, tender, and flaky. A flaky pastry crust has many thin layers of dough.

Pastry dough is made with flour, salt, water, and fat. The ingredients for pastry dough are combined using the biscuit method. (This is described in Chapter 18.) Pastry dough is rolled out on a lightly floured surface. It's easiest to roll if you start at the center and work outward using short, light strokes. As you roll, try to keep the dough in the shape of a circle. The dough is ready when it's ⅛-inch thick and 4 inches bigger than your pie pan (2 inches on each side).

Lift the dough by rolling it onto the rolling pin. Dough tears easily, so handle it with care. Place the rolling pin over the edge of the pan and unroll the dough into the pan. Be careful not to stretch the dough. The next steps depend on whether you are making a one-crust or two-crust pie.

One-Crust Pies

One-crust pies have a crust only on the bottom to hold the pie filling. Once the dough for a one-crust pie is in the pan, you'll need to shape the edge with a fork or your fingers. Then, trim off the excess dough. If the pie filling is to be baked, pour it into the crust. Bake it according to the recipe. If the filling isn't baked, prick the bottom and sides of the crust with a fork. This keeps the crust from puffing up during cooking. Bake and cool. Add the filling and serve.

Two-Crust Pies

Two-crust pies have a crust on the bottom to hold the filling and a crust on the top to cover the filling. The filling of two-crust pies is baked along with the pie crusts. After the dough for the bottom crust is placed in the pan, the filling is poured into the crust. Then, a second crust is rolled out, rolled onto the rolling pin, and placed on top of the pie filling. The edges of the top crust should overlap the edge of the pie pan 1 to 2 inches. To seal the edges of the bottom and top crust, moisten the edge of the bottom crust with water or a beaten egg. Then, press the two crusts together with your finger or a fork. Trim off the excess dough. Gently cut four or five short (1-inch) slashes in the top pie crust. These slashes will let the steam that forms during baking escape. Bake, cool, and serve.

Some two-crust pies have a *lattice top.* See 23-11. Lattice tops are made by weaving dough strips on top of the pie filling.

23-11 This two-crust pie has a lattice top.

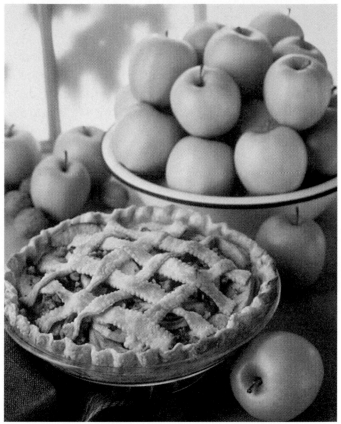

Washington Apple Commission

Storing Pies

Most pies taste best the day they are made. Leftovers will stay fresh for a day or two. Wrap pies loosely and keep them in a cool place. If pies are covered tightly, the crust will become soggy. Pies containing meat, eggs, or milk need to be refrigerated.

Pastry dough can be frozen. You can freeze it in a ball or you can roll out into a pie pan and freeze it in the pie pan. Wrapped tightly, frozen pastry dough stays fresh for up to six months. Thaw it at room temperature.

Fruit pies can be frozen before or after they are baked. Thaw baked pies at room temperature. Unbaked pies can go directly from the freezer to the oven. Fruit pies can be frozen for six months. Chiffon pies can be frozen for a few weeks. Cream and custard pies don't freeze well. Their fillings tend to become watery when they are thawed.

Convenience Desserts

Supermarkets sell many convenience dessert items. You can buy canned and frozen pie fillings. Ready-to-fill crumb crusts are sold, too. Supermarkets also sell mixes for cakes, cookies, pie fillings, and pie crusts. These mixes are simple to prepare. Often, you only need to add liquid and eggs. The directions are easy to follow, and the desserts can be prepared quickly. Their quality may be close to homemade desserts.

÷ Math in the Kitchen

Comparing Cookie Cost and Appeal

This activity will give you a chance to compare the appeal and cost of six types of chocolate chip cookies. For this activity, you'll need to prepare chocolate chip cookies in each of the following ways:

Cookie Type A: From scratch using a recipe from a cookbook.
Cookie Type B: From refrigerated dough.
Cookie Type C: From a mix.

You'll also need to obtain the following:

Cookie Type D: A package of ready-to-eat chocolate chip cookies from a supermarket.
Cookie Type E: Six ready-to-eat chocolate chip cookies from a bakery.
Cookie Type F: Six ready-to-eat chocolate chip cookies from a specialty cookie store.

Record and total the costs of all the ingredients used to make *Cookie Types A, B,* and *C.* Also, record the prices of *Cookie Types D, E,* and *F.*

After all the cookies are baked or purchased, weigh all the cookies of each type. Record the weights.

Now, calculate the cost per ounce of each cookie type. Here's the equation for calculating cost per ounce:

$$\text{Total cost} \div \begin{matrix}\text{Weight} \\ \text{in ounces} \\ \text{of all cookies}\end{matrix} = \begin{matrix}\text{Cost per ounce} \\ \text{of a} \\ \text{cookie type}\end{matrix}$$

For instance, suppose all the ingredients for *Cookie Type A* cost $3.20. Also, suppose all the *Type A* cookies together weighed 16 ounces. Using the equation above, you would find *Cookie Type A* costs 20 cents per ounce.

$$\$3.20 \div 16 \text{ ounces} = \$0.20$$

Set up a taste panel. Compare the color, taste, and texture of each type of cookie. Which cookie looked the best? Which cookie tasted the best? Which cookie had the best texture? Did the cookie that cost the most seem worth the higher price? Why or why not? Which cookie took the most time to prepare? Did the cookie that took the longest to prepare seem worth the extra time? Why or why not? How can you use this information?

Refrigerated and frozen cakes, cookies, pies, and pastry crusts are other convenience items. Most of these are heat-and-eat foods. They only require baking. Just pop them into the oven and serve. Some frozen cakes and pies are ready to serve, they don't need baking at all.

Ready-to-eat desserts need no preparation, 23-12. Just open the package and serve. You can buy ready-to-eat cakes, pies, and cookies at supermarkets and bakeries.

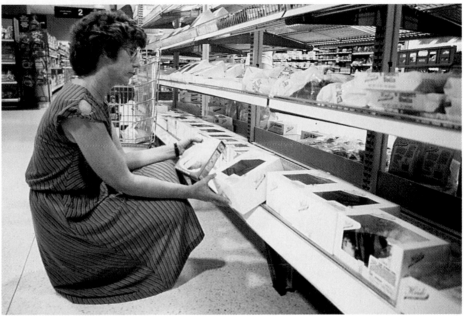

USDA

23-12 Convenience dessert items can save busy cooks time.

Convenience dessert items often cost much more than homemade desserts. Mixes tend to be the least costly convenience dessert items. Ready-to-eat pies, cakes, and cookies are the most costly convenience dessert items. Convenience desserts may cost more than homemade desserts, but they save you time and energy. Convenience desserts help you to serve appealing, sweet treats even when you are in a hurry.

Focus on Food

Chocolate, 1,000 Years of Delight

Chocolate is a popular food. It's so well liked that the average person in the United States eats about 10 pounds per year! People have been enjoying chocolate for at least 1,000 years. The Aztec Indians living in Central America were some of the first people to eat it. They made a cocoa drink called chocolatl. They served it to their ruler, Montezuma, in a golden cup. It is said that he drank 50 cups of chocolatl each day!

In the early 1500s, Spanish explorers learned about cocoa from the Aztecs. They took this new food back to Europe. Cocoa quickly became a hit.

It may surprise you to learn that chocolate grows on trees. It is made from the beans of the *cacao* tree. These trees grow in hot, humid regions near the equator. Cacao beans are a major crop in West African countries, such as Ghana, Ivory Coast, and Nigeria. Other major growers are the Latin American countries of Mexico, Venezuela, Ecuador, and Brazil. Cacao beans aren't all the same. The types vary from region to region. Each type has its own special flavor.

If you ate a plain cacao bean, you might be surprised that it doesn't taste anything like a candy bar. The beans are very bitter. They must go through a long process before they become chocolate. The process begins by harvesting the ripe bean pods. The beans are removed from the pods. After resting for about a week, the beans are dried. The next step is to

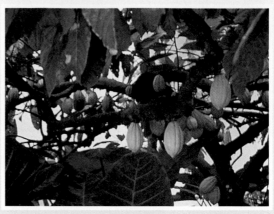

Doug Furtek, American Cocoa Research, Institute Molecular Biology Lab, Penn State

The yellow fruit hanging on this tree contains cacao beans.

ship them to chocolate makers in the United States or Europe.

The chocolate makers roast the beans to develop their flavor and aroma. Next, the chocolate makers remove the skins from the beans. Then they crush the beans. The crushed pieces are called nibs. Nibs look like dark brown pebbles. They are very bitter and dry. Nibs from beans grown in different regions are blended. Each chocolate maker has a secret recipe for blending the nibs. That is why each brand of chocolate has a unique flavor. Some brands have a mild flavor. Others are strong.

The blended nibs are ground. They become warm during grinding, which causes the fat in the bean to melt. This fat is called *cocoa butter.* The grinding produces a thick, bitter liquid. This liquid may be

- dried to make cocoa
- poured into molds to make blocks of unsweetened chocolate
- sweetened and used to make chocolate bars and candy

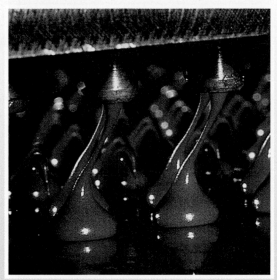

Doug Furtek, American Cocoa Research,
Institute Molecular Biology Lab, Penn State

Sweetened liquid chocolate is used to make chocolate candy.

Large amounts of sugar are needed to make this liquid taste sweet. Chocolate may be 20 to 80 percent sugar. Semisweet, bittersweet, and sweet chocolate are made by adding more and more sugar to the liquid. Milk chocolate is made by adding milk to sweet chocolate.

The best chocolate has a silky sheen and a rich, brown color. It breaks firmly and crisply. The broken edges are clean and don't crumble. It smells good and melts like butter in your mouth. It has a fine, pleasing flavor. Top quality chocolate doesn't stick to your mouth, feel gritty, or leave an after taste.

It's important to store chocolate in a cool, dry place. If it gets warmer than 78°F (25°C), the cocoa butter melts and rises to the top. This makes the surface of the chocolate turn gray. The gray color doesn't affect the quality or flavor of the chocolate. It is still safe to eat, but it doesn't look as nice. Chocolate can be stored in the refrigerator, too. It is likely to turn gray if refrigerated. Cocoa powder can be stored at room temperature in a tightly sealed container. Unopened chocolate syrup can be stored at room temperature, too. Once it's open, store it in the refrigerator. Properly stored chocolate and cocoa will keep for a year or more.

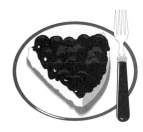

What's the difference between a desert and dessert? A desert is a hot, dry place. A dessert is a tasty, sweet food. Desert has only one s and dessert has two. To keep the spelling straight, just remember that many people like to have two servings of desserts!

In a Nutshell

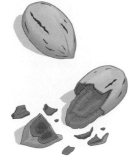

- The nutrient content of desserts depends on the ingredients used to make them.
- The two types of cakes are shortened cakes and foam cakes.
- Ingredients in shortened cakes can be blended using the conventional or quick-mix method.
- Store cakes, cookies, and pies in a cool, dry place. Refrigerate them if they contain pudding or cream.
- Cakes, cookies, and fruit pies can be frozen for long-term storage.
- Cookies can be put into six groups: drop, bar, molded, rolled, pressed, and refrigerator.
- Cookie ingredients are blended using the conventional method.
- Pies are any food baked in a crust.
- There are four types of dessert pies: fruit, custard, cream, and chiffon.
- Most pie crusts are made with pastry dough.
- Supermarkets sell many convenience dessert items.

In the Know

1. Which is a shortened cake?
   A. Angel food cake.
   B. Chocolate layer cake.
   C. Chiffon cake.
   D. Sponge cake.
2. True or false? A shortened cake is fat free.
3. Put the steps for the quick-mix method of making a cake in order.
   ___ A. Put the fat, flavoring, and liquid into the mixing bowl and beat two minutes.
   ___ B. Sift all the dry ingredients into the mixing bowl.
   ___ C. Put the eggs into the mixing bowl and beat two minutes.
4. True or false? After baking a shortened cake, leave it in the pan until it is completely cool.
5. Which type of cookie is not baked on a cookie sheet?
   A. Drop cookie.
   B. Rolled cookie.
   C. Pressed cookie.
   D. Bar cookie.

6. _____ cookies are made by forcing the dough through a cookie press.
7. The best cookies are baked on a _____.
   A. hot pan in a preheated oven
   B. cool, dark pan in a preheated oven
   C. cool, light pan in a unpreheated oven
   D. cool, light pan in a preheated oven
8. If crisp cookies become soft, explain how you can make them crisp again.
9. A _____ is any food baked in a crust.
10. A _____ pie contains gelatin and beaten eggs.
    A. fruit
    B. custard
    C. chiffon
    D. cream

What Would You Do?

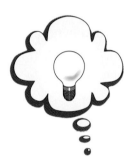

You want to make a special dessert for your sister's high school graduation party. She is watching her weight and doesn't eat many sweets. What type of low-calorie desserts could you make?

Expanding Your Knowledge

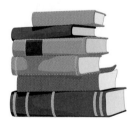

1. Visit a bakery. Observe how desserts are made in large quantities. Note how cakes are decorated. What type of equipment is used? How are the ingredients measured? How often are desserts made? How long do they stay fresh? Do some research to find out how you can become a baker.
2. Plan a bake sale. Prepare a variety of cupcakes, tarts, and cookies.
3. Make a cookie recipe file. Group the recipes according to the six types of cookies.
4. Gather favorite pie, cake, and cookie recipes from your friends. Combine them into a cookbook.

5. Visit a supermarket. Record the cost of a cake mix, frozen cake, and ready-to-eat cake. Find a cake recipe in a cookbook and compute the cost of the ingredients. Which form is the best buy? How much time does it take to prepare each?

6. Find a pie crust recipe in a cookbook. Practice making it. Write a script on making pie crusts for a cooking show. Have someone videotape your presentation.

7. Design a bulletin board about cakes, cookies, and pies from around the world. Use a world map for the background. You can place a picture of a Black Forest Cake near Germany or an eclair near France. Use string and tacks to connect the picture of the dessert with its country of origin.

8. Compare the effects of pans on cookies. Find a recipe in a cookbook for sugar cookies. Bake a third of the dough on a light, shiny cookie sheet. Bake a third of the dough in a light, shiny pan with sides such as a cake pan. Bake a third of the dough in a dark pan with sides. Compare the color and texture of the cookies.

9. Do some research to find more details on chocolate processing. Make a poster that shows how cacao beans become a candy bar.

Chapter 24

A Career to Consider

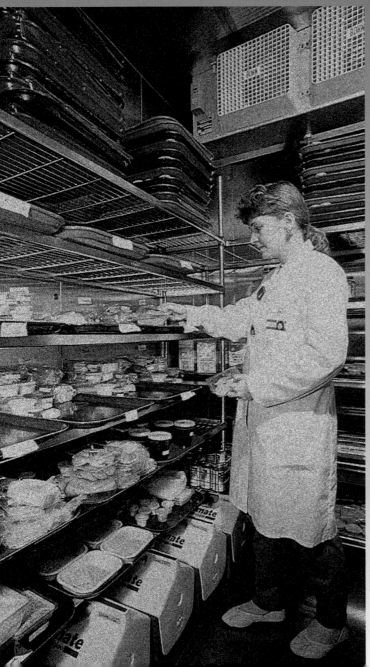

Objectives

After reading this chapter, you will be able to
- describe how to choose a career path that suits you.
- list characteristics employers expect employees to have.
- describe career opportunities in food and nutrition.
- explain how to find a job.

New Terms

career: the work in a certain field that you do for a long period of time.
values: beliefs and ideas that are important to you.
goals: aims you want to achieve.
career ladder: a series of jobs in the same field to which you can advance.
references: people an employer can call to ask about your abilities as a worker.

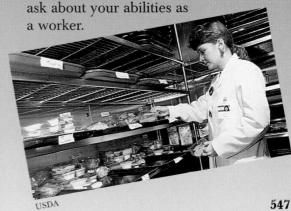

USDA

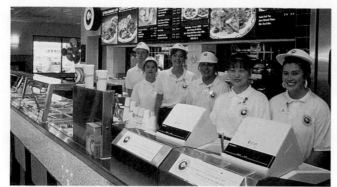

Food service workers

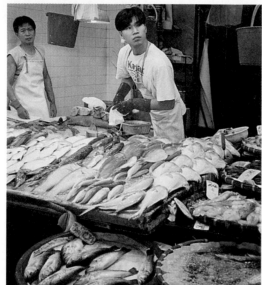

Fish seller USDA

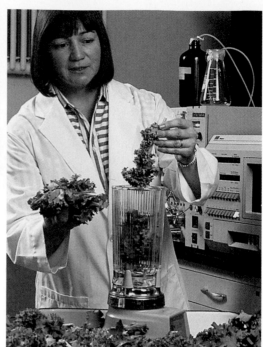

Food scientist USDA

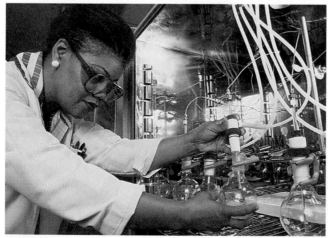

Nutrition research technician USDA

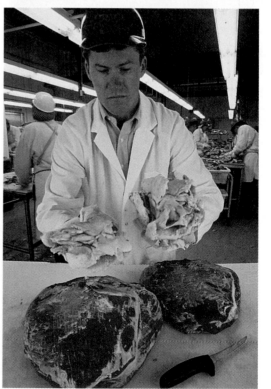

Butcher USDA

24-1 Career paths can lead in many different directions.

"What do you want to be when you grow up?" You have probably answered this question many times since you were a small child. As you got older, your answer may have changed. Your answer may change a few more times before you actually begin your career. These changes may occur because you learn more about yourself. These changes often occur because you learn about new career possibilities. A *career* is the work you do for a long period of time in a certain field.

Finding a career that you will enjoy is important. This is because your career will affect every aspect of your lifestyle. For instance, your career is likely to affect the way you feel about yourself. It may affect how others see you. The career you choose also will affect who you meet. It will affect when you work. It may affect where you live. Your career will have a strong influence on you. This is why you'll want to find a career that will give you the lifestyle and enjoyment you want. To find such a career, you will need to think about your personal characteristics. You'll also need to learn about different types of careers. This chapter will help you do just that. It will also help you learn about the many careers in foods and nutrition. See 24-1.

Thinking About Yourself

One of the first steps in choosing a career is to think about your personal qualities. What are your personality traits? What are your interests? What are your talents? Answers to questions like these can help you find a career that is right for you. For instance, if you have an outgoing personality, you might do well in sales. If you enjoy helping people, you might choose a career that lets you counsel people. If your hobby is cooking and you do it well, you would probably be successful in a food preparation career. If you enjoy studying chemistry at school, you may want to pursue a career in science.

Your values also play an important part in a career search. *Values* are beliefs and ideas that are important to you. Answering questions like those listed in 24-2 can help you identify some of your personal values. Your answers will also help you identify what you want from your career. Your answers can help you find a career that suits you. If you value creativity, you may be happy in a career that lets you develop new recipes. If you like spending a great deal of time with your family, you may not want a career that requires frequent travel.

Personal Values	
Independence	Do you like to work on your own or as part of a group?
Money	Are you concerned more about your income or enjoying your work?
Helping others	Do you enjoy doing things for other people?
Variety	Do you like to work on one project or several different projects?
Job security	Do you prefer to work where you don't have to worry about losing your job?
Status	Do you want to have a prestigious career?
Creativity	Do you like to create new items or discover new ways to do tasks?
Power	Do you like having authority over others?
Competition	Do you like to compete with others?
Fame	Do you want to be publicly recognized for your work?
Family and friends	Do you like to spend time with your family and friends every day?
Education	Do you enjoy learning new information? Do you enjoy going to school?

24-2 These questions can help you identify your personal values.

You also need to think about your goals when choosing a career. *Goals* are the aims you want to achieve. They describe what you want to do with your life. A person who wants to pursue a career as a dietitian might have the goals listed below.

- I want to become an officer in the Family and Consumer Sciences Club next year.
- I want to take a nutrition course in high school.
- I want to volunteer to work in the dietary department at the local hospital.
- I want to talk to my family and consumer sciences teacher about becoming a dietitian.
- I want to earn a college degree in nutrition.
- After college, I want to get a nutrition counseling job at a large hospital.

It's important to be realistic when setting your goals. Do you really want to reach a certain goal? How much time will it take to achieve it? How much money will it cost? Do you have the ability to achieve it? Is the goal in keeping with your values? Well-defined, realistic goals can help you choose a career. They can also help you get ready to begin your career.

Exploring Careers

Learning about different careers is interesting. It will help you decide which type of career you might want to pursue. You may have already identified a career that interests you. If you haven't, now is a good time to begin exploring career choices. You can learn about careers by talking to your school counselor and teachers. Your parents and people in your community can help you explore career paths, too. You can also get career information at the library.

When you are exploring a career choice, be sure to get answers to the questions in 24-3. These answers will give you a good idea of what a certain career involves. Your answers will also help you decide whether a certain career is right for you.

Exploring Careers
What is the daily routine of people working in this career?
What responsibilities do they have?
What would the working conditions be like?
What hours do people in this career work?
Where do they work?
How much do they travel?
What income can people in this career expect to earn?
Are job opportunities expected to increase or decrease in the future?
How much training or education is needed to enter this career?
How much training or education and experience are needed to move up the career ladder?
What are the opportunities for advancing up the career ladder?
How much self-satisfaction will I get from this career?
What other careers are related to this one? Would I enjoy pursuing a related career?

24-3 When exploring careers, ask yourself and others these questions.

Preparing for a Career

Learning about careers helps you identify steps you can take now to prepare for them. For example, you may learn that a certain career requires further education. If so, you can begin to research colleges that provide the education needed. If you discover that experience is needed, you could get a summer job. If you learn that a specific skill is needed, you could take a course in high school to learn that skill. The more you prepare yourself, the more likely you are to make a satisfying career choice.

Preparing yourself will also put you at an advantage when it's time to apply for the job you want. Preparing yourself helps you move up the career ladder, too. A *career ladder* is a series of jobs in the same field, 24-4. It shows you the jobs to which you can advance. The bottom of the career ladder represents entry-level jobs. The middle represents mid-level jobs. The upper rungs represent high-level jobs. Entry-level jobs usually do not require experience or a college degree. Each job on a career ladder builds on the skills learned in the jobs below. To climb up the career ladder, you need to gain skill and experience in entry-level jobs. You also need to begin developing the skills needed to succeed in upper-level jobs. You may need to earn a college degree to climb the career ladder.

24-4 These are the jobs you might have as you advance in a food preparation career.

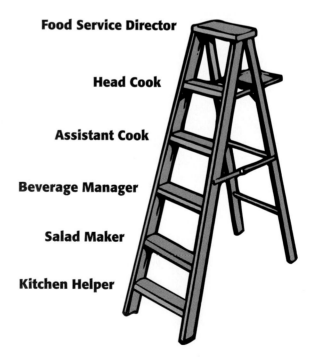

Food Service Director

Head Cook

Assistant Cook

Beverage Manager

Salad Maker

Kitchen Helper

An important part of preparing yourself for any career is to work hard in school. Employers like to hire good students because good students usually become good employees. Also, education will play a key role in your future career.

For success in almost any job, you must be able to read, write, do math, and communicate well. Suppose you wanted to apply for work in a restaurant as a food server. To fill out the job application, you would need to know how to read and write. You would also need these skills to read the menu and take food orders. Math skills are important because you would be handling money. You would also need to be able to listen, understand, and speak clearly to customers and your employer.

Education beyond high school is required for some careers. Further education is always helpful. The more education a person has, the better his or her chances are of moving up the career ladder. Technology is rapidly changing our world. To stay up-to-date and keep moving up the career ladder, you need to learn new skills. It is important to continue learning throughout your life.

Careers in Foods and Nutrition

Have you ever thought about a career related to foods and nutrition? There are enough choices to suit almost every interest. For instance, do you like to bake cakes and cookies? If so, you might consider becoming a baker. If you like to meet people, think about being a host in a restaurant. Do you dream about working under the wide-open sky? If so, you might become a farmer. If the bustling business world appeals to you, you might enjoy a supermarket career. Do you enjoy experimenting with new recipes in the kitchen? You might think about working in a test kitchen. You might want to be a dietitian if promoting good health is important to you. If you have an artistic flair, food styling may be the career for you.

Many people in the United States work in careers related to food and nutrition. The number of job opportunities in this field is growing rapidly. There are jobs in this field for people of all educational backgrounds. Some jobs require a high school diploma.

Others require further education. Sometimes you can be trained on the job. There are many opportunities for moving up the career ladder. Careers related to food and nutrition can be divided into four main groups

- food service careers
- food producing and processing careers
- food marketing careers
- health care, education, communication, and research careers
  This chapter takes a look at each of these career paths.

Food Service Careers

Restaurants, snack bars, fast-food chains, cruise ships, hotels, and hospitals are just some of the places people in food service careers work. There are four main areas in food service

- food preparation
- sanitation
- customer service
- management

To be successful in food service careers, people need to be healthy and able to work hard. They also need to be able to work quickly under pressure.

Food service workers have many opportunities to work their way up the career ladder. Many people learn their skills on the job. Those in the food preparation and management areas may need special training. They may get this special training in vocational or technical school. A company may teach special classes. They can also get special training in college.

If you are interested in a food service career, think about getting some experience soon. You might get an after-school job at a fast-food restaurant. You might consider working in the kitchen at a camp during the summer. You could also take foods and business courses in school.

Food Preparation

Food preparation involves preparing food to be sold. Salad makers, sandwich makers, bakers, and chefs are examples of people who work in the food preparation area, 24-5.

24-5 People working in food service prepare foods to be sold in restaurants.

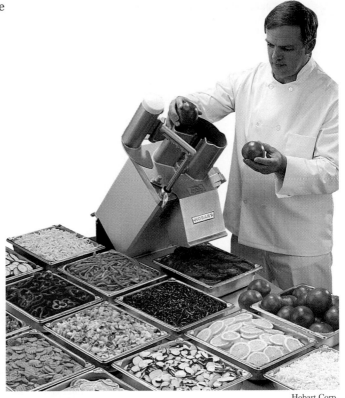

Hobart Corp.

Sanitation

Sanitation involves keeping the restaurant and its supplies clean. Dishwashers are responsible for keeping the tableware, pots, and pans clean and sanitary. Maintenance people work to keep the rest of the restaurant clean, safe, and sanitary. They clean the kitchen, appliances, and dining area.

Customer Service

Customer service involves working with customers. Those who work in the customer service area might be food servers, table busers, or restaurant hosts. Cashiers also work in the customer service area.

Management

Management involves working with both customers and employees. Managers, executive chefs, and business owners work in the management area.

Food Producing and Processing Careers _____

People in food producing and processing careers are responsible for most of the food supply. They learn many of their skills on the job. Some workers, such as government inspectors, may require special training. Managers of large farms may need a college education. Some food company managers may need a college education, too. Employees at other companies may become managers through hard work and experience. Soil scientists, agricultural researchers, and veterinarians are other workers in the food production field who need college degrees. See 24-6.

24-6 This agricultural researcher is trying to determine why these leaves died.

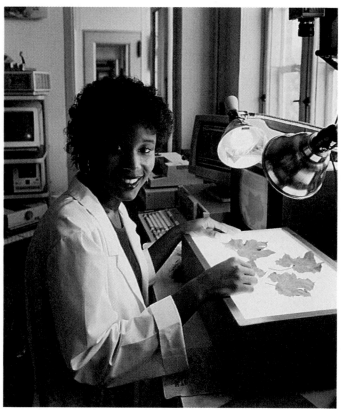

USDA

Students interested in food producing and processing careers may want to explore the opportunities to learn more about these career areas by becoming involved in 4-H, the National FFA Organization, and high school agriculture programs.

Food Producing Careers

People in *food producing careers* usually work outdoors. See 24-7. Farmers produce most of our food. They grow crops such as oats, tomatoes, and oranges. They may also raise livestock such as cows and chickens or even fish and shellfish. People best suited to food producing careers enjoy working outdoors in all types of weather. They are able to respond quickly to events that affect the food they produce.

To obtain experience in food producing careers, you could work after school at a local nursery, farm, or fish hatchery.

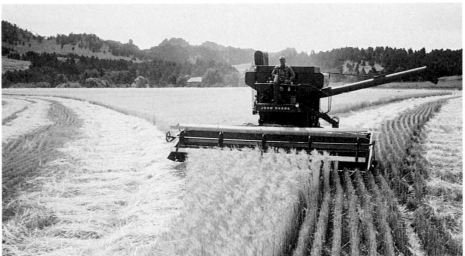

USDA

24-7 Farmers work under the wide-open sky in all types of weather.

Food Processing Careers

People in *food processing* careers often handle the foods that food producers provide before the foods are sold to consumers. People in food processing careers must know about sanitation and good food preparation practices. After harvest, most food products are taken to processing plants. Many jobs at food processing plants are very similar to food preparation jobs. This is because food processors help to get food ready to be sold. For example, some foods, like vegetables, are washed, pared, cooked, and canned. Other foods undergo other processing steps. For example, to make ice cream, the cream is pasteurized, blended with sugar and other ingredients, and frozen.

There are also management and sanitation jobs at food processing plants. *Government inspectors* check to be sure sanitary food preparation practices are followed, 24-8. After processing, foods are transported to the location where they will be marketed. Trucks, trains, planes, and ships are the main ways foods are transported.

If you're interested in food processing, look for a job at a food processing plant or dairy. You might consider working in a food warehouse, too.

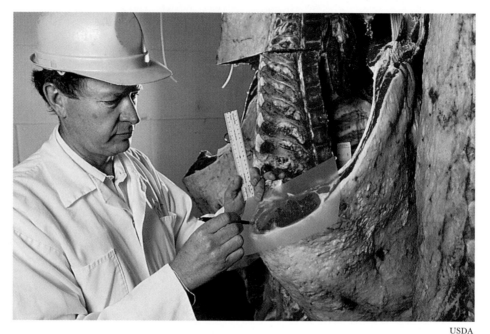

USDA

24-8 This government inspector is checking to be sure this meat meets government standards.

Food Marketing Careers

Think of the hundreds of foods in your supermarket. Who decides which foods will be sold there? How did the foods get from the farmers and processors to your food store? People in *food marketing* careers are responsible for getting foods to your food store. They also decide which foods will be sold in your store. People who pursue food marketing careers buy and sell the foods that food producers and processors provide.

Are you interested in sales? If so, a food marketing career may be right for you. To gain experience, you could get a summer job at a farmer's market. You may want to get a weekend job at a local supermarket. You could also take business, consumer economics, and agriculture courses in high school.

People who are successful in food marketing careers are able to judge the quality of foods. They also are able to predict how much they can sell. They are able to work under pressure and make good decisions quickly. They work well with people, too. Many of the skills needed in food marketing careers can be learned on the job. Management positions may require special training. Brokers who work for large companies often need a college education.

There are four main career paths in food marketing

- brokers
- distributors
- wholesalers
- retailers

Food Brokers

Food brokers purchase extremely large amounts of foods directly from food producers and processors. They may buy a million cases of yogurt from a dairy processor. Often, they store the food in a single, central location. Most brokers specialize in just one type of food, such as wheat or beef. Food brokers sell their food to a few food distributors.

Food Distributors

Food distributors buy a large amount of food from a broker. For instance, one food distributor may buy 200,000 cases of yogurt. Food distributors move the food they buy from one central location to several different regional locations. They also may put brand name labels on the foods they buy. Many food distributors specialize in one type of food. A food distributor sells food to many food wholesalers.

Food Wholesalers

Food wholesalers buy moderate amounts of food from a food distributor. One wholesaler might buy 20,000 cases of yogurt. Food wholesalers move the food they buy from a regional location to many nearby cities. A food wholesaler sells food to many, many food retailers. Food wholesalers often carry several types of food.

Food Retailers

Food retailers buy small amounts of food from wholesalers. For example, a retailer might buy 75 cases of yogurt. Retailers move the food to their food stores. They sell the food directly to consumers. For example, a consumer might buy two cartons of yogurt. Most food retailers sell hundreds of types of food.

You may be wondering why food passes through so many hands before it gets to food stores. See 24-9. The main reason is the volume of food that brokers, distributors, wholesalers, and retailers can sell before it spoils. Distributors are unlikely to sell the amount of food that brokers buy before it spoils. Likewise, wholesalers aren't likely to be able to sell the amounts that distributors buy. Retailers are unlikely to sell the quantity of food wholesalers buy. You are unlikely to be able to use the amount of food a retailer buys before it spoils.

Health Care, Education, Communication, and Research Careers

There are many food and nutrition careers in health care, education, communication, and research. People in these careers all work to help people improve their diets and health. Most of the jobs in these career paths require a college education.

Health Care

Dietetics is the health care career path that combines health and nutrition. Dietitians, dietetic technicians, and diet clerks work in the dietetics field. They may work in hospitals, schools, community centers, health departments, and businesses.

Dietitians plan healthful diets and provide nutrition advice. See 24-10. They counsel people and help them choose healthful diets and develop good eating habits. They prescribe diets for people with health problems. Those who work in hospitals and nursing homes supervise food preparation and menu planning. Dietitians need a four-year college degree in nutrition. They also must do an internship and pass a national exam.

Food Distribution

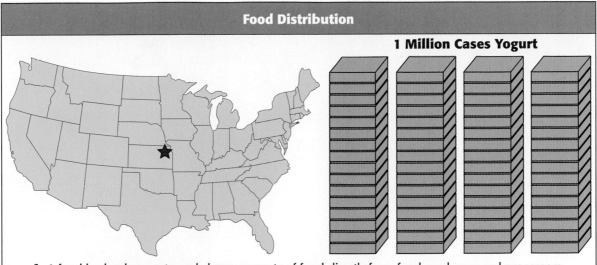

1 Million Cases Yogurt

1. A food broker buys extremely large amounts of food directly from food producers and processors.

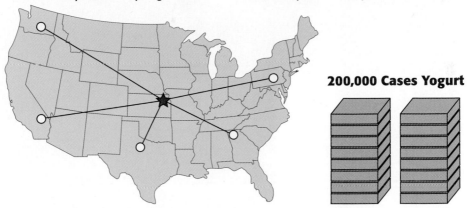

200,000 Cases Yogurt

2. Several food distributors then buy large amounts of food from the food broker.

75 Cases Yogurt

4. Hundreds of food retailers buy small amounts from food wholesalers.

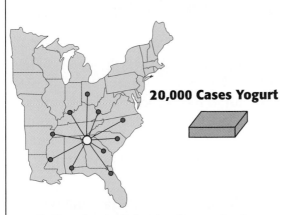

20,000 Cases Yogurt

3. Many food wholesalers buy moderate amounts from the food distributor.

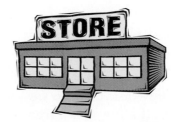

2 Cartons Yogurt

5. A food retailer sells you the amount of food you need.

24-9 The marketing of food goes something like this.

24-10 These dietitians are planning nutritious meals.

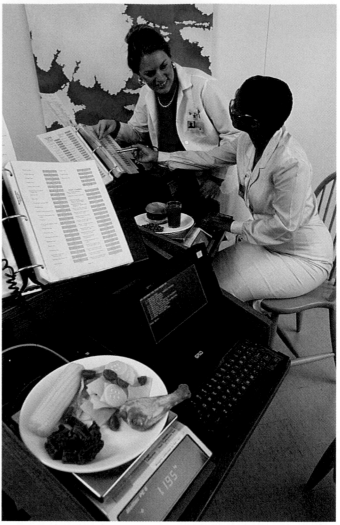

Dietetic technicians assist dietitians who work in hospitals. They may check meal trays to be sure each patient is served the right diet. Dietetic technicians also may record which foods each patient eats. Dietetic technicians need a two-year degree from a vocational school or college. *Diet clerks* assist dietetic technicians and dietitians. Diet clerks are sometimes called nutrition aides. They often learn needed skills on the job.

People best suited to the health care field enjoy helping people. They also need to be patient, understanding, and flexible. To find out if a dietetics career is for you, you could volunteer to work at a local hospital or nursing home. Get to know the dietitians there and ask them about this career path. Think about joining a health careers club and taking health, nutrition, and science courses in high school. After graduating from high school, you could get a job as a diet clerk.

Education

People who pursue careers in education may teach at any education level. See 24-11. Some teach in preschools or elementary schools. Others teach middle and high school. Still others teach in colleges. Food and nutrition teachers teach students about nutrition, health, food safety, and sanitation. They also teach food preparation and meal management.

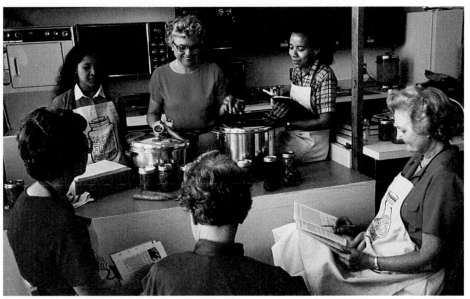

USDA

24-11 Teachers may teach people of all ages.

Most teachers work in schools. There are some teaching jobs in companies, too. Teachers working for companies may teach consumers how to use and care for a product the company makes. They may go to supermarkets to demonstrate how to prepare the company's food products. They also may teach other employees in the company how to plan, prepare, and eat a nutritious diet. Sometimes they develop teaching materials for school teachers.

To be successful in education careers, people need to be able to communicate well. They need to be able to explain ideas clearly. They need leadership skills, too. Teachers in schools need at least a four-year college degree. Most teachers working for companies need the same type of degree.

To learn more about being a food and nutrition teacher, talk to your family and consumer science or home economics teacher. You can start getting teaching experience now by joining a future teachers club at school. You can also volunteer to help your teachers prepare materials like bulletin boards, posters, and reports. Becoming a club officer or scout leader will help you develop teaching skills, too. Jobs at child care centers provide teaching experience. Summer camp counselor jobs also provide good experience for future teachers.

Communications

People who enjoy writing may choose a career in communications. If they have an expertise in food and nutrition, they may become food and nutrition writers or editors for newspapers and/or magazines. Some write nutrition textbooks, cookbooks, or care manuals that come with kitchen appliances. Others may write recipes and directions on food packages. Still others may produce radio and television shows on food, nutrition, and cooking. Food and nutrition experts who have an artistic flair may pursue careers in food advertising. They may become food stylists who prepare food to be photographed.

People who work in communications may work for a company. Many are self-employed. Those who pursue a communications career need well-developed speaking and writing skills. They also need to be well-organized and able to meet deadlines. They usually need a four-year college degree. Often, they need several years of teaching or health care experience before pursuing a communications career. If you are interested in a communications career, think about taking speech, journalism, and art classes at school. Join clubs that help you develop communication skills. For instance, you may want to join the school newspaper or debate team. Do a lot of reading to find out how other people express themselves in writing. You could get a summer job at a local newspaper.

Research

People who enjoy solving puzzles and making new discoveries may enjoy a career in research. For example, a nutrition researcher might study the links between diet and health. A nutrition researcher also may conduct studies designed to determine how a vitamin works in the body. Researchers working in test kitchens find new ways to prepare foods and test new kitchen appliances. See 24-12. Food scientists develop new products and food packages. They may create new food additives and study how the additives work. Food scientists also may develop new techniques for keeping foods fresh and safe to eat. See 24-13.

24-12 This test kitchen researcher is testing new bread recipes.

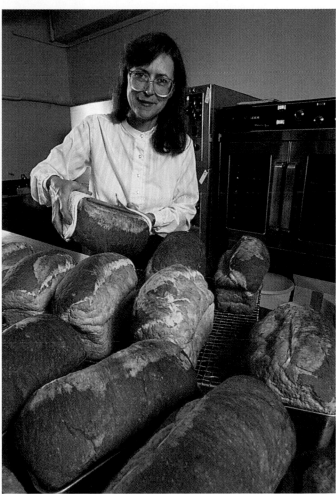

USDA

24-13 These food scientists are researching new ways to keep tomato juice fresh.

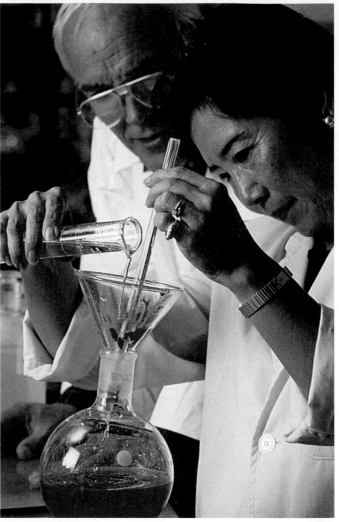

USDA

Most researchers work in colleges, government, and companies. Food and nutrition research jobs require at least a four-year degree in nutrition, food science, food technology, or chemistry. Most research jobs require advanced college degrees and many years of experience. Those who pursue a research career must be curious and inquisitive. They also must be creative so that they can solve problems. If you are interested in a research career, you could take science, nutrition, and health courses in school. You may be able to find a summer job in a test kitchen or hospital lab, 24-14. You can also try some of the experiments described in the Science in the Kitchen features in this book.

24-14 A summer job in a lab can help you determine if a research career is right for you.

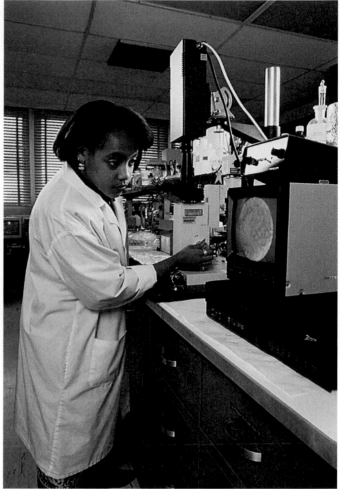

Finding a Job

If you are interested in a food and nutrition-related career, you might want to begin with a part-time job while you are in high school. Think about all the food-related businesses in your area. There are food stores and restaurants. There may be other food-related businesses, too. These companies often have entry-level positions available to high school students. Getting experience while you're still in high school can help you learn more about a career. Experience may also help you climb the career ladder to higher level jobs in the future.

Focus on Careers

A Test Kitchen Researcher at Work

Test kitchen researchers develop new recipes for foods. They also may test new appliances and create recipes especially for those appliances. For instance, test kitchen researchers who work for companies that make microwave ovens develop recipes that work well in these ovens. They also experiment with foods to discover the best way to prepare the foods in a microwave oven.

Several years ago, a company was thinking about adding a turntable to their microwave ovens. They thought a turntable that rotates when the oven is on would help food cook more evenly. They weren't sure, so they asked their test kitchen researchers to find out. This is one of the experiments the researchers tried. By trying the experiment yourself, you can learn more about their work.

For this experiment, you'll need one chocolate cake mix. Prepare the batter according to the directions on the box. Use waxed paper to line the bottom of three 6-inch ovenproof glass dishes that are the same size. Pour equal amounts of batter into each dish. Be sure not to fill the dishes more than half full.

Bake one dish in a conventional oven preheated to 325°F (160°C) for 20 to 25 minutes. The cake is done when a toothpick inserted in the center comes out clean. This cake is the one the microwave oven-baked cake should look and taste like.

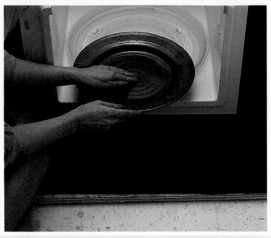

Sharp Electronics Corporation

In developing turntables for microwave ovens, researchers at appliance companies tested a variety of materials. They performed tests on prototypes (models) such as this one. They then tested turntables by performing experiments using food.

Loosely cover each of the other two dishes with a paper towel. Place the second dish in a microwave oven and cook on high for one minute. Turn the dish a quarter turn and cook on high for another minute. Test for doneness with a toothpick. If the cake is not done, cook on high for 10 seconds more and test again. When the cake is done, remove the paper towel.

Wind up a microwave oven rotating turntable and place it in the microwave oven. Put the third dish on the turntable and microwave on high for two minutes. Test for doneness as you did with the second dish. Remove the paper towel.

When each cake is done, let it cool for five minutes. Run a knife around the inside edge of each dish to loosen the cake. Then invert each onto a separate plate. Remove the waxed paper. Cut the cakes in half.

How did each cake look? How much did each cake rise? What were their textures like? How did they taste? Were they moist? Which microwave cake looked and tasted most like the cake baked in the conventional oven? What effect did the turntable have on the cake? How can you use the information gained from this experiment? Would you recommend that the company add turntables? Explain your answer.

You can find job openings by looking at the help wanted ads in your local newspaper. Some businesses put help wanted signs in their windows. Your school counselor may know of businesses that have job openings. Friends, neighbors, and family members also may know of businesses that are hiring.

When you hear about a job that interests you, contact the employer. You may contact an employer by letter or phone or in person. If the job is still open, the employer may ask you to fill out an *application form*. When filling out applications, be sure to write neatly and complete every item accurately. You will need to write your name, address, phone number, and Social Security number. You will also need to list the name of your school and any other jobs you have had. You may need to give references. **References** are people the employer can call to ask about your abilities as a worker. You should not list friends and family members as references. Teachers, school counselors, coaches, scout leaders, and former employers are good to use as references. Ask these people if you can use them as references before listing them on an application form. On some applications, you may also need to specify when you can start to work. You may need to indicate the position for which you are applying and the wages you expect to earn.

After you turn in the application, the employer will review it. If the employer thinks you may be suited to the job, you may be interviewed. During the *interview*, the employer will ask you about your interests and skills. The employer also will ask you about your previous jobs and your qualifications for this job. In food and nutrition-related jobs be sure to tell employers about your family and consumer sciences classes at school. Much of what you have learned from this book can be applied to a food and nutrition-related job. During the interview, you will have a chance to discuss the job with the employer, too. To make a good impression, be sure you and your clothes look neat and clean. Be sure to arrive on time. Also remember to have a good attitude and speak clearly.

If your interview goes well, you may be offered the job. Keep in mind the employer may be interviewing others. Therefore, you may not know if you got the job for a week or two. During the interview, you could ask the employer when you might expect to hear whether you got the job. After the interview, it is a good idea to write a follow-up letter. In this letter, you should thank the interviewer for talking with you and express your interest in the job.

If you are offered the job, let the employer know as soon as possible if you will take the job. Also find out when you should report to work. Ask about other items such as training classes and uniforms. If you are not offered a job, think about why this occurred. Ask yourself these questions.

- Was my application neat and accurate?
- Did I arrive at the interview on time?
- Did I look neat and clean at the interview?
- Did I show an interest in the job?
- Did I appear willing to learn and work hard?
- Did I seem friendly and able to get along with other workers and customers?

If your answer to all of these questions is yes, you may have done everything right. The employer may have just felt that another person was more qualified for the job. If you answer no to a question, this might help you see why you were not offered the job. Think about how you can improve for the next interview. Once you get a job, you're well on your way to exploring a career path!

What Employers Expect from Employees

Imagine you are an employer. What qualities would your best employees have? How would they behave? Knowing what employers expect helps you meet their expectations and do your best on the job. Doing your best gives you a feeling of pride and self-confidence. It also helps the company increase its output and profits.

Always try to be the best employee you can be. Guidelines in 24-15 describe how employers want employees to think and act. As you can see, employers want employees to be responsible and on time. They want employees who follow company rules and policies. They also want employees who are honest, loyal, and courteous.

What Employers Expect from Employees
• To come to work on time every day. • To work hard and do the job to the best of their abilities. • To follow company rules and policies. • To carry out the orders of supervisors. • To be honest and courteous. • To be loyal and not discuss the company's business outside work. • To have a neat, clean personal appearance. • To do work correctly and complete it on time. • To take pride in their work and the company. • To make an effort to improve their skills and knowledge. • To have a good attitude. • To accept responsibility for their work. • To appreciate job privileges and not abuse them. • To get along with coworkers and be a team player • To pitch in and lend a helping hand whenever asked.

24-15 Knowing your employer's expectations will help you be a model employee.

Companies appreciate employees who are willing to learn. You can show your willingness to learn by doing each task you are given to the best of your ability. You can also show your willingness to learn by looking for ways to learn new skills. You could volunteer for extra training. You also could let your employer know you want to try new work assignments.

Employers value employees who have a good attitude. A good attitude shows a person is willing to try hard. People who have good attitudes are pleasant and want to please. They are willing to listen to suggestions and show respect for the opinions of others. They accept responsibility for their work. People with good attitudes don't make excuses or blame others for mistakes they make.

Getting along with others is important to employers, too. Companies function best when every employee cooperates and is a team player. When employees work as a team, all workers do their share of the work. They pitch in to do a little extra when special needs arise. Teamwork gets all the tasks done on time. Cooperative employees are friendly and respect their coworkers. They try hard to do a good job. They have a positive attitude and don't cause arguments. Employers appreciate and reward cooperative employees. Employees who aren't cooperative reduce company output and service. Uncooperative employees make working conditions unpleasant. Companies can't afford to keep employees who don't get along with others.

Focus on Careers

Smart Cookies Make Dough

Have you ever thought about going into business for yourself? If so, you may want to become an entrepreneur. An *entrepreneur* is a person who organizes, manages, and assumes responsibility for a business. Entrepreneurs need good imaginations. They need to be able to look at problems and find better ways to solve them. Then they must sell their ideas to others.

Entrepreneurs can be any age. Even teens can become entrepreneurs! Take Louise Kramer and Lizzie Denis, for example. When they were 11 years old, they were on their school's Grandparent's Day committee. Their job was to make chocolate chip cookies for the event. They baked tray after tray of cookies. It seemed to take forever to bake all those cookies because the oven would only hold two cookie sheets. "Why can't we do this faster?" asked Louise. They began to brainstorm about how they could speed up the process.

They imagined a rack that could hold four cookie sheets at once. This rack would let them bake twice as many cookies at one time. They drew a sketch of

the rack and made a trip to a local hardware store. A store employee welded pieces of scrap metal together. The first Double Decker Cookie Baker was born! They took their invention home and tried it. They found that they could bake up to 10 dozen cookies at once! Louise and Lizzie also found that the cookies browned evenly and baked in the same amount of

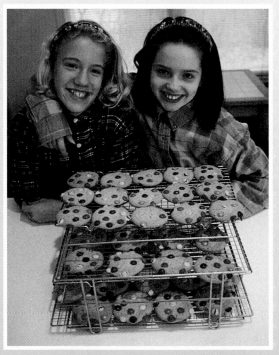

L & L Products, Inc.

Entrepreneurs, Louise Kramer and Lizzie Denis, developed the Double Decker Baking Rack.

time as the recipe stated. (In some ovens, rotating the pans about half-way through the baking time may be necessary. However, time and energy are still conserved.)

A few weeks later, Louise and Lizzie entered their invention in a school contest. It won first place! The girls and their parents decided to apply for a patent. A *patent* is a government document that permits only the inventor to make, use, and sell his or her invention. A patent prevents others from profiting from an inventor's idea. After patenting their invention, the girls and their parents hired a manufacturing company to make the baking rack. Now, the Double Decker Cookie Baker is being sold all over the United States. By the time the girls were 14, they had sold more than 10,000 racks! They plan to use their earnings to pay for college.

To make their company grow, the girls and their families are working on other inventions. Lizzie has good advice for entrepreneurs. "If you have an idea, you may not think it's very good, but you should check it out. You never know!"

In a Nutshell

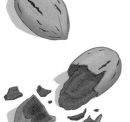

- Careers affect every aspect of your lifestyle.
- Your personality, interests, talents, values, and goals can help you find a career that suits you.
- Learning about career choices can help you identify the type of career that is right for you.
- Preparing yourself for your career will help you move up the career ladder.
- Working hard in school helps you prepare for any career.
- People in food service careers prepare and serve foods in restaurants, hotels, and hospitals.
- People in food producing and processing careers produce food and get it ready for sale to consumers.
- People in food marketing careers are responsible for getting foods to your food store.
- People in food and nutrition-related health care, education, communication, and research careers help people improve their eating habits and health.
- A neat, accurate application and successful interview help you get the job you want.
- Knowing what employers expect of employees helps you do your best on the job.

In the Know

1. Explain why it is important to find a career you will enjoy.
2. _____ are beliefs and ideas that are important to you.
3. Name a career that you think you might enjoy. Write three goals that you might achieve in the next year that would help you learn more about this career.
4. List five questions you should ask when investigating a specific career.
5. Explain why a supermarket cashier must be able to read, write, do math, and communicate well.
6. True or false? Managers in food service careers work with both customers and employees.
7. A food _____ purchases extremely large amounts of foods directly from food producers and processors.
8. Name the health care career path that combines nutrition and health.
9. Describe the skills people who want to pursue a career in communications need.
10. Name three people you could list as references on a job application.
11. Describe five qualities an employer wants an employee to have.

What Would You Do?

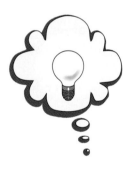

Your friend is interested in studying nutrition in college. He doesn't know what types of jobs are available in nutrition. He also isn't sure what type of job he really wants. What advice would you give him? How could he get the information he needs to learn more about careers in nutrition? What could he do to learn more about himself and the type of job that will best suit him?

Expanding Your Knowledge

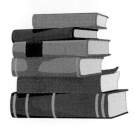

1. Invite a school counselor to talk to your class about careers. Ask the school counselor to explain how you can learn more about careers. Also find out how the counselor can help you match your interests, talents, and skills with a career.

2. Interview a person who has a job in a career area that interests you. Ask the questions listed in 24-3. If possible, arrange to go to work for one day with the person. Prepare a report on the interview and your observations. Share your findings with your class.

3. Attend a careers day at a local college or vocational school. Talk to the counselors about careers that interest you. Ask them to explain the training programs they offer.

4. Invite a job recruiter or human resources manager to visit your class. Ask the recruiter to talk about how to prepare for interviews. Also ask the recruiter for tips that will help you do well in interviews. You could ask the recruiter to conduct practice interviews with the class.

5. Read the help wanted ads in the local newspaper. What jobs in food and nutrition are open? Identify the jobs that interest you. Do you have the qualifications required for the jobs? What could you do to become qualified for the jobs?

6. Select a career related to food and nutrition. Research the career in the library. Make a poster that describes the career. Display the poster in the school cafeteria.

7. Invite your school's cafeteria manager or dietitian to speak to your class. Ask the manager or dietitian to describe his or her job. You could ask the questions listed in 24-3.

8. Interview for a summer job. You could practice for the interview by writing down questions you think the employer might ask. Have a friend or family member ask the questions. Answer them as though you were actually in the interview.

Appendix

Food Composition Table

Food Item	Serving Size	Weight (g)	Cal- ories	Pro- tein (g)	Fat (g)	Satu- rated Fat (g)	Mono- unsat- urated Fat (g)	Poly- unsat- urated Fat (g)	Cho- les- terol (g)	Car- bohy- drate (g)	Cal- cium (mg)	Iron (mg)	Sod- ium (mg)	Vita- min A (µg)	Vita- min C (mg)
Beverages															
Carbonated:															
Club soda	12 ounces	355	0	0	0	0	0	0	0	0	18	0	78	0	0
Cola, regular	12 ounces	369	160	0	0	0	0	0	0	41	11	0.2	18	0	0
Cola, diet	12 ounces	355	0	0	0	0	0	0	0	0	14	0.2	23	0	0
Ginger ale	12 ounces	366	125	0	0	0	0	0	0	32	11	0.1	29	0	0
Grape soda	12 ounces	372	180	0	0	0	0	0	0	46	15	0.4	48	0	0
Lemon-lime soda	12 ounces	372	155	0	0	0	0	0	0	39	7	0.4	33	0	0
Orange soda	12 ounces	372	180	0	0	0	0	0	0	46	15	0.3	52	0	0
Pepper-type soda	12 ounces	369	160	0	0	0	0	0	0	41	11	0.1	37	0	0
Root beer	12 ounces	370	165	0	0	0	0	0	0	42	15	0.2	48	0	0
Coffee:															
Coffee, brewed	6 ounces	180	0	0	0	0	0	0	0	0	4	0	2	0	0
Coffee, instant, prepared	6 ounces	182	0	0	0	0	0	0	0	1	2	0.1	0	0	0
Fruit Drinks, Noncarbonated:															
Fruit punch drink, canned	6 ounces	190	85	0	0	0	0	0	0	22	15	0.4	15	2	61
Grape drink, canned	6 ounces	187	100	0	0	0	0	0	0	26	2	0.3	11	0	64
Pineapple-grapefruit juice drink	6 ounces	187	90	0	0	0	0	0	0	23	13	0.9	24	6	110
Lemonade, frozen concentrate	6 ounces	219	425	0	0	0	0	0	0	112	9	0.4	4	4	66
Lemonade, from frozen concentrate	6 ounces	185	80	0	0	0	0	0	0	21	2	0.1	1	1	13
Limeade, frozen concentrate	6 ounces	218	410	0	0	0	0	0	0	108	11	0.2	0	0	26
Limeade, from frozen concentrate	6 ounces	185	75	0	0	0	0	0	0	20	2	0	0	0	4
Fruit Juices: see Fruits and Fruit Juices															
Milk Beverages: see Dairy Products															
Tea:															
Tea, brewed	8 ounces	240	0	0	0	0	0	0	0	0	0	0	1	0	0
Tea, instant, unsweetened	8 ounces	241	0	0	0	0	0	0	0	1	1	0	1	0	0
Tea, instant, sweetened	8 ounces	262	85	0	0	0	0	0	0	22	1	0	0	0	0
Condiments															
Catsup	1 tbsp.	15	15	0	0	0	0	0	0	4	3	0.1	156	21	2
Olives, canned, green	4 medium	13	15	0	2	0.2	1.2	0.1	0	0	8	0.2	312	4	0
Olives, canned, ripe, mission	3 small	9	15	0	2	0.3	1.3	0.2	0	0	10	0.2	68	1	0
Pickles, cucumber, dill	1 pickle	65	5	0	0	0	0	0.1	0	1	17	0.7	928	7	4
Pickles, cucumber, fresh pack	2 slices	15	10	0	0	0	0	0	0	3	5	0.3	101	2	1
Pickles, cucumber, sweet gherkin	1 pickle	15	20	0	0	0	0	0	0	5	2	0.2	107	1	1
Relish, sweet	1 tbsp.	15	20	0	0	0	0	0	0	5	3	0.1	107	2	1
Vinegar, cider	1 tbsp.	15	0	0	0	0	0	0	0	1	1	0.1	0	0	0

Dairy Products

Butter: see Fats and Oils

Cheese:

Food Item	Serving Size	Weight (g)	Calories	Protein (g)	Fat (g)	Saturated Fat (g)	Monounsaturated Fat (g)	Polyunsaturated Fat (g)	Cholesterol (g)	Carbohydrate (g)	Calcium (mg)	Iron (mg)	Sodium (mg)	Vitamin A (µg)	Vitamin C (mg)
Blue cheese	1 ounce	28.35	100	6	8	5.3	2.2	0.2	21	1	150	0.1	396	65	0
Camembert cheese	1 wedge	38	115	8	9	5.8	2.7	0.3	27	0	147	0.1	320	96	0
Cheddar cheese	1 ounce	28.35	115	7	9	6.0	2.7	0.3	30	0	204	0.2	176	86	0
Cheddar cheese	1 cubic inch	17	70	4	6	3.6	1.6	0.2	18	0	123	0.1	105	52	0
Cheddar cheese, shredded	1 cup	113	455	28	37	23.8	10.6	1.1	119	1	815	0.8	701	342	0
Cottage cheese, creamed	1 cup	210	215	26	9	6.0	2.7	0.3	31	6	126	0.3	850	101	0
Cottage cheese, lowfat 2%	1 cup	226	205	31	4	2.8	1.2	0.1	19	8	155	0.4	918	45	0
Cottage cheese, uncreamed	1 cup	145	125	25	1	0.4	0.2	0	10	3	46	0.3	19	12	0
Cream cheese	1 ounce	28.35	100	2	10	6.2	2.8	0.4	31	1	23	0.3	84	124	0
Feta cheese	1 ounce	28.35	75	4	6	4.2	1.3	0.2	25	1	140	0.2	316	36	0
Mozzarella cheese, whole milk	1 ounce	28.35	80	6	6	3.7	1.9	0.2	22	1	147	0.1	106	68	0
Mozzarella cheese, part skim	1 ounce	28.35	80	8	5	3.1	1.4	0.1	15	1	207	0.1	150	54	0
Muenster cheese	1 ounce	28.35	105	7	9	5.4	2.5	0.2	27	0	203	0.1	178	90	0
Parmesan cheese, grated	1 cup	100	455	42	30	19.1	8.7	0.7	79	4	1376	1.0	1861	173	0
Parmesan cheese, grated	1 tbsp.	5	25	2	2	1.0	0.4	0	4	0	69	0	93	9	0
Parmesan cheese, grated	1 ounce	28.35	130	12	9	5.4	2.5	0.2	22	1	390	0.3	528	49	0
Provolone cheese	1 ounce	28.35	100	7	8	4.8	2.1	0.2	20	1	214	0.1	248	75	0
Ricotta cheese, whole milk	1 cup	246	430	28	32	20.4	8.9	0.9	124	7	509	0.9	207	330	0
Ricotta cheese, part skim milk	1 cup	246	340	28	19	12.1	5.7	0.6	76	13	669	1.1	307	278	0
Swiss cheese	1 ounce	28.35	105	8	8	5.0	2.1	0.3	26	1	272	0	74	72	0
Processed cheese, American	1 ounce	28.35	105	6	9	5.6	2.5	0.3	27	0	174	0.1	406	82	0
Processed cheese, Swiss	1 ounce	28.35	95	7	7	4.5	2.0	0.2	24	1	219	0.2	388	65	0
Processed cheese food	1 ounce	28.35	95	6	7	4.4	2.0	0.2	18	2	163	0.2	337	62	0
Processed cheese spread	1 ounce	28.35	80	5	6	3.8	1.8	0.2	16	2	159	0.1	381	54	0
Cream, Sweet:															
Half and half, cream	1 cup	242	315	7	28	17.3	8.0	1.0	89	10	254	0.2	98	259	2
Half and half, cream	1 tbsp.	15	20	0	2	1.1	0.5	0.1	6	1	16	0	6	16	0
Light cream	1 cup	240	470	6	46	28.8	13.4	1.7	159	9	231	0.1	95	437	2
Light cream	1 tbsp.	15	30	0	3	1.8	0.8	0.1	10	1	14	0	6	27	0
Whipping cream, unwhipped, light	1 cup	239	700	5	74	46.2	21.7	2.1	265	7	166	0.1	82	705	1
Whipping cream, unwhipped, light	1 tbsp.	15	45	0	5	2.9	1.4	0.1	17	0	10	0	5	44	0
Whipping cream, unwhipped, heavy	1 cup	238	820	5	88	54.8	25.4	3.3	326	7	154	0.1	89	1002	1
Whipping cream, unwhipped, heavy	1 tbsp.	15	50	0	6	3.5	1.6	0.2	21	0	10	0	6	63	0
Whipped topping, pressurized	1 cup	60	155	2	13	8.3	3.9	0.5	46	7	61	0	78	124	0
Whipped topping, pressurized	1 tbsp.	3	10	0	1	0.4	0.2	0	2	0	3	0	4	6	0
Cream, Sour:															
Sour cream	1 cup	230	495	7	48	30	13.9	1.8	102	10	268	0.1	123	448	2
Sour cream	1 tbsp.	12	25	0	3	1.6	0.7	0.1	5	1	14	0	6	23	0

Food Composition Table (continued)

Food Item	Serving Size	Weight (g)	Calories	Protein (g)	Fat (g)	Saturated Fat (g)	Mono-unsaturated Fat (g)	Poly-unsaturated Fat (g)	Cholesterol (g)	Carbohydrate (g)	Calcium (mg)	Iron (mg)	Sodium (mg)	Vitamin A (µg)	Vitamin C (mg)
Cream Products, Imitation:															
Imitation creamers, frozen	1 tbsp.	15	20	0	1	1.4	0	0	0	2	1	0	12	1	0
Imitation creamers, powdered	1 tsp.	2	10	0	1	0.7	0	0	0	1	0	0	4	0	0
Imitation whipped topping, frozen	1 cup	75	240	1	19	16.3	1.2	0.4	0	17	5	0.1	19	65	0
Imitation whipped topping, frozen	1 tbsp.	4	15	0	1	0.9	0.1	0	0	1	0	0	1	3	0
Imitation whipped topping, powdered	1 cup	80	150	3	10	8.5	0.7	0.2	8	13	72	0	53	39	1
Imitation whipped topping, powdered	1 tbsp.	4	10	0	0	0.4	0	0	0	1	4	0	3	2	0
Imitation whipped topping, pressurized	1 cup	70	185	1	16	13.2	1.3	0.2	0	11	4	0	43	33	0
Imitation whipped topping, pressurized	1 tbsp.	4	10	0	1	0.8	0.1	0	0	1	0	0	2	2	0
Imitation sour dressing	1 cup	235	415	8	39	31.2	4.6	1.1	13	11	266	0.1	113	5	2
Imitation sour dressing	1 tbsp.	12	20	0	2	1.6	0.2	0.1	1	1	14	0	6	0	0
Milk:															
Milk, whole, 3.3% fat	1 cup	244	150	8	8	5.1	2.4	0.3	33	11	291	0.1	120	76	2
Milk, lowfat, 2%	1 cup	244	120	8	5	2.9	1.4	0.2	18	12	297	0.1	122	139	2
Milk, lowfat, 1%	1 cup	244	100	8	3	1.6	0.7	0.1	10	12	300	0.1	123	144	2
Milk, skim	1 cup	245	85	8	0	0.3	0.1	0	4	12	302	0.1	126	149	2
Buttermilk, fluid	1 cup	245	100	8	2	1.3	0.6	0.1	9	12	285	0.1	257	20	2
Sweetened condensed milk, canned	1 cup	306	980	24	27	16.8	7.4	1.0	104	166	868	0.6	389	248	8
Evaporated milk, whole, canned	1 cup	252	340	17	19	11.6	5.9	0.6	74	25	657	0.5	267	136	5
Evaporated milk, skim, canned	1 cup	255	200	19	1	0.3	0.2	0	9	29	738	0.7	293	298	3
Buttermilk, dried	1 cup	120	465	41	7	4.3	2.0	0.3	83	59	1421	0.4	621	65	7
Nonfat dry milk	1 cup	68	245	24	0	0.3	0.1	0	12	35	837	0.2	373	483	4
Chocolate milk, regular	1 cup	250	210	8	8	5.3	2.5	0.3	31	26	280	0.6	149	73	2
Chocolate milk, lowfat 2%	1 cup	250	180	8	5	3.1	1.5	0.2	17	26	284	0.6	151	143	2
Chocolate milk, lowfat 1%	1 cup	250	160	8	3	1.5	0.8	0.1	7	26	287	0.6	152	148	2
Chocolate milk, skim	1 cup	250	140	8	1	0.75	0.25	0	7	25	290	0.6	175	150	2
Eggnog	1 cup	254	340	10	19	11.3	5.7	0.9	149	34	330	0.5	138	203	4
Malted milk, chocolate, powder	3/4 ounce	21	85	1	2	0.5	0.3	0.1	1	18	13	0.4	49	5	0
Malted milk, natural, powder	3/4 ounce	21	85	3	2	0.9	0.5	0.3	4	15	56	0.2	96	17	0
Shakes, thick, chocolate	10 ounces	283	335	9	8	4.8	2.2	0.3	30	60	374	0.9	314	59	0
Shakes, thick, vanilla	10 ounces	283	315	11	9	5.3	2.5	0.3	33	50	413	0.3	270	79	0
Milk Desserts:															
Ice cream, vanilla, regular	1 cup	133	270	5	14	8.9	4.1	0.5	59	32	176	0.1	116	133	1
Ice cream, vanilla, soft serve	1 cup	173	375	7	23	13.5	6.7	1.0	153	38	236	0.4	153	199	1
Ice cream, vanilla, rich	1 cup	148	350	4	24	14.7	6.8	0.9	88	32	151	0.1	108	219	1
Ice milk, vanilla	1 cup	131	185	5	6	3.5	1.6	0.2	18	29	176	0.2	105	52	1

Food Item	Serving Size	Weight (g)	Calories	Protein (g)	Fat (g)	Saturated Fat (g)	Mono-unsaturated Fat (g)	Poly-unsaturated Fat (g)	Cholesterol (g)	Carbohydrate (g)	Calcium (mg)	Iron (mg)	Sodium (mg)	Vitamin A (µg)	Vitamin C (mg)
Ice milk, vanilla, soft serve	1 cup	175	225	8	5	2.9	1.3	0.2	13	38	274	0.3	163	44	1
Sherbet	1 cup	193	270	2	4	2.4	1.1	0.1	14	59	103	0.3	88	39	4
Yogurt:															
Yogurt, lowfat with fruit	8 ounces	227	230	10	2	1.6	0.7	0.1	10	43	345	0.2	133	25	1
Yogurt, lowfat, plain	8 ounces	227	145	12	4	2.3	1.0	0.1	14	16	415	0.2	159	36	2
Yogurt, nonfat	8 ounces	227	125	13	0	0.3	0.1	0	4	17	452	0.2	174	5	2
Yogurt, whole milk	8 ounces	227	140	8	7	4.8	2.0	0.2	29	11	274	0.1	105	68	1
Eggs															
Eggs, raw, whole	1 egg	50	75	6	5	1.6	1.9	0.7	213	1	25	0.7	63	95	0
Eggs, raw, white	1 white	33	15	4	0	0	0	0	0	0	2	0	55	0	0
Eggs, raw, yolk	1 yolk	17	60	3	5	1.6	1.9	0.7	213	0	23	0.6	7	97	0
Eggs, cooked, fried	1 egg	46	90	6	7	1.9	2.7	1.3	211	1	25	0.7	162	114	0
Eggs, cooked, hard-cooked	1 egg	50	75	6	5	1.6	2.0	0.7	213	1	25	0.6	62	84	0
Eggs, cooked, poached	1 egg	50	75	6	5	1.5	1.9	0.7	212	1	25	0.7	140	95	0
Eggs, cooked, scrambled/omelet	1 egg	61	100	7	7	2.2	2.9	1.3	215	1	44	0.7	171	119	0
Fast Foods															
Cheeseburger, regular	1 burger	112	300	15	15	7.3	5.6	1.0	44	28	135	2.3	672	65	1
Cheeseburger, 4 oz patty	1 large burger	194	525	30	31	15.1	12.2	1.4	104	40	236	4.5	1224	128	3
Enchilada	1 enchilada	230	235	20	16	7.7	6.7	0.6	19	24	97	3.3	1332	352	0
English muffin with egg, cheese & bacon	1 sandwich	138	360	18	18	8.0	8.0	0.7	213	31	197	3.1	832	160	1
Fish sandwich with cheese, regular	1 sandwich	140	420	16	23	6.3	6.9	7.7	56	39	132	1.8	667	25	2
Fish sandwich, no cheese, large	1 sandwich	170	470	18	27	6.3	8.7	9.5	91	41	61	2.2	621	15	1
Hamburger, regular	1 burger	98	245	12	11	4.4	5.3	0.5	32	28	56	2.2	463	14	1
Hamburger, 4 oz patty	1 large burger	174	445	25	21	7.1	11.7	0.6	71	38	75	4.8	763	28	1
Pizza, cheese	1 slice	120	290	15	9	4.1	2.6	1.3	56	39	220	1.6	699	106	2
Roast beef sandwich	1 sandwich	150	345	22	13	3.5	6.9	1.8	55	34	60	4.0	757	32	2
Taco	1 taco	81	195	9	11	4.1	5.5	0.8	21	15	109	1.2	456	57	1
Fats and Oils															
Butter:															
Butter, salted	1 tbsp.	14	100	0	11	7.1	3.3	0.4	31	0	3	0	116	106	0
Butter, unsalted	1 tbsp.	14	100	0	11	7.1	3.3	0.4	31	0	3	0	2	106	0
Fats:															
Vegetable shortening	1 tbsp.	13	115	0	13	3.3	5.8	3.4	0	0	0	0	0	0	0
Lard	1 tbsp.	13	115	0	13	5.1	5.9	1.5	12	0	0	0	0	0	0
Margarine:															
Margarine, reduced fat	1 tbsp.	14	50	0	5	1.1	2.2	1.9	0	0	2	0	134	139	0
Margarine, regular	1 tbsp.	14	100	0	11	2.2	5.0	3.6	0	0	4	0	132	139	0
Margarine, regular, soft	1 tbsp.	14	100	0	11	1.9	4.0	4.8	0	0	4	0	151	139	0
Margarine, spread	1 tbsp.	14	75	0	9	2.0	3.6	2.5	0	0	3	0	139	139	0
Oils:															
Corn oil	1 tbsp.	14	125	0	14	1.8	3.4	8.2	0	0	0	0	0	0	0

Food Composition Table (continued)

Food Item	Serving Size	Weight (g)	Calories	Protein (g)	Fat (g)	Saturated Fat (g)	Monounsaturated Fat (g)	Polyunsaturated Fat (g)	Cholesterol (g)	Carbohydrate (g)	Calcium (mg)	Iron (mg)	Sodium (mg)	Vitamin A (µg)	Vitamin C (mg)
Olive oil	1 tbsp.	14	125	0	14	1.9	10.3	1.2	0	0	0	0	0	0	0
Peanut oil	1 tbsp.	14	125	0	14	2.4	6.5	4.5	0	0	0	0	0	0	0
Safflower oil	1 tbsp.	14	125	0	14	1.3	1.7	10.4	0	0	0	0	0	0	0
Soybean oil, hydrogenated	1 tbsp.	14	125	0	14	2.1	6.0	5.3	0	0	0	0	0	0	0
Soybean-cottonseed oil, hydrogenated	1 tbsp.	14	125	0	14	2.5	4.1	6.7	0	0	0	0	0	0	0
Sunflower oil	1 tbsp.	14	125	0	14	1.4	2.7	9.2	0	0	0	0	0	0	0
Salad Dressings:															
Blue cheese salad dressing	1 tbsp.	15	75	1	8	1.5	1.8	4.2	3	1	12	0	164	10	0
French salad dressing	1 tbsp.	16	85	0	9	1.4	4.0	3.5	0	1	2	0	188	0	0
French salad dressing, low calorie	1 tbsp.	16	25	0	2	0.2	0.3	1.0	0	2	6	0	306	0	0
Italian salad dressing	1 tbsp.	15	80	0	9	1.3	3.7	3.2	0	1	1	0	162	3	0
Italian salad dressing, low calorie	1 tbsp.	15	5	0	0	0	0	0	0	2	1	0	136	0	0
Mayonnaise	1 tbsp.	14	100	0	11	1.7	3.2	5.8	8	0	3	0.1	80	12	0
Mayonnaise, imitation	1 tbsp.	15	35	0	3	0.5	0.7	1.6	4	2	0	0	75	0	0
Mayonnaise type salad dressing	1 tbsp.	15	60	0	5	0.7	1.4	2.7	4	4	2	0	107	13	0
Tartar sauce	1 tbsp.	14	75	0	8	1.2	2.6	3.9	4	1	3	0.1	182	9	0
1000 Island salad dressing	1 tbsp.	16	60	0	6	1.0	1.3	3.2	4	2	2	0.1	112	15	0
1000 Island salad dressing, low calorie	1 tbsp.	15	25	0	2	0.2	0.4	0.9	2	2	2	0.1	150	14	0
Vinegar and oil salad dressing	1 tbsp.	16	70	0	8	1.5	2.4	3.9	0	0	0	0	0	0	0
Fish and Shellfish															
Clams, raw	3 ounces	85	65	11	1	0.3	0.3	0.3	43	2	59	2.6	102	26	9
Clams, canned, drained	3 ounces	85	85	13	2	0.5	0.5	0.4	54	2	47	3.5	102	26	3
Crabmeat, canned	1 cup	135	135	23	3	0.5	0.8	1.4	135	1	61	1.1	1350	14	0
Fish sticks, frozen, reheated	1 stick	28	70	6	3	0.8	1.4	0.8	26	4	11	0.3	53	5	0
Flounder or sole, baked with butter	3 ounces	85	120	16	6	3.2	1.5	0.5	68	0	13	0.3	145	54	1
Flounder or sole, baked with margarine	3 ounces	85	120	16	6	1.2	2.3	1.9	55	0	14	0.3	151	69	1
Flounder or sole, baked with no fat	3 ounces	85	80	17	1	0.3	0.2	0.4	59	0	13	0.3	101	10	1
Haddock, breaded, fried	3 ounces	85	175	17	9	2.4	3.9	2.4	75	7	34	1.0	123	20	0
Halibut, broiled with butter	3 ounces	85	140	20	6	3.3	1.6	0.7	62	0	14	0.7	103	174	1
Herring, pickled	3 ounces	85	190	17	13	4.3	4.6	3.1	85	0	29	0.9	850	33	0
Ocean perch, breaded, fried	3 ounces	85	185	16	11	2.6	4.6	2.8	66	7	31	1.2	138	20	0
Oysters, raw	1 cup	240	160	20	4	1.4	0.5	1.4	120	8	226	15.6	175	223	24
Oysters, breaded, fried	1 oyster	45	90	5	5	1.4	2.1	1.4	35	5	49	3.0	70	44	4
Salmon, canned	3 ounces	85	120	17	5	0.9	1.5	2.1	34	0	167	0.7	443	18	0
Salmon, baked	3 ounces	85	140	21	5	1.2	2.4	1.4	60	0	26	0.5	55	87	0
Salmon, smoked	3 ounces	85	150	18	8	2.6	3.9	0.7	51	0	12	0.8	1700	77	0

Food Item	Serving Size	Weight (g)	Cal-ories	Pro-tein (g)	Fat (g)	Satu-rated Fat (g)	Mono-unsat-urated Fat (g)	Poly-unsat-urated Fat (g)	Cho-les-terol (g)	Car-bohy-drate (g)	Cal-cium (mg)	Iron (mg)	Sod-ium (mg)	Vita-min A (µg)	Vita-min C (mg)
Sardines, canned in oil	3 ounces	85	175	20	9	2.1	3.7	2.9	85	0	371	2.6	425	56	0
Scallops, breaded, frozen	6 scallops	90	195	15	10	2.5	4.1	2.5	70	10	39	2.0	298	21	0
Shrimp, canned	3 ounces	85	100	21	1	0.2	0.2	0.4	128	1	98	1.4	1955	15	0
Shrimp, french fried	3 ounces	85	200	16	10	2.5	4.1	2.6	168	11	61	2.0	384	26	0
Trout, broiled with butter	3 ounces	85	175	21	9	4.1	2.9	1.6	71	0	26	1.0	122	60	1
Tuna, canned in oil	3 ounces	85	165	24	7	1.4	1.9	3.1	55	0	7	1.6	303	20	0
Tuna, canned in water	3 ounces	85	135	30	1	0.3	0.2	0.3	48	0	17	0.6	468	32	0
Tuna salad	1 cup	205	375	33	19	3.3	4.9	9.2	80	19	31	2.5	877	53	6
Fruits and Fruit Juices															
Apples, raw, unpeeled	1 medium apple	138	80	0	0	0.1	0	0.1	0	21	10	0.2	0	7	8
Apples, raw, peeled, sliced	1 cup	110	65	0	0	0.1	0	0.1	0	16	4	0.1	0	5	4
Apples, dried	10 rings	64	155	1	0	0	0	0.1	0	42	9	0.9	56	0	2
Apple juice, canned	1 cup	248	115	0	0	0	0	0.1	0	29	17	0.9	7	0	2
Applesauce, canned, sweetened	1 cup	255	195	0	0	0.1	0	0.1	0	51	10	0.9	8	3	4
Applesauce, canned, unsweetened	1 cup	244	105	0	0	0	0	0.1	0	28	7	0.3	5	7	3
Apricots, raw	3 apricots	106	50	1	0	0	0.2	0.1	0	12	15	0.6	1	277	11
Apricot, canned, heavy syrup	1 cup	258	215	1	0	0	0.1	0	0	55	23	0.8	10	317	8
Apricots, canned, juice pack	1 cup	248	120	2	0	0	0	0	0	31	30	0.7	10	419	12
Apricots, dried	1 cup	130	310	5	1	0	0.3	0.1	0	80	59	6.1	13	941	3
Apricot nectar	1 cup	251	140	1	0	0	0.1	0.1	0	36	18	1.0	8	330	2
Avocados, California	1 avocado	173	305	4	30	4.5	19.4	3.5	0	12	19	2.0	21	106	14
Avocados, Florida	1 avocado	304	340	5	27	5.3	14.8	4.5	0	27	33	1.6	15	186	24
Bananas	1 banana	114	105	1	1	0.2	0	0.1	0	27	7	0.4	1	9	10
Blackberries, raw	1 cup	144	75	1	1	0.2	0.1	0.1	0	18	46	0.8	0	24	30
Blueberries, raw	1 cup	145	80	1	1	0	0.1	0.3	0	20	9	0.2	9	15	19
Blueberries, frozen, sweetened	1 cup	230	185	1	0	0	0	0.1	0	50	14	0.9	2	10	2
Cherries, sour, red, canned in water	1 cup	244	90	2	0	0.1	0.1	0.1	0	22	27	3.3	17	184	5
Cherries, sweet, raw	10 cherries	68	50	1	1	0.1	0.2	0.2	0	11	10	0.3	0	15	5
Cranberry juice cocktail	1 cup	253	145	0	0	0	0	0.1	0	38	8	0.4	10	1	108
Cranberry sauce, canned	1 cup	277	420	1	0	0	0.1	0.2	0	108	11	0.6	80	6	6
Dates	10 dates	83	230	2	0	0.1	0.1	0	0	61	27	1.0	2	4	0
Dates, chopped	1 cup	178	490	4	1	0.3	0.2	0	0	131	57	2.0	5	9	0
Figs, dried	10 figs	187	475	6	2	0.4	0.5	1.0	0	122	269	4.2	21	25	1
Fruit cocktail, canned in heavy syrup	1 cup	255	185	1	0	0	0	0.1	0	48	15	0.7	15	52	5
Fruit cocktail, canned in juice	1 cup	248	115	1	0	0	0	0	0	29	20	0.5	10	76	7
Grapefruit, raw, white	1/2 fruit	120	40	1	0	0	0	0	0	10	14	0.1	0	1	41
Grapefruit, raw, pink	1/2 fruit	120	40	1	0	0	0	0	0	10	14	0.1	0	31	41
Grapefruit, canned in syrup	1 cup	254	150	1	0	0	0	0.1	0	39	36	1.0	5	0	54
Grapefruit juice, raw	1 cup	247	95	1	0	0	0.1	0.1	0	23	22	0.5	2	2	94
Grapefruit juice, canned, unsweetened	1 cup	247	95	1	0	0	0	0.1	0	22	17	0.5	2	2	72

Food Composition Table (continued)

Food Item	Serving Size	Weight (g)	Calories	Protein (g)	Fat (g)	Saturated Fat (g)	Mono-unsaturated Fat (g)	Poly-unsaturated Fat (g)	Cholesterol (g)	Carbohydrate (g)	Calcium (mg)	Iron (mg)	Sodium (mg)	Vitamin A (µg)	Vitamin C (mg)
Grapefruit juice, canned, sweetened	1 cup	250	115	1	0	0	0	0.1	0	28	20	0.9	5	2	67
Grapefruit juice, frozen concentrate	6 ounces	207	300	4	1	0.1	0.1	0.2	0	72	56	1.0	6	6	248
Grapefruit juice, from frozen concentrate	1 cup	247	100	1	0	0	0	0.1	0	24	20	0.3	2	2	83
Grapes, raw, Thompson (green)	10 grapes	50	35	0	0	0.1	0	0.1	0	9	6	0.1	1	4	5
Grapes, raw, Tokay (red or purple)	10 grapes	57	40	0	0	0.1	0	0.1	0	10	6	0.1	1	4	6
Grape juice, canned	1 cup	253	155	1	0	0.1	0	0.1	0	38	23	0.6	8	2	0
Grape juice, frozen concentrate	6 ounces	216	385	1	1	0.2	0	0.2	0	96	28	0.8	15	6	179
Grape juice, from frozen concentrate	1 cup	250	125	0	0	0.1	0	0.1	0	32	10	0.3	5	2	60
Kiwifruit, raw	1 kiwifruit	76	45	1	0	0	0.1	0.1	0	11	20	0.3	4	13	74
Lemons, raw	1 lemon	58	15	1	0	0	0	0.1	0	5	15	0.3	1	2	31
Lemon juice, raw	1 cup	244	60	1	0	0	0	0	0	21	17	0.1	2	5	112
Lemon juice, canned	1 cup	244	50	1	1	0.1	0	0.2	0	16	27	0.3	51	4	61
Lemon juice, canned	1 tbsp.	15	5	0	0	0	0	0	0	1	2	0	3	0	4
Lemon juice, frozen	6 ounces	244	55	1	1	0.1	0	0.2	0	16	20	0.3	2	3	77
Lime juice, raw	1 cup	246	65	1	0	0	0	0.1	0	22	22	0.1	2	2	72
Lime juice, canned	1 cup	246	50	1	1	0.1	0.1	0.2	0	16	30	0.6	39	4	16
Mangos, raw	1 mango	207	135	1	1	0.1	0.2	0.1	0	35	21	0.3	4	806	57
Cantaloupe, raw	1/2 melon	267	95	2	1	0	0.1	0.3	0	22	29	0.6	24	861	113
Honeydew melon, raw	1/10 melon	129	45	1	0	0	0	0.1	0	12	8	0.1	13	5	32
Nectarines, raw	1 nectarine	136	65	1	1	0.1	0.2	0.3	0	16	7	0.2	0	100	7
Oranges, raw	1 orange	131	60	1	0	0	0	0	0	15	52	0.1	0	27	70
Oranges, raw, sections	1 cup	180	85	2	0	0	0	0	0	21	72	0.2	0	37	96
Orange juice, fresh	1 cup	248	110	2	0	0.1	0.1	0.1	0	26	27	0.5	2	50	124
Orange juice, canned	1 cup	249	105	1	0	0	0.1	0.1	0	25	20	1.1	5	44	86
Orange juice, frozen concentrate	6 ounces	213	340	5	0	0.1	0.1	0.1	0	81	68	0.7	6	59	294
Orange juice, from frozen concentrate	1 cup	249	110	2	0	0	0	0	0	27	22	0.2	2	19	97
Orange & grapefruit juice, canned	1 cup	247	105	1	0	0	0	0	0	25	20	1.1	7	29	72
Papayas, raw	1 cup	140	65	1	0	0.1	0.1	0	0	17	35	0.3	9	40	92
Peaches, raw	1 peach	87	35	1	0	0	0	0	0	10	4	0.1	0	47	6
Peaches, raw, sliced	1 cup	170	75	1	0	0	0.1	0.1	0	19	9	0.2	0	91	11
Peaches, canned, heavy syrup	1 cup	256	190	1	0	0	0.1	0.1	0	51	8	0.7	15	85	7
Peaches, canned in heavy syrup	1 half	81	60	0	0	0	0	0	0	16	2	0.2	5	27	2
Peaches, canned in juice	1 cup	248	110	2	0	0	0	0	0	29	15	0.7	10	94	9
Peaches, canned in juice	1 half	77	35	0	0	0	0	0	0	9	5	0.2	3	29	3
Peaches, dried	1 cup	160	380	6	1	0.1	0.4	0.6	0	98	45	6.5	11	346	8

Food Item	Serving Size	Weight (g)	Calories	Protein (g)	Fat (g)	Saturated Fat (g)	Monounsaturated Fat (g)	Polyunsaturated Fat (g)	Cholesterol (g)	Carbohydrate (g)	Calcium (mg)	Iron (mg)	Sodium (mg)	Vitamin A (μg)	Vitamin C (mg)
Peaches, frozen, sweetened	1 cup	250	235	2	0	0	0.1	0.2	0	60	8	0.9	15	71	236
Pears, raw, Bartlett	1 pear	166	100	1	1	0	0.1	0.2	0	25	18	0.4	0	3	7
Pears, raw, Bosc	1 pear	141	85	1	1	0	0.1	0.1	0	21	16	0.4	0	3	6
Pears, raw, D'anjou	1 pear	200	120	1	1	0	0.2	0.2	0	30	22	0.5	0	4	8
Pears, canned in heavy syrup	1 cup	255	190	1	0	0	0.1	0.1	0	49	13	0.6	13	1	3
Pears, canned in heavy syrup	1 half	79	60	0	0	0	0	0	0	15	4	0.2	4	0	1
Pears, canned in juice	1 cup	248	125	1	0	0	0	0	0	32	22	0.7	10	1	4
Pears, canned in juice	1 half	77	40	0	0	0	0	0	0	10	7	0.2	3	0	1
Pineapple, raw, diced	1 cup	155	75	1	1	0	0.1	0.2	0	19	11	0.6	2	4	24
Pineapple, canned in heavy syrup	1 cup	255	200	1	0	0	0	0.1	0	52	36	1.0	3	4	19
Pineapple, canned in juice	1 slice	58	45	0	0	0	0	0	0	12	8	0.2	1	1	4
Pineapple, canned in juice	1 cup	250	150	1	0	0	0	0.1	0	39	35	0.7	3	10	24
Pineapple, canned in juice	1 slice	58	35	0	0	0	0	0	0	9	8	0.2	1	2	6
Pineapple juice, canned	1 cup	250	140	1	0	0	0	0.1	0	34	43	0.7	3	1	27
Plantains, raw	1 plantain	179	220	2	1	0.3	0.1	0.1	0	57	5	1.1	7	202	33
Plantains, cooked	1 cup	154	180	1	0	0.1	0	0.1	0	48	3	0.9	8	140	17
Plums, raw	1 medium	28	15	0	0	0	0.1	0	0	4	1	0	0	9	3
Plums, canned in heavy syrup	1 cup	258	230	1	0	0	0.2	0.1	0	60	23	2.2	49	67	1
Plums, canned in heavy syrup	3 plums	133	120	0	0	0	0.1	0	0	31	12	1.1	25	34	1
Plums, canned in juice	1 cup	252	145	1	0	0	0	0	0	38	25	0.9	3	254	7
Plums, canned in juice	3 plums	95	55	0	0	0	0	0	0	14	10	0.3	1	96	3
Prunes, dried	5 large	49	115	1	0	0	0.2	0.1	0	31	25	1.2	2	97	2
Prune juice, canned	1 cup	256	180	2	0	0	0.1	0	0	45	31	3.0	10	1	10
Raisins	1 cup	145	435	5	1	0.2	0	0.2	0	115	71	3.0	17	1	5
Raspberries, raw	1 cup	123	60	1	1	0	0.1	0.4	0	14	27	0.7	0	16	31
Raspberries, frozen, sweetened	1 cup	250	255	2	0	0	0	0.2	0	65	38	1.6	3	15	41
Rhubarb, cooked with added sugar	1 cup	240	280	1	0	0	0	0.1	0	75	348	0.5	2	17	8
Strawberries, raw	1 cup	149	45	1	1	0	0.1	0.3	0	10	21	0.6	1	4	84
Strawberries, frozen, sweetened	1 cup	255	245	1	0	0	0	0.2	0	66	28	1.5	8	6	106
Tangerines, raw	1 tangerine	84	35	1	0	0	0	0	0	9	12	0.1	1	77	26
Tangerines, canned in light syrup	1 cup	252	155	1	0	0	0	0.1	0	41	18	0.9	15	212	50
Tangerine juice, canned, sweetened	1 cup	249	125	1	0	0	0	0.1	0	30	45	0.5	2	105	55
Watermelon, raw	1 piece	482	155	3	2	0.3	0.2	1.0	0	35	39	0.8	10	176	46
Watermelon, raw, diced	1 cup	160	50	1	1	0.1	0.1	0.3	0	11	13	0.3	3	59	15

Grain Products

Bagels:

Food Item	Serving Size	Weight (g)	Calories	Protein (g)	Fat (g)	Saturated Fat (g)	Monounsaturated Fat (g)	Polyunsaturated Fat (g)	Cholesterol (g)	Carbohydrate (g)	Calcium (mg)	Iron (mg)	Sodium (mg)	Vitamin A (μg)	Vitamin C (mg)
Bagels, plain	1 bagel	68	200	7	2	0.3	0.5	0.7	0	38	29	1.8	245	0	0
Bagels, egg	1 bagel	68	200	7	2	0.3	0.5	0.7	44	38	29	1.8	245	7	0

Biscuits:

Food Item	Serving Size	Weight (g)	Calories	Protein (g)	Fat (g)	Saturated Fat (g)	Monounsaturated Fat (g)	Polyunsaturated Fat (g)	Cholesterol (g)	Carbohydrate (g)	Calcium (mg)	Iron (mg)	Sodium (mg)	Vitamin A (μg)	Vitamin C (mg)
Baking powder biscuits, home-made	1 biscuit	28	100	2	5	1.2	2.0	1.3	0	13	47	0.7	195	3	0

Food Composition Table (continued)

Food Item	Serving Size	Weight (g)	Calories	Protein (g)	Fat (g)	Saturated Fat (g)	Monounsaturated Fat (g)	Polyunsaturated Fat (g)	Cholesterol (g)	Carbohydrate (g)	Calcium (mg)	Iron (mg)	Sodium (mg)	Vitamin A (µg)	Vitamin C (mg)
Baking powder biscuits, from mix	1 biscuit	28	95	2	3	0.8	1.4	0.9	0	14	58	0.7	262	4	0
Baking powder biscuits, from dough	1 biscuit	200	65	1	2	0.6	0.9	0.6	1	10	4	0.5	249	0	0
Bread:															
Bread crumbs, dry, grated	1 cup	100	390	13	5	1.5	1.6	1.0	5	73	122	4.1	736	0	0
Boston brown bread	1 slice	45	95	2	1	0.3	0.1	0.1	3	21	41	0.9	113	3	0
Cracked-wheat bread	1 loaf	454	1190	42	16	3.1	4.3	5.7	0	227	295	12.1	1966	0	0
Cracked-wheat bread	1 slice	25	65	2	1	0.2	0.2	0.3	0	12	16	0.7	106	0	0
Cracked-wheat bread, toasted	1 slice	21	65	2	1	0.2	0.2	0.3	0	12	16	0.7	106	0	0
French or Vienna bread	1 loaf	454	1270	43	18	3.8	5.7	5.9	0	230	499	14.0	2633	0	0
French bread	1 slice	35	100	3	1	0.3	0.4	0.5	0	18	39	1.1	203	0	0
Vienna bread	1 slice	25	70	2	1	0.2	0.3	0.3	0	13	28	0.8	145	0	0
Italian bread	1 loaf	454	1255	41	4	0.6	0.3	1.6	0	256	77	12.7	2656	0	0
Italian bread	1 slice	30	85	3	0	0	0	0.1	0	17	5	0.8	176	0	0
Mixed grain bread	1 loaf	454	1165	45	17	3.2	4.1	6.5	0	212	472	14.8	1870	0	0
Mixed grain bread	1 slice	25	65	2	1	0.2	0.2	0.4	0	12	27	0.8	106	0	0
Mixed grain bread, toasted	1 slice	23	65	2	1	0.2	0.2	0.4	0	12	27	0.8	106	0	0
Oatmeal bread	1 loaf	454	1145	38	20	3.7	7.1	8.2	0	212	267	12.0	2231	0	0
Oatmeal bread	1 slice	25	65	2	1	0.2	0.4	0.5	0	12	15	0.7	124	0	0
Oatmeal bread, toasted	1 slice	23	65	2	1	0.2	0.4	0.5	0	12	15	0.7	124	0	0
Pita bread	1 pita	60	165	6	1	0.1	0.1	0.4	0	33	49	1.4	339	0	0
Pumpernickel bread	1 loaf	454	1160	42	16	2.6	3.6	6.4	0	218	322	12.4	2461	0	0
Pumpernickel bread	1 slice	32	80	3	1	0.2	0.3	0.5	0	16	23	0.9	177	0	0
Pumpernickel bread, toasted	1 slice	29	80	3	1	0.2	0.3	0.5	0	16	23	0.9	177	0	0
Raisin bread	1 loaf	454	1260	37	18	4.1	6.5	6.7	0	239	463	14.1	1657	0	0
Raisin bread	1 slice	25	65	2	1	0.2	0.3	0.4	0	13	25	0.8	92	0	0
Raisin bread, toasted	1 slice	21	65	2	1	0.2	0.3	0.4	0	13	25	0.8	92	0	0
Rye bread, light	1 loaf	454	1190	38	17	3.3	5.2	5.5	0	218	363	12.3	3164	0	0
Rye bread, light	1 slice	25	65	2	1	0.2	0.3	0.3	0	12	20	0.7	175	0	0
Rye bread, light, toasted	1 slice	22	65	2	1	0.2	0.3	0.3	0	12	20	0.7	175	0	0
Wheat bread	1 loaf	454	1160	43	19	3.9	7.3	4.5	0	213	572	15.8	2447	0	0
Wheat bread	1 slice	25	65	2	1	0.2	0.4	0.3	0	12	32	0.9	138	0	0
Wheat bread, toasted	1 slice	23	65	3	1	0.2	0.4	0.3	0	12	32	0.9	138	0	0
White bread	1 loaf	454	1210	38	18	5.6	6.5	4.2	0	222	572	12.9	2334	0	0
White bread	1 slice	25	65	2	1	0.3	0.4	0.2	0	12	32	0.7	129	0	0
White bread, toasted	1 slice	22	65	2	1	0.3	0.4	0.2	0	12	32	0.7	129	0	0
White bread, sliced thinly	1 thin slice	20	55	2	1	0.2	0.3	0.2	0	10	25	0.6	101	0	0
White bread, sliced thinly, toasted	1 thin slice	17	55	2	1	0.2	0.3	0.2	0	10	25	0.6	101	0	0
White bread cubes	1 cup	30	80	2	1	0.4	0.4	0.3	0	15	38	0.9	154	0	0
White bread crumbs, soft	1 cup	45	120	4	2	0.6	0.6	0.4	0	22	57	1.3	231	0	0
Whole-wheat bread	1 loaf	454	1110	44	20	5.8	6.8	5.2	0	206	327	15.5	2887	0	0
Whole-wheat bread	1 slice	28	70	3	1	0.4	0.4	0.3	0	13	20	1.0	180	0	0

Food Item	Serving Size	Weight (g)	Cal-ories	Pro-tein (g)	Fat (g)	Satu-rated Fat (g)	Mono-unsat-urated Fat (g)	Poly-unsat-urated Fat (g)	Cho-les-terol (g)	Car-bohy-drate (g)	Cal-cium (mg)	Iron (mg)	Sod-ium (mg)	Vita-min A (µg)	Vita-min C (mg)
Whole-wheat bread, toasted	1 slice	25	70	3	1	0.4	0.4	0.3	0	13	20	1.0	180	0	0
Bread stuffing, from mix, dry	1 cup	140	500	9	31	6.1	13.3	9.6	0	50	92	2.2	1254	273	0
Bread stuffing, from mix, moist	1 cup	203	420	9	26	5.3	11.3	8.0	67	40	81	2.0	1023	256	0
Breakfast Cereals, Cooked:															
Corn grits, cooked, white	1 cup	242	145	3	0	0	0.1	0.2	0	31	0	1.5	0	0	0
Corn grits, cooked, yellow	1 cup	242	145	3	0	0	0.1	0.2	0	31	0	1.5	0	14	0
Corn grits, cooked, instant	1 packet	137	80	2	0	0	0	0.1	0	18	7	1.0	343	0	0
Cream of wheat, cooked, instant	1 cup	244	140	4	0	0.1	0	0.2	0	29	54	10.9	5	0	0
Cream of wheat, cooked, quick	1 cup	244	140	4	0	0.1	0	0.2	0	29	54	10.9	142	0	0
Cream of wheat, cooked, mix & eat	1 packet	142	100	3	0	0	0	0.1	0	21	20	8.1	241	376	0
Oatmeal, cooked	1 cup	234	145	6	2	0.4	0.8	1.0	0	25	19	1.6	2	5	0
Oatmeal, cooked, instant, plain	1 packet	177	105	4	2	0.3	0.6	0.7	0	18	163	6.3	285	453	0
Oatmeal, cooked, instant, flavored	1 packet	164	160	5	2	0.3	0.7	0.8	0	31	168	6.7	254	460	0
Breakfast Cereals, Ready-to-Eat:															
Bran cereal	1 ounce	28.35	70	4	1	0.1	0.1	0.3	0	21	23	4.5	320	375	15
Bran flakes	1 ounce	28.35	90	4	1	0.1	0.1	0.3	0	22	14	8.1	264	375	0
Corn flakes	1 ounce	28.35	110	2	0	0	0	0	0	24	1	1.8	351	375	15
Crisped rice cereal	1 ounce	28.35	110	2	0	0	0	0.1	0	25	4	1.8	340	375	15
Frosted wheat flakes	1 ounce	28.35	110	1	0	0	0	0	0	26	1	1.8	230	375	15
Graham cereal	1 ounce	28.35	110	2	1	0.7	0.1	0.2	0	24	17	4.5	346	375	15
Granola cereal	1 ounce	28.35	125	3	5	3.3	0.7	0.7	0	19	18	0.9	58	2	0
Oat cereal	1 ounce	28.35	110	4	2	0.3	0.6	0.7	0	20	48	4.5	307	375	15
Raisin bran	1 ounce	28.35	90	3	1	0.1	0.1	0.3	0	21	10	3.5	207	288	0
Shredded wheat	1 ounce	28.35	100	3	1	0.1	0.1	0.3	0	23	11	1.2	3	0	0
Sweetened corn cereal	1 ounce	28.35	120	1	3	1.7	0.3	0.4	0	23	5	7.5	213	4	0
Sweetened oat cereal	1 ounce	28.35	105	3	1	0.1	0.3	0.3	0	23	20	4.5	257	375	15
Sweetened wheat cereal	1 ounce	28.35	105	2	1	0.1	0.1	0.2	0	25	3	1.8	75	375	15
Wheat flakes	1 ounce	28.35	100	3	0	0.1	0	0.2	0	23	43	4.5	354	375	15
Cakes:															
Angel food cake	1 piece	53	125	3	0	0	0	0.1	0	29	44	0.2	269	0	0
Coffee cake, crumb	1 piece	72	230	5	7	2.0	2.8	1.6	47	38	44	1.2	310	32	0
Devil's food cake with chocolate frosting	1 piece	69	235	3	8	3.5	3.2	1.2	37	40	41	1.4	181	31	0
Devil's food cake with chocolate frosting	1 cupcake	35	120	2	4	1.8	1.6	0.6	19	20	21	0.7	92	16	0
Gingerbread cake	1 piece	63	175	2	4	1.1	1.8	1.2	1	32	57	1.2	192	0	0
Yellow cake with chocolate frosting	1 piece	69	235	3	8	3.0	3.0	1.4	36	40	63	1.0	157	29	0
Carrot cake with cream cheese frosting	1 piece	96	385	4	21	4.1	8.4	6.7	74	48	44	1.3	279	15	1

Food Composition Table *(continued)*

Food Item	Serving Size	Weight (g)	Cal-ories	Pro-tein (g)	Fat (g)	Satu-rated Fat (g)	Mono-unsat-urated Fat (g)	Poly-unsat-urated Fat (g)	Cho-les-terol (g)	Car-bohy-drate (g)	Cal-cium (mg)	Iron (mg)	Sod-ium (mg)	Vita-min A (µg)	Vita-min C (mg)
Fruitcake, dark	1 piece	43	165	2	7	1.5	3.6	1.6	20	25	41	1.2	67	13	16
Sheet cake, with no frosting	1 piece	86	315	4	12	3.3	5.0	2.8	61	48	55	1.3	258	41	0
Sheet cake, with white frosting	1 piece	121	445	4	14	4.6	5.6	2.9	70	77	61	1.2	275	71	0
Pound cake, home-made	1 slice	30	120	2	5	1.2	2.4	1.6	32	15	20	0.5	96	60	0
Pound cake, commercial	1 slice	29	110	2	5	3.0	1.7	0.2	64	15	8	0.5	108	41	0
Snack cakes, chocolate & creme filling	1 small	28	105	1	4	1.7	1.5	0.6	15	17	21	1.0	105	4	0
Snack cakes, sponge with creme filling	1 small	42	155	1	5	2.3	2.1	0.5	7	27	14	0.6	155	9	0
White cake with white frosting	1 piece	71	260	3	9	2.1	3.8	2.6	3	42	33	1.0	176	12	0
Yellow cake with chocolate frosting	1 piece	69	245	2	11	5.7	3.7	0.6	38	39	23	1.2	192	30	0
Cheesecake	1 piece	92	280	5	18	9.9	5.4	1.2	170	26	52	0.4	204	69	5
Cookies:															
Brownies with nuts & frosting, commercial	1 brownie	25	100	1	4	1.6	2.0	0.6	14	16	13	0.6	59	18	0
Brownies with nuts, home-made	1 brownie	20	95	1	6	1.4	2.8	1.2	18	11	9	0.4	51	6	0
Chocolate chip cookies, commercial	4 cookies	42	180	2	9	2.9	3.1	2.6	5	28	13	0.8	140	15	0
Chocolate chip cookies, home-made	4 cookies	40	185	2	11	3.9	4.3	2.0	18	26	13	1.0	82	5	0
Chocolate chip cookies, refrig dough	4 cookies	48	225	2	11	4.0	4.4	2.0	22	32	13	1.0	173	8	0
Fig bars	4 cookies	56	210	2	4	1.0	1.5	1.0	27	42	40	1.4	180	6	0
Oatmeal raisin cookies	4 cookies	52	245	3	10	2.5	4.5	2.8	2	36	18	1.1	148	12	0
Peanut butter cookies, home-made	4 cookies	48	245	4	14	4.0	5.8	2.8	22	28	21	1.1	142	5	0
Sandwich type cookies	4 cookies	40	195	2	8	2.0	3.6	2.2	0	29	12	1.4	189	0	0
Shortbread cookies, commercial	4 cookies	32	155	2	8	2.9	3.0	1.1	27	20	13	0.8	123	8	0
Shortbread cookies, home-made	2 cookies	28	145	2	8	1.3	2.7	3.4	0	17	6	0.6	125	89	0
Sugar cookies, from refrig dough	4 cookies	48	235	2	12	2.3	5.0	3.6	29	31	50	0.9	261	11	0
Vanilla wafers	10 cookies	40	185	2	7	1.8	3.0	1.8	25	29	16	0.8	150	14	0
Crackers:															
Cheese crackers, plain	10 crackers	10	50	1	3	0.9	1.2	0.3	6	6	11	0.3	112	5	0
Cheese crackers with peanut butter	1 sandwich	8	40	1	2	0.4	0.8	0.3	1	5	7	0.3	90	1	0
Graham cracker, plain	2 crackers	14	60	1	1	0.4	0.6	0.4	0	11	6	0.4	86	0	0
Melba toast, plain	1 piece	5	20	1	0	0.1	0.1	0.1	0	4	6	0.1	44	0	0
Rye wafers, whole-grain	2 wafers	14	55	1	1	0.3	0.4	0.3	0	10	7	0.5	115	0	0
Saltines	4 crackers	12	50	1	1	0.5	0.4	0.2	4	9	3	0.5	165	0	0

Food Item	Serving Size	Weight (g)	Cal- ories	Pro- tein (g)	Fat (g)	Satu- rated Fat (g)	Mono- unsat- urated Fat (g)	Poly- unsat- urated Fat (g)	Cho- les- terol (g)	Car- bohy- drate (g)	Cal- cium (mg)	Iron (mg)	Sod- ium (mg)	Vita- min A (µg)	Vita- min C (mg)
Snack type crackers	1 cracker	3	15	0	1	0.2	0.4	0.1	0	2	3	0.1	30	0	0
Wheat, thin crackers	4 crackers	8	35	1	1	0.5	0.5	0.4	0	5	3	0.3	69	1	0
Whole-wheat wafers, crackers	2 crackers	8	35	1	2	0.5	0.6	0.4	0	5	3	0.2	59	0	0
Flour and Meals:															
Buckwheat flour, light, sifted	1 cup	98	340	6	1	0.2	0.4	0.4	0	78	11	1.0	2	0	0
Cornmeal, enriched, dry	1 cup	138	500	11	2	0.2	0.4	0.9	0	108	8	5.9	1	61	0
Cornmeal, enriched, cooked	1 cup	240	120	3	0	0	0.1	0.2	0	26	2	1.4	0	14	0
Wheat flour, all-purpose	1 cup	115	420	12	1	0.2	0.1	0.5	0	88	18	5.1	2	0	0
Wheat flour, cake or pastry	1 cup	96	350	7	1	0.1	0.1	0.3	0	76	16	4.2	2	0	0
Wheat flour, self-rising	1 cup	125	440	12	1	0.2	0.1	0.5	0	93	331	5.5	1349	0	0
Whole-wheat flour	1 cup	120	400	16	2	0.3	0.3	1.1	0	85	49	5.2	4	0	0
Grains:															
Barley, light, uncooked	1 cup	200	700	16	2	0.3	0.2	0.9	0	158	32	4.2	6	0	0
Bulgur, uncooked	1 cup	170	600	19	3	1.2	0.3	1.2	0	129	49	9.5	7	0	0
Rice, brown, cooked	1 cup	195	230	5	1	0.3	0.3	0.4	0	50	23	1.0	0	0	0
Rice, white, raw	1 cup	185	670	12	1	0.2	0.2	0.3	0	149	44	5.4	9	0	0
Rice, white, cooked	1 cup	205	225	4	0	0.1	0.1	0.1	0	50	21	1.8	0	0	0
Rice, white, instant, cooked	1 cup	165	180	4	0	0.1	0.1	0.1	0	40	5	1.3	0	0	0
Rice, white, parboiled, raw	1 cup	185	685	14	1	0.1	0.1	0.2	0	150	111	5.4	17	0	0
Rice, white, parboiled, cooked	1 cup	175	185	4	0	0	0	0.1	0	41	33	1.4	0	0	0
Grain snacks:															
Corn chips	1 ounce	28	155	2	9	1.4	2.4	3.7	0	16	35	0.5	233	11	1
Popcorn, air-popped, unsalted	1 cup	8	30	1	0	0	0.1	0.2	0	6	1	0.2	0	1	0
Popcorn, popped in oil, salted	1 cup	11	55	1	3	0.5	1.4	1.2	0	6	3	0.3	86	2	0
Popcorn, sugar syrup coated	1 cup	35	135	2	1	0.1	0.3	0.6	0	30	2	0.5	0	3	0
Pretzels, stick	10 pretzels	3	10	0	0	0	0	0	0	2	1	0.1	48	0	0
Pretzels, twisted, Dutch	1 pretzel	16	65	2	1	0.1	0.2	0.2	0	13	4	0.3	258	0	0
Pretzels, twisted, thin	10 pretzels	60	240	6	2	0.4	0.8	0.6	0	48	16	1.2	966	0	0
Muffins:															
Blueberry muffins, home-made	1 muffin	45	135	3	5	1.5	2.1	1.2	19	20	54	0.9	198	9	1
Blueberry muffins, from mix	1 muffin	45	140	3	5	1.4	2.0	1.2	45	22	15	0.9	225	11	0
Bran muffins, home-made	1 muffin	45	125	3	6	1.4	1.6	2.3	24	19	60	1.4	189	30	3
Bran muffins, from mix	1 muffin	45	140	3	4	1.3	1.6	1.0	28	24	27	1.7	385	14	0
Corn muffins, home-made	1 muffin	45	145	3	5	1.5	2.2	1.4	23	21	66	0.9	169	15	0
Corn muffins, from mix	1 muffin	45	145	3	6	1.7	2.3	1.4	42	22	30	1.3	291	16	0
English muffins, plain	1 muffin	57	140	5	1	0.3	0.2	0.3	0	27	96	1.7	378	0	0
English muffins, plain, toasted	1 muffin	50	140	5	1	0.3	0.2	0.3	0	27	96	1.7	378	0	0
Noodles and Pasta:															
Macaroni, cooked, firm	1 cup	130	190	7	1	0.1	0.1	0.3	0	39	14	2.1	1	0	0
Macaroni, cooked, tender	1 cup	105	115	4	0	0.1	0.1	0.2	0	24	8	1.3	1	0	0
Noodles, egg, cooked	1 cup	160	200	7	2	0.5	0.6	0.6	50	37	16	2.6	3	34	0
Noodles, chow mein, canned	1 cup	45	220	6	11	2.1	7.3	0.4	5	26	14	0.4	450	0	0
Spaghetti, cooked, firm	1 cup	130	190	7	1	0.1	0.1	0.3	0	39	14	2.0	1	0	0
Spaghetti, cooked, tender	1 cup	140	155	5	1	0.1	0.1	0.2	0	32	11	1.7	1	0	0

Food Composition Table (continued)

Food Item	Serving Size	Weight (g)	Calories	Protein (g)	Fat (g)	Saturated Fat (g)	Monounsaturated Fat (g)	Polyunsaturated Fat (g)	Cholesterol (g)	Carbohydrate (g)	Calcium (mg)	Iron (mg)	Sodium (mg)	Vitamin A (µg)	Vitamin C (mg)
Pancakes, Waffles, and French Toast:															
French toast, home-made	1 slice	65	155	6	7	1.6	2.0	1.6	112	17	72	1.3	257	32	0
Pancakes, buckwheat, from mix	1 pancake	27	55	2	2	0.9	0.9	0.5	20	6	59	0.4	125	17	0
Pancakes, plain, home-made	1 pancake	27	60	2	2	0.5	0.8	0.5	16	9	27	0.5	115	10	0
Pancakes, plain, from mix	1 pancake	27	60	2	2	0.5	0.9	0.5	16	8	36	0.7	160	7	0
Waffles, home-made	1 waffle	75	245	7	13	4.0	4.9	2.6	102	26	154	1.5	445	39	0
Waffles, from mix	1 waffle	75	205	7	8	2.7	2.9	1.5	59	27	179	1.2	515	49	0
Pastries:															
Croissants	1 croissant	57	235	5	12	3.5	6.7	1.4	13	27	20	2.1	452	13	0
Danish pastry, plain, no nuts	1 ring	340	1305	21	71	21.8	28.6	15.6	292	152	360	6.5	1302	99	0
Danish pastry, plain, no nuts	1 pastry	57	220	4	12	3.6	4.8	2.6	49	26	60	1.1	218	17	0
Danish pastry, fruit	1 pastry	65	235	4	13	3.9	5.2	2.9	56	28	17	1.3	233	11	0
Doughnuts, cake type, plain	1 doughnut	50	210	3	12	2.8	5.0	3.0	20	24	22	1.0	192	5	0
Doughnuts, glazed	1 doughnut	60	235	4	13	5.2	5.5	0.9	21	26	17	1.4	222	0	0
Pie crust, home-made	1 shell	180	900	11	60	14.8	25.9	15.7	0	79	25	4.5	1100	0	0
Pie crust, from mix	2 crust	320	1485	20	93	22.7	41.0	25.0	0	141	131	9.3	2602	0	0
Toaster pastries	1 pastry	54	210	2	6	1.7	3.6	0.4	0	38	104	2.2	248	52	4
Pies:															
Apple pie	1 piece	158	405	3	18	4.6	7.4	4.4	0	60	13	1.6	476	5	2
Blueberry pie	1 piece	158	380	4	17	4.3	7.4	4.6	0	55	17	2.1	423	14	6
Cherry pie	1 piece	158	410	4	18	4.7	7.7	4.6	0	61	22	1.6	480	70	0
Creme pie	1 piece	152	455	3	23	15.0	4.0	1.1	8	59	46	1.1	369	65	0
Custard pie	1 piece	152	330	9	17	5.6	6.7	3.2	169	36	146	1.5	436	96	0
Lemon meringue pie	1 piece	140	355	5	14	4.3	5.7	2.9	143	53	20	1.4	395	66	4
Peach pie	1 piece	158	405	4	17	4.1	7.3	4.4	0	60	16	1.9	423	115	5
Pecan pie	1 piece	138	575	7	32	4.7	17.0	7.9	95	71	65	4.6	305	54	0
Pumpkin pie	1 piece	152	320	6	17	6.4	6.7	3.0	109	37	78	1.4	325	416	0
Fried pie, apple	1 pie	85	255	2	14	5.8	6.6	0.6	14	31	12	0.9	326	3	1
Fried pie, cherry	1 pie	85	250	2	14	5.8	6.7	0.6	13	32	11	0.7	371	19	1
Rolls:															
Rolls, dinner	1 roll	28	85	2	2	0.5	0.8	0.6	0	14	33	0.8	155	0	0
Rolls, frankfurter or hamburger	1 roll	40	115	3	2	0.5	0.8	0.6	0	20	54	1.2	241	0	0
Rolls, hard	1 roll	50	155	5	2	0.4	0.5	0.6	0	30	24	1.4	313	0	0
Rolls, hoagie or submarine	1 roll	135	400	11	8	1.8	3.0	2.2	0	72	100	3.8	683	0	0
Rolls, dinner, home-made	1 roll	35	120	3	3	0.8	1.2	0.9	12	20	16	1.1	98	8	0
Tortillas:															
Tortillas, corn	1 tortilla	30	65	2	1	0.1	0.3	0.6	0	13	42	0.6	1	8	0
Legumes, Nuts & Seeds															
Beans and Other Legumes:															
Black beans, dry, cooked	1 cup	171	225	15	1	0.1	0.1	0.5	0	41	47	2.9	1	0	0
Great northern beans, dry, cooked	1 cup	180	210	14	1	0.1	0.1	0.6	0	38	90	4.9	13	0	0

Food Item	Serving Size	Weight (g)	Calories	Protein (g)	Fat (g)	Saturated Fat (g)	Mono-unsaturated Fat (g)	Poly-unsaturated Fat (g)	Cholesterol (g)	Carbohydrate (g)	Calcium (mg)	Iron (mg)	Sodium (mg)	Vitamin A (μg)	Vitamin C (mg)
Lima beans, dry, cooked	1 cup	190	260	16	1	0.2	0.1	0.5	0	49	55	5.9	4	0	0
Pea beans, dry, cooked	1 cup	190	225	15	1	0.1	0.1	0.7	0	40	95	5.1	13	0	0
Pinto beans, dry, cooked	1 cup	180	265	15	1	0.1	0.1	0.5	0	49	86	5.4	3	0	0
Beans, dry, canned with frankfurters	1 cup	255	365	19	18	7.4	8.8	0.7	30	32	94	4.8	1374	33	0
Beans, dry, canned with pork	1 cup	255	310	16	7	2.4	2.7	0.7	10	48	138	4.6	1181	33	5
Beans, dry, canned without pork	1 cup	255	385	16	12	4.3	4.9	1.2	10	54	161	5.9	969	33	5
Red kidney beans, dry, canned	1 cup	255	230	15	1	0.1	0.1	0.6	0	42	74	4.6	968	1	0
Black-eyed peas, dry, cooked	1 cup	250	190	13	1	0.2	0	0.3	0	35	43	3.3	20	3	0
Chickpeas, cooked, drained	1 cup	163	270	15	4	0.4	0.9	1.9	0	45	80	4.9	11	0	0
Lentils, dry, cooked	1 cup	200	215	16	1	0.1	0.2	0.5	0	38	50	4.2	26	4	0
Peanuts, oil roasted, salted	1 cup	145	840	39	71	9.9	35.5	22.6	0	27	125	2.8	626	0	0
Peanuts, oil roasted, unsalted	1 cup	145	840	39	71	9.9	35.5	22.6	0	27	125	2.8	22	0	0
Peanuts, oil roasted, salted	1 ounce	28.35	165	8	14	1.9	6.9	4.4	0	5	24	0.5	122	0	0
Peanuts, oil roasted, unsalted	1 ounce	28.35	165	8	14	1.9	6.9	4.4	0	5	24	0.5	4	0	0
Peanut butter	1 tbsp.	16	95	5	8	1.4	4.0	2.5	0	3	5	0.3	75	0	0
Peas, split, dry, cooked	1 cup	200	230	16	1	0.1	0.1	0.3	0	42	22	3.4	26	8	0
Refried beans, canned	1 cup	290	295	18	3	0.4	0.6	1.4	0	51	141	5.1	1228	0	17
Soybeans, dry, cooked, drained	1 cup	180	235	20	10	1.3	1.9	5.3	0	19	131	4.9	4	5	0
Miso	1 cup	276	470	29	13	1.8	2.6	7.3	0	65	188	4.7	8142	11	0
Tofu	1 piece	120	85	9	5	0.7	1.0	2.9	0	3	108	2.3	8	0	0
Nuts:															
Almonds, slivered	1 cup	135	795	27	70	6.7	45.8	14.8	0	28	359	4.9	15	0	1
Almonds, whole	1 ounce	28.35	165	6	15	1.4	9.6	3.1	0	6	75	1.0	3	0	0
Brazil nuts	1 ounce	28.35	185	4	19	4.6	6.5	6.8	0	4	50	1.0	1	0	0
Cashew nuts, dry roasted, salted	1 ounce	28.35	165	4	13	2.6	7.7	2.2	0	9	13	1.7	181	0	0
Cashew nuts, dry roasted, unsalted	1 ounce	28.35	165	4	13	2.6	7.7	2.2	0	9	13	1.7	4	0	0
Cashew nuts, oil roasted, salted	1 ounce	28.35	165	5	14	2.7	8.1	2.3	0	8	12	1.2	177	0	0
Cashew nuts, oil roasted, unsalted	1 ounce	28.35	165	5	14	2.7	8.1	2.3	0	8	12	1.2	5	0	0
Chestnuts, roasted	1 cup	143	350	5	3	0.6	1.1	1.2	0	76	41	1.3	3	3	37
Coconut, raw, pieces	1 piece	45	160	1	15	13.4	0.6	0.2	0	7	6	1.1	9	0	1
Coconut, raw, shredded	1 cup	80	285	3	27	23.8	1.1	0.3	0	12	11	1.9	16	0	3
Coconut, dried, sweetened, shredded	1 cup	93	470	3	33	29.3	1.4	0.4	0	44	14	1.8	244	0	1
Filberts, (hazelnuts) chopped	1 ounce	28.35	180	4	18	1.3	13.9	1.7	0	4	53	0.9	1	2	0
Macadamia nuts, oil roasted, salted	1 ounce	28.35	205	2	22	3.2	17.1	0.4	0	4	13	0.5	74	0	0
Macadamia nuts, oil roasted, unsalted	1 ounce	28.35	205	2	22	3.2	17.1	0.4	0	4	13	0.5	2	0	0
Mixed nuts, dry roasted, salted	1 ounce	28.35	170	5	15	2.0	8.9	3.1	0	7	20	1.0	190	0	0

Food Composition Table (continued)

Food Item	Serving Size	Weight (g)	Cal- ories	Pro- tein (g)	Fat (g)	Satu- rated Fat (g)	Mono- unsat- urated Fat (g)	Poly- unsat- urated Fat (g)	Cho- les- terol (g)	Car- bohy- drate (g)	Cal- cium (mg)	Iron (mg)	Sod- ium (mg)	Vita- min A (μg)	Vita- min C (mg)
Mixed nuts, dry roasted, unsalted	1 ounce	28.35	170	5	15	2.0	8.9	3.1	0	7	20	1.0	3	0	0
Mixed nuts, oil roasted, salted	1 ounce	28.35	175	5	16	2.5	9.0	3.8	0	6	31	0.9	185	1	0
Mixed nuts, oil roasted, unsalted	1 ounce	28.35	175	5	16	2.5	9.0	3.8	0	6	31	0.9	3	1	0
Pecans, halves	1 ounce	28.35	190	2	19	1.5	12.0	4.7	0	5	10	0.6	0	4	1
Pine nuts	1 ounce	28.35	160	3	17	2.7	6.5	7.3	0	5	2	0.9	20	1	1
Pistachio nuts	1 ounce	28.35	165	6	14	1.7	9.3	2.1	0	7	38	1.9	2	7	0
Walnuts, black, chopped	1 ounce	28.35	170	7	16	1.0	3.6	10.6	0	3	16	0.9	0	8	0
Walnuts, English, chopped	1 ounce	28.35	180	4	18	1.6	4.0	11.1	0	5	27	0.7	3	4	1
Seeds:															
Pumpkin and squash kernels	1 ounce	28.35	155	7	13	2.5	4.0	5.9	0	5	12	4.2	5	11	0
Sesame seeds	1 tbsp.	8	45	2	4	0.6	1.7	1.9	0	1	11	0.6	3	1	0
Sunflower seeds	1 ounce	28.35	160	6	14	1.5	2.7	9.3	0	5	33	1.9	1	1	0
Tahini	1 tbsp.	15	90	3	8	1.1	3.0	3.5	0	3	21	0.7	5	1	1
Meat and Meat Products															
Beef:															
Beef, cooked, chuck blade, lean & fat	3 ounces	85	325	22	26	10.8	11.7	0.9	87	0	11	2.5	53	0	0
Beef, cooked, chuck blade, lean only	2.2 ounces	62	170	19	9	3.9	4.2	0.3	66	0	8	2.3	44	0	0
Beef, cooked, bottom round, lean & fat	3 ounces	85	220	25	13	4.8	5.7	0.5	81	0	5	2.8	43	0	0
Beef, cooked, bottom round, lean only	2.8 ounces	78	175	25	8	2.7	3.4	0.3	75	0	4	2.7	40	0	0
Ground beef, broiled, lean	3 ounces	85	230	21	16	6.2	6.9	0.6	74	0	9	1.8	65	0	0
Ground beef, broiled, regular	3 ounces	85	245	20	18	6.9	7.7	0.7	76	0	9	2.1	70	0	0
Beef heart, braised	3 ounces	85	150	24	5	1.2	0.8	1.6	164	7	5	6.4	54	0	5
Beef liver, fried	3 ounces	85	185	23	7	2.5	3.6	1.3	410	7	9	5.3	90	9120	23
Beef roast, rib, lean & fat	3 ounces	85	315	19	26	10.8	11.4	0.9	72	0	8	2.0	54	0	0
Beef roast, rib, lean only	2.2 ounces	61	150	17	9	3.6	3.7	0.3	49	0	5	1.7	45	0	0
Beef roast, eye of round, lean & fat	3 ounces	85	205	23	12	4.9	5.4	0.5	62	0	5	1.6	50	0	0
Beef roast, eye of round, lean only	2.6 ounces	75	135	22	5	1.9	2.1	0.2	52	0	3	1.5	46	0	0
Beef steak, sirloin, broiled, lean & fat	3 ounces	85	240	23	15	6.4	6.9	0.6	77	0	9	2.6	53	0	0
Beef steak, sirloin, broiled, lean only	2.5 ounces	72	150	22	6	2.6	2.8	0.3	64	0	8	2.4	48	0	0
Beef, canned, corned	3 ounces	85	185	22	10	4.2	4.9	0.4	80	0	17	3.7	802	0	0
Beef, dried, chipped	2.5 ounces	72	145	24	4	1.8	2.0	0.2	46	0	14	2.3	3053	0	0
Lamb:															
Lamb, chops, arm, braised, lean & fat	2.2 ounces	63	220	20	15	6.9	6.0	0.9	77	0	16	1.5	46	0	0

Food Item	Serving Size	Weight (g)	Cal-ories	Pro-tein (g)	Fat (g)	Satu-rated Fat (g)	Mono-unsat-urated Fat (g)	Poly-unsat-urated Fat (g)	Cho-les-terol (g)	Car-bohy-drate (g)	Cal-cium (mg)	Iron (mg)	Sod-ium (mg)	Vita-min A (μg)	Vita-min C (mg)
Lamb, chops, arm, braised, lean only	1.7 ounces	48	135	17	7	2.9	2.6	0.4	59	0	12	1.3	36	0	0
Lamb, chops, loin, broil, lean & fat	2.8 ounces	80	235	22	16	7.3	6.4	1.0	78	0	16	1.4	62	0	0
Lamb, chops, loin, broil, lean only	2.3 ounces	64	140	19	6	2.6	2.4	0.4	60	0	12	1.3	54	0	0
Lamb, leg, roasted, lean & fat	3 ounces	85	205	22	13	5.6	4.9	0.8	78	0	8	1.7	57	0	0
Lamb, leg, roasted, lean only	2.6 ounces	73	140	20	6	2.4	2.2	0.4	65	0	6	1.5	50	0	0
Lamb, rib, roasted, lean & fat	3 ounces	85	315	18	26	12.1	10.6	1.5	77	0	19	1.4	60	0	0
Lamb, rib, roasted, lean only	2 ounces	57	130	15	7	3.2	3.0	0.5	50	0	12	1.0	46	0	0
Pork:															
Pork, cured, bacon, cooked	3 slices	19	110	6	9	3.3	4.5	1.1	16	0	2	0.3	303	0	6
Pork, cured, bacon, Canadian, cooked	2 slices	46	85	11	4	1.3	1.9	0.4	27	1	5	0.4	711	0	10
Pork, cured, ham, roasted, lean & fat	3 ounces	85	205	18	14	5.1	6.7	1.5	53	0	6	0.7	1009	0	0
Pork, cured, ham, roasted, lean	2.4 ounces	68	105	17	4	1.3	1.7	0.4	37	0	5	0.6	902	0	0
Pork, cured, ham, canned	3 ounces	85	140	18	7	2.4	3.5	0.8	35	0	6	0.9	908	0	19
Pork chop, loin, broiled, lean & fat	3.1 ounce	87	275	24	19	7.0	8.8	2.2	84	0	3	0.7	61	3	0
Pork chop, loin, broiled, lean only	2.5 ounces	72	165	23	8	2.6	3.4	0.9	71	0	4	0.7	56	1	0
Pork chop, loin, pan fried, lean & fat	3.1 ounce	89	335	21	27	9.8	12.5	3.1	92	0	4	0.7	64	3	0
Pork chop, loin, pan fried, lean only	2.4 ounces	67	180	19	11	3.7	4.8	1.3	72	0	3	0.7	57	1	0
Pork fresh ham, roasted, lean & fat	3 ounces	85	250	21	18	6.4	8.1	2.0	79	0	5	0.9	50	2	0
Pork fresh ham, roasted, lean only	2.5 ounces	72	160	20	8	2.7	3.6	1.0	68	0	5	0.8	46	1	0
Pork fresh rib, roasted, lean & fat	3 ounces	85	270	21	20	7.2	9.2	2.3	69	0	9	0.8	37	3	0
Pork fresh rib, roasted, lean only	2.5 ounces	71	175	20	10	3.4	4.4	1.2	56	0	8	0.7	33	2	0
Pork shoulder, braised, lean & fat	3 ounces	85	295	23	22	7.9	10	2.4	93	0	6	1.4	75	3	0
Pork shoulder, braised, lean only	2.4 ounces	67	165	22	8	2.8	3.7	1.0	76	0	5	1.3	68	1	0
Sausage and Luncheon Meats:															
Bologna	2 slices	57	180	7	16	6.1	7.6	1.4	31	2	7	0.9	581	0	12
Braunschweiger	2 slices	57	205	8	18	6.2	8.5	2.1	89	2	5	5.3	652	2405	6
Brown and serve sausage	1 link	13	50	2	5	1.7	2.2	0.5	9	0	1	0.1	105	0	0
Frankfurter, cooked	1 frank	45	145	5	13	4.8	6.2	1.2	23	1	5	0.5	504	0	12

Food Composition Table (continued)

Food Item	Serving Size	Weight (g)	Calories	Protein (g)	Fat (g)	Saturated Fat (g)	Monounsaturated Fat (g)	Polyunsaturated Fat (g)	Cholesterol (g)	Carbohydrate (g)	Calcium (mg)	Iron (mg)	Sodium (mg)	Vitamin A (µg)	Vitamin C (mg)
Pork, link, cooked	1 link	13	50	3	4	1.4	1.8	0.5	11	0	4	0.2	168	0	0
Pork, canned luncheon meat	2 slices	42	140	5	13	4.5	6.0	1.5	26	1	3	0.3	541	0	0
Pork, chopped ham luncheon meat	2 slices	42	95	7	7	2.4	3.4	0.9	21	0	3	0.3	576	0	8
Pork, cooked ham luncheon meat	2 slices	57	105	10	6	1.9	2.8	0.7	32	2	4	0.6	751	0	16
Pork, lean cooked ham luncheon meat	2 slices	57	75	11	3	0.9	1.3	0.3	27	1	4	0.4	815	0	15
Salami, cooked	2 slices	57	145	8	11	4.6	5.2	1.2	37	1	7	1.5	607	0	7
Salami, dry	2 slices	20	85	5	7	2.4	3.4	0.6	16	1	2	0.3	372	0	5
Sandwich spread, pork & beef	1 tbsp.	15	35	1	3	0.9	1.1	0.4	6	2	2	0.1	152	1	0
Vienna sausage	1 sausage	16	45	2	4	1.5	2.0	0.3	8	0	2	0.1	152	0	0
Veal:															
Veal cutlet, braised or broiled	3 ounces	85	185	23	9	4.1	4.1	0.6	86	0	9	0.8	56	0	0
Veal rib, roasted	3 ounces	85	230	23	14	6.0	6.0	1.0	109	0	10	0.7	57	0	0
Mixed Dishes															
Beef and vegetable stew, home-made	1 cup	245	220	16	11	4.4	4.5	0.5	71	15	29	2.9	292	568	17
Beef potpie, home-made	1 piece	210	515	21	30	7.9	12.9	7.4	42	39	29	3.8	596	517	6
Chicken a la king, home-made	1 cup	245	470	27	34	12.9	13.4	6.2	221	12	127	2.5	760	272	12
Chicken and noodles, home-made	1 cup	240	365	22	18	5.1	7.1	3.9	103	26	26	2.2	600	130	0
Chicken chow mein, canned	1 cup	250	95	7	0	0.1	0.1	0.8	8	18	45	1.3	725	28	13
Chicken chow mein, home-made	1 cup	250	255	31	10	4.1	4.9	3.5	75	10	58	2.5	718	50	10
Chicken potpie, home-made	1 piece	232	545	23	31	10.3	15.5	6.6	56	42	70	3.0	594	735	5
Chili con carne with beans, canned	1 cup	255	340	19	16	5.8	7.2	1.0	28	31	82	4.3	1354	15	8
Chop suey with beef & pork, home-made	1 cup	250	300	26	17	4.3	7.4	4.2	68	13	60	4.8	1053	60	33
Macaroni and cheese, canned	1 cup	240	230	9	10	4.7	2.9	1.3	24	26	199	1.0	730	72	0
Macaroni and cheese, home-made	1 cup	200	430	17	22	9.8	7.4	3.6	44	40	362	1.8	1086	232	1
Quiche Lorraine	1 slice	176	600	13	48	23.2	17.8	4.1	285	29	211	1.0	653	454	0
Spaghetti, canned	1 cup	250	190	6	2	0.4	0.4	0.5	3	39	40	2.8	955	120	10
Spaghetti, home-made	1 cup	250	260	9	9	3.0	3.6	1.2	8	37	80	2.3	955	140	13
Spaghetti with meatballs, canned	1 cup	250	260	12	10	2.4	3.9	3.1	23	29	53	3.3	1220	100	5
Spaghetti with meatballs, home-made	1 cup	248	330	19	12	3.9	4.4	2.2	89	39	124	3.7	1009	159	22
Poultry															
Chicken:															
Chicken, canned, boneless	5 ounces	142	235	31	11	3.1	4.5	2.5	88	0	20	2.2	714	48	3
Chicken, fried, batter, breast	4.9 ounces	140	365	35	18	4.9	7.6	4.3	119	13	28	1.8	385	28	0

Food Item	Serving Size	Weight (g)	Cal-ories	Pro-tein (g)	Fat (g)	Satu-rated Fat (g)	Mono-unsat-urated Fat (g)	Poly-unsat-urated Fat (g)	Cho-les-terol (g)	Car-bohy-drate (g)	Cal-cium (mg)	Iron (mg)	Sod-ium (mg)	Vita-min A (µg)	Vita-min C (mg)
Chicken, fried, batter, drumstick	2.5 ounces	72	195	16	11	3.0	4.6	2.7	62	6	12	1.0	194	19	0
Chicken, fried, flour, breast	3.5 ounces	98	220	31	9	2.4	3.4	1.9	87	2	16	1.2	74	15	0
Chicken, fried, flour, drumstick	1.7 ounces	49	120	13	7	1.8	2.7	1.6	44	1	6	0.7	44	12	0
Chicken, roasted, breast	3.0 ounces	86	140	27	3	0.9	1.1	0.7	73	0	13	0.9	64	5	0
Chicken, roasted, drumstick	1.6 ounces	44	75	12	2	0.7	0.8	0.6	41	0	5	0.6	42	8	0
Chicken, stewed, light & dark	1 cup	140	250	38	9	2.6	3.3	2.2	116	0	20	1.6	98	21	0
Chicken frankfurter	1 frank	45	115	6	9	2.5	3.8	1.8	45	3	43	0.9	616	17	0
Chicken liver, cooked	1 liver	20	30	5	1	0.4	0.3	0.2	126	0	3	1.7	10	983	3
Chicken roll, light	2 slices	57	90	11	4	1.1	1.7	0.9	28	1	24	0.6	331	14	0
Duck:															
Duck, roasted, flesh only	1/2 duck	221	445	52	25	9.2	8.2	3.2	197	0	27	6.0	144	51	0
Turkey:															
Turkey, roasted, dark meat	4 pieces	85	160	24	6	2.1	1.4	1.8	72	0	27	2.0	67	0	0
Turkey, roasted, light meat	2 pieces	85	135	25	3	0.9	0.5	0.7	59	0	16	1.1	54	0	0
Turkey, roasted, light & dark	1 cup	140	240	41	7	2.3	1.4	2.0	106	0	35	2.5	98	0	0
Turkey, roasted, light & dark	3 pieces	85	145	25	4	1.4	0.9	1.2	65	0	21	1.5	60	0	0
Gravy and turkey, frozen	5 ounces	142	95	8	4	1.2	1.4	0.7	26	7	20	1.3	787	18	0
Turkey ham, cured turkey thigh	2 slices	57	75	11	3	1.0	0.7	0.9	32	0	6	1.6	565	0	0
Turkey loaf, breast meat	2 slices	42	45	10	1	0.2	0.2	0.1	17	0	3	0.2	608	0	0
Turkey patties, breaded, fried	1 patty	64	180	9	12	3.0	4.8	3.0	40	10	9	1.4	512	7	0
Turkey roast, frozen, cooked	3 ounces	85	130	18	5	1.6	1.0	1.4	45	3	4	1.4	578	0	0

Soups, Sauces, and Gravies

Canned Soup:

Food Item	Serving Size	Weight (g)	Cal-ories	Pro-tein (g)	Fat (g)	Satu-rated Fat (g)	Mono-unsat-urated Fat (g)	Poly-unsat-urated Fat (g)	Cho-les-terol (g)	Car-bohy-drate (g)	Cal-cium (mg)	Iron (mg)	Sod-ium (mg)	Vita-min A (µg)	Vita-min C (mg)
Clam chowder, New England with milk	1 cup	248	165	9	7	3.0	2.3	1.1	22	17	186	1.5	992	40	3
Cream of chicken soup with milk, canned	1 cup	248	190	7	11	4.6	4.5	1.6	27	15	181	0.7	1047	94	1
Cream of mushroom soup with milk, canned	1 cup	248	205	6	14	5.1	3.0	4.6	20	15	179	0.6	1076	37	2
Tomato soup with milk, canned	1 cup	248	160	6	6	2.9	1.6	1.1	17	22	159	1.8	932	109	68
Bean with bacon soup, canned	1 cup	253	170	8	6	1.5	2.2	1.8	3	23	81	2.0	951	89	2
Beef broth, bouillon, consomme, canned	1 cup	240	15	3	1	0.3	0.2	0	0	0	14	0.4	782	0	0
Beef noodle soup, canned	1 cup	244	85	5	3	1.1	1.2	0.5	5	9	15	1.1	952	63	0
Chicken noodle soup, canned	1 cup	241	75	4	2	0.7	1.1	0.6	7	9	17	0.8	1106	71	0
Chicken rice soup, canned	1 cup	241	60	4	2	0.5	0.9	0.4	7	7	17	0.7	815	66	0
Clam chowder, Manhattan, canned	1 cup	244	80	4	2	0.4	0.4	1.3	2	12	34	1.9	1808	92	3
Cream of chicken soup with water, canned	1 cup	244	115	3	7	2.1	3.3	1.5	10	9	34	0.6	986	56	0
Cream of mushroom soup with water, canned	1 cup	244	130	2	9	2.4	1.7	4.2	2	9	46	0.5	1032	0	1

Food Composition Table (continued)

Food Item	Serving Size	Weight (g)	Calories	Protein (g)	Fat (g)	Saturated Fat (g)	Monounsaturated Fat (g)	Polyunsaturated Fat (g)	Cholesterol (g)	Carbohydrate (g)	Calcium (mg)	Iron (mg)	Sodium (mg)	Vitamin A (μg)	Vitamin C (mg)
Minestrone soup, canned	1 cup	241	80	4	3	0.6	0.7	1.1	2	11	34	0.9	911	234	1
Pea, green, soup, canned	1 cup	250	165	9	3	1.4	1.0	0.4	0	27	28	2.0	988	20	2
Tomato soup with water, canned	1 cup	244	85	2	2	0.4	0.4	1.0	0	17	12	1.8	871	69	66
Vegetable beef soup, canned	1 cup	244	80	6	2	0.9	0.8	0.1	5	10	17	1.1	956	189	2
Vegetarian soup, canned	1 cup	241	70	2	2	0.3	0.8	0.7	0	12	22	1.1	822	301	1
Dry soup:															
Bouillon, dry	1 packet	6	15	1	1	0.3	0.2	0	1	1	4	0.1	1019	0	0
Onion soup, dry	1 packet	7	20	1	0	0.1	0.2	0	0	4	10	0.1	627	0	0
Chicken noodle soup, dry, prepared	1 packet	188	40	2	1	0.2	0.4	0.3	2	6	24	0.4	957	5	0
Onion soup, dry, prepared	1 packet	184	20	1	0	0.1	0.2	0.1	0	4	9	0.1	635	0	0
Tomato vegetable soup, dry, prepared	1 packet	189	40	1	1	0.3	0.2	0.1	0	8	6	0.5	856	14	5
Sauces:															
Barbecue sauce	1 tbsp.	16	10	0	0	0	0.1	0.1	0	2	3	0.1	130	14	1
Cheese sauce with milk, mix	1 cup	279	305	16	17	9.3	5.3	1.6	53	23	569	0.3	1565	117	2
Hollandaise sauce with water, mix	1 cup	259	240	5	20	11.6	5.9	0.9	52	14	124	0.9	1564	220	0
Soy sauce	1 tbsp.	18	10	2	0	0	0	0	0	2	3	0.5	1029	0	0
White sauce with milk, mix	1 cup	264	240	10	13	6.4	4.7	1.7	34	21	425	0.3	797	92	3
White sauce, medium, home-made	1 cup	250	395	10	30	9.1	11.9	7.2	32	24	292	0.9	888	340	2
Gravies:															
Beef gravy, canned	1 cup	233	125	9	5	2.7	2.3	0.2	7	11	14	1.6	1305	0	0
Chicken gravy, canned	1 cup	238	190	5	14	3.4	6.1	3.6	5	13	48	1.1	1373	264	0
Mushroom gravy, canned	1 cup	238	120	3	6	1.0	2.8	2.4	0	13	17	1.6	1357	0	0
Brown gravy from dry mix	1 cup	261	80	3	2	0.9	0.8	0.1	2	14	66	0.2	1147	0	0
Chicken gravy from dry mix	1 cup	260	85	3	2	0.5	0.9	0.4	3	14	39	0.3	1134	0	3

Spices and Herbs

Food Item	Serving Size	Weight (g)	Calories	Protein (g)	Fat (g)	Saturated Fat (g)	Monounsaturated Fat (g)	Polyunsaturated Fat (g)	Cholesterol (g)	Carbohydrate (g)	Calcium (mg)	Iron (mg)	Sodium (mg)	Vitamin A (μg)	Vitamin C (mg)
Celery seed	1 tsp.	2	10	0	1	0	0.3	0.1	0	1	35	0.9	3	0	0
Chili powder	1 tsp.	2.60	10	0	0	0.1	0.1	0.2	0	1	7	0.4	26	91	2
Cinnamon	1 tsp.	2.30	5	0	0	0	0	0	0	2	28	0.9	1	1	1
Curry powder	1 tsp.	2	5	0	0	0	0	0	0	1	10	0.6	1	2	0
Garlic powder	1 tsp.	2.80	10	0	0	0	0	0	0	2	2	0.1	1	0	0
Mustard, prepared, yellow	1 tsp.	5	5	0	0	0	0.2	0	0	0	4	0.1	63	0	0
Onion powder	1 tsp.	2.10	5	0	0	0	0	0	0	2	8	0.1	1	0	0
Oregano	1 tsp.	1.50	5	0	0	0	0	0	0	1	24	0.7	0	10	1
Paprika	1 tsp.	2.10	5	0	0	0	0	0.1	0	1	4	0.5	1	127	1
Pepper, black	1 tsp.	2.10	5	0	0	0	0	0.2	0	1	9	0.6	1	0	0
Salt	1 tsp.	5.50	0	0	0	0	0	0	0	0	14	0	2132	0	0

Sugars and Sweets

Food Item	Serving Size	Weight (g)	Calories	Protein (g)	Fat (g)	Saturated Fat (g)	Monounsaturated Fat (g)	Polyunsaturated Fat (g)	Cholesterol (g)	Carbohydrate (g)	Calcium (mg)	Iron (mg)	Sodium (mg)	Vitamin A (μg)	Vitamin C (mg)
Candy:															
Caramels, plain or chocolate	1 ounce	28.35	115	1	3	2.2	0.3	0.1	1	22	42	0.4	64	0	0
Chocolate, bitter or baking	1 ounce	28.35	145	3	15	9.0	4.9	0.5	0	8	22	1.9	1	1	0
Chocolate, milk, plain	1 ounce	28.35	145	2	9	5.4	3.0	0.3	6	16	50	0.4	23	10	0
Chocolate, milk, with almonds	1 ounce	28.35	150	3	10	4.8	4.1	0.7	5	15	65	0.5	23	8	0
Chocolate, milk, with peanuts	1 ounce	28.35	155	4	11	4.2	3.5	1.5	5	13	49	0.4	19	8	0
Chocolate, milk, with rice cereal	1 ounce	28.35	140	2	7	4.4	2.5	0.2	6	18	48	0.2	46	8	0
Chocolate, semisweet	1 cup	170	860	7	61	36.2	19.9	1.9	0	97	51	5.8	24	3	0
Chocolate, sweet (dark)	1 ounce	28.35	150	1	10	5.9	3.3	0.3	0	16	7	0.6	5	1	0
Fondant, uncoated	1 ounce	28.35	105	0	0	0	0	0	0	27	2	0.1	57	0	0
Fudge, chocolate, plain	1 ounce	28.35	115	1	3	2.1	1.0	0.1	1	21	22	0.3	54	0	0
Gum drops	1 ounce	28.35	100	0	0	0	0	0.1	0	25	2	0.1	10	0	0
Hard candy	1 ounce	28.35	110	0	0	0	0	0.1	0	28	0	0.1	7	0	0
Jelly beans	1 ounce	28.35	105	0	0	0	0	0.1	0	26	1	0.3	7	0	0
Marshmallows	1 ounce	28.35	90	1	0	0	0	0	0	23	1	0.5	25	0	0
Desserts:															
Custard, baked	1 cup	265	305	14	15	6.8	5.4	0.7	278	29	297	1.1	209	146	1
Gelatin dessert, prepared	1/2 cup	120	70	2	0	0	0	0	0	17	2	0	55	0	0
Popsicle	1 popsicle	95	70	0	0	0	0	0	0	18	0	0	11	0	0
Pudding, chocolate, canned	5 ounces	142	205	3	11	9.5	0.5	0.1	1	30	74	1.2	285	31	0
Pudding, tapioca, canned	5 ounces	142	160	3	5	4.8	0	0	0	28	119	0.3	252	0	0
Pudding, vanilla, canned	5 ounces	142	220	2	10	9.5	0.2	0.1	1	33	79	0.2	305	0	0
Pudding, chocolate, instant, mix	1/2 cup	130	155	4	4	2.3	1.1	0.2	14	27	130	0.3	440	33	1
Pudding, chocolate, mix	1/2 cup	130	150	4	4	2.4	1.1	0.1	15	25	146	0.2	167	34	1
Pudding, rice, mix	1/2 cup	132	155	4	4	2.3	1.1	0.1	15	27	133	0.5	140	33	1
Pudding, tapioca, mix	1/2 cup	130	145	4	4	2.3	1.1	0.1	15	25	131	0.1	152	34	1
Pudding, vanilla, instant, mix	1/2 cup	130	150	4	4	2.2	1.1	0.2	15	27	129	0.1	375	33	1
Pudding, vanilla, mix	1/2 cup	130	145	4	4	2.3	1.0	0.1	15	25	132	0.1	178	34	1
Sugars and Sweeteners:															
Honey	1 tbsp.	21	65	0	0	0	0	0	0	17	1	0.1	1	0	0
Jams and preserves	1 tbsp.	20	55	0	0	0	0	0	0	14	4	0.2	2	0	0
Jellies	1 tbsp.	18	50	0	0	0	0	0	0	13	2	0.1	5	0	1
Molasses, cane, blackstrap	2 tbsp.	40	85	0	0	0	0	0	0	22	274	10.1	38	0	0
Sugar, brown	1 cup	220	820	0	0	0	0	0	0	212	187	4.8	97	0	0
Sugar, white, granulated	1 cup	200	770	0	0	0	0	0	0	199	3	0.1	5	0	0
Sugar, white, granulated	1 tbsp.	12	45	0	0	0	0	0	0	12	0	0	0	0	0
Sugar, powdered	1 cup	100	385	0	0	0	0	0.1	0	100	1	0	2	0	0
Syrup, chocolate flavored thin	2 tbsp.	38	85	1	0	0.2	0.1	0.1	0	22	6	0.8	36	0	0
Syrup, chocolate flavored, fudge	2 tbsp.	38	125	2	5	3.1	1.7	0.2	0	21	38	0.5	42	13	0
Table syrup (corn and maple)	2 tbsp.	42	122	0	0	0	0	0	0	32	1	0	19	0	0

Food Composition Table (continued)

Vegetables and Vegetable Products

Food Item	Serving Size	Weight (g)	Calories	Protein (g)	Fat (g)	Saturated Fat (g)	Monounsaturated Fat (g)	Polyunsaturated Fat (g)	Cholesterol (g)	Carbohydrate (g)	Calcium (mg)	Iron (mg)	Sodium (mg)	Vitamin A (µg)	Vitamin C (mg)
Alfalfa seeds, sprouted, raw	1 cup	33	10	1	0	0	0	0.1	0	1	11	0.3	2	5	3
Artichokes, globe, cooked	1 artichoke	120	55	3	0	0	0	0.1	0	12	47	1.6	79	17	9
Asparagus, cooked from raw, pieces	1 cup	180	45	5	1	0.1	0	0.2	0	8	43	1.2	7	149	49
Asparagus, cooked from raw, spears	4 spears	60	15	2	0	0	0	0.1	0	3	14	0.4	2	50	16
Asparagus, cooked from frozen, pieces	1 cup	180	50	5	1	0.2	0	0.3	0	9	41	1.2	7	147	44
Asparagus, cooked from frozen, spears	4 spears	60	15	2	0	0.1	0	0.1	0	3	14	0.4	2	49	15
Asparagus, canned, spears	4 spears	80	10	1	0	0	0	0.1	0	2	11	0.5	278	38	13
Bamboo shoots, canned, drained	1 cup	131	25	2	1	0.1	0	0.2	0	4	10	0.4	9	1	1
Beans, lima, thick seeds, frozen, cooked	1 cup	170	170	10	1	0.1	0	0.3	0	32	37	2.3	90	32	22
Beans lima, baby, cooked from frozen	1 cup	180	190	12	1	0.1	0	0.2	0	35	50	3.5	52	30	10
Beans, snap, raw, cooked, green	1 cup	125	45	2	0	0.1	0	0.2	0	10	58	1.6	4	83	12
Beans, snap, cooked from raw, yellow	1 cup	125	45	2	0	0	0	0.1	0	10	58	1.6	4	10	12
Beans, snap, cooked from frozen, green	1 cup	135	35	2	0	0	0	0.1	0	8	61	1.1	18	71	11
Beans, snap, cooked from frozen, yellow	1 cup	135	35	2	0	0	0	0.1	0	8	61	1.1	18	15	11
Beans, snap, canned, green	1 cup	135	25	2	0	0	0	0.1	0	6	35	1.2	339	47	6
Beans, snap, canned, yellow	1 cup	135	25	2	0	0	0	0.1	0	6	35	1.2	339	14	6
Bean sprouts, mung, raw	1 cup	104	30	3	0	0	0	0	0	6	14	0.9	6	2	14
Bean sprouts, mung, cooked	1 cup	124	25	3	0	0	0	0	0	5	15	0.8	12	2	14
Beets, cooked, diced	1 cup	170	55	2	0	0	0	0	0	11	19	1.1	83	2	9
Beets, cooked, whole	2 beets	100	30	1	0	0	0	0.1	0	7	11	0.6	49	1	6
Beets, canned	1 cup	170	55	2	0	0	0	0.1	0	12	26	3.1	466	2	7
Beet greens, cooked	1 cup	144	40	4	0	0	0.1	0.6	0	8	164	2.7	347	734	36
Blackeye peas, cooked from raw	1 cup	165	180	13	1	0.3	0.1	0.5	0	30	46	2.4	7	105	3
Blackeye peas, cooked from frozen	1 cup	170	225	14	1	0.3	0.1	0.3	0	40	39	3.6	9	13	4
Broccoli, raw	1 spear	151	40	4	1	0.1	0.1	0.2	0	8	72	1.3	41	233	141
Broccoli, cooked from raw, spears	1 spear	180	50	5	1	0.1	0	0.2	0	10	82	2.1	20	254	113
Broccoli, cooked from raw, pieces	1 cup	155	45	5	0	0.1	0	0	0	9	71	1.8	17	218	97
Broccoli, cooked from frozen, spears	1 piece	30	10	1	0	0	0	0	0	2	15	0.2	7	57	12

Food Item	Serving Size	Weight (g)	Calories	Protein (g)	Fat (g)	Saturated Fat (g)	Mono-unsaturated Fat (g)	Poly-unsaturated Fat (g)	Cholesterol (g)	Carbohydrate (g)	Calcium (mg)	Iron (mg)	Sodium (mg)	Vitamin A (µg)	Vitamin C (mg)
Broccoli, cooked from frozen, pieces	1 cup	185	50	6	0	0	0	0.1	0	10	94	1.1	44	350	74
Brussels sprouts, cooked from raw	1 cup	155	60	4	1	0.2	0.1	0.4	0	13	56	1.9	33	111	96
Brussels sprouts, cooked from frozen	1 cup	155	65	6	1	0.1	0	0.3	0	13	37	1.1	36	91	71
Cabbage, raw	1 cup	70	15	1	0	0	0	0.1	0	4	33	0.4	13	9	33
Cabbage, cooked	1 cup	150	30	1	0	0	0	0.2	0	7	50	0.6	29	13	36
Cabbage, Chinese, pak-choi, cooked	1 cup	170	20	3	0	0	0	0.1	0	3	158	1.8	58	437	44
Cabbage, Chinese, pe-tsai, raw	1 cup	76	10	1	0	0	0	0.1	0	2	59	0.2	7	91	21
Cabbage, red, raw	1 cup	70	20	1	0	0	0	0.1	0	4	36	0.3	8	3	40
Cabbage, savoy, raw	1 cup	70	20	1	0	0	0	0	0	4	25	0.3	20	70	22
Carrots, raw, whole	1 carrot	72	30	1	0	0	0	0.1	0	7	19	0.4	25	2025	7
Carrots, raw, grated	1 cup	110	45	1	0	0	0	0.1	0	11	30	0.6	39	3094	10
Carrots, cooked from raw	1 cup	156	70	2	0	0.1	0	0.1	0	16	48	1.0	103	3830	4
Carrots, cooked from frozen	1 cup	146	55	2	0	0	0	0.1	0	12	41	0.7	86	2585	4
Carrots, canned	1 cup	146	35	1	0	0.1	0	0.1	0	8	37	0.9	352	2011	4
Cauliflower, raw	1 cup	100	25	2	0	0	0	0.1	0	5	29	0.6	15	2	72
Cauliflower, cooked from raw	1 cup	125	30	2	0	0	0	0.1	0	6	34	0.5	8	2	69
Cauliflower, cooked from frozen	1 cup	180	35	3	0	0.1	0	0.2	0	7	31	0.7	32	4	56
Celery, pascal type, raw, stalk	1 stalk	40	5	0	0	0	0	0	0	1	14	0.2	35	5	3
Celery, pascal type, raw, pieces	1 cup	120	20	1	0	0	0	0.1	0	4	43	0.6	106	15	8
Collards, cooked from raw	1 cup	190	25	2	0	0.1	0	0.2	0	5	148	0.8	36	422	19
Collards, cooked from frozen	1 cup	170	60	5	1	0.1	0.1	0.4	0	12	357	1.9	85	1017	45
Corn, cooked from raw, yellow	1 ear	77	85	3	1	0.2	0.3	0.5	0	19	2	0.5	13	17	5
Corn, cooked from raw, white	1 ear	77	85	3	1	0.2	0.3	0.5	0	19	2	0.5	13	0	5
Corn, cooked from frozen, yellow	1 ear	63	60	2	1	0.1	0.1	0.2	0	14	2	0.4	3	13	3
Corn, cooked from frozen, white	1 ear	63	60	2	1	0.1	0.1	0.2	0	14	2	0.4	3	0	4
Corn, cooked from frozen, yellow	1 cup	165	135	5	1	0	0	0.1	0	34	3	0.5	8	41	4
Corn, cooked from frozen, white	1 cup	165	135	5	1	0	0	0.1	0	34	3	0.5	8	0	4
Corn, canned, cream style, yellow	1 cup	256	185	4	1	0.2	0.3	0.5	0	46	8	1.0	730	25	12
Corn, canned, cream style, white	1 cup	256	185	4	1	0.2	0.3	0.5	0	46	8	1.0	730	0	12
Corn, canned, whole kernel, yellow	1 cup	210	165	5	1	0.2	0.3	0.5	0	41	11	0.9	571	51	17
Corn, canned, whole kernel, white	1 cup	210	165	5	1	0.2	0.3	0.5	0	41	8	0.9	571	0	17
Cucumber with peel	6 slices	28	5	0	0	0	0	0	0	1	4	0.1	1	1	1
Dandelion greens, cooked	1 cup	105	35	2	1	0.1	0	0.3	0	7	147	1.9	46	1229	19
Eggplant, cooked, steamed	1 cup	96	25	1	0	0	0	0.1	0	6	6	0.3	3	6	1
Endive, curly, raw	1 cup	50	10	1	0	0	0	0	0	2	26	0.4	11	103	3
Jerusalem-artichoke, raw	1 cup	150	115	3	0	0	0	0	0	26	21	5.1	6	3	6
Kale, cooked from raw	1 cup	130	40	2	1	0.1	0	0.3	0	7	94	1.2	30	962	53
Kale, cooked from frozen	1 cup	130	40	4	1	0.1	0	0.3	0	7	179	1.2	20	826	33
Kohlrabi, cooked	1 cup	165	50	3	0	0	0	0.1	0	11	41	0.7	35	6	89

Food Composition Table (continued)

Food Item	Serving Size	Weight (g)	Calories	Protein (g)	Fat (g)	Saturated Fat (g)	Mono-unsaturated Fat (g)	Poly-unsaturated Fat (g)	Cholesterol (g)	Carbohydrate (g)	Calcium (mg)	Iron (mg)	Sodium (mg)	Vitamin A (µg)	Vitamin C (mg)
Lettuce, butterhead, raw, head	1 head	163	20	2	0	0	0	0.2	0	4	52	0.5	8	158	13
Lettuce, butterhead, raw, leaves	1 leaf	15	0	0	0	0	0	0	0	0	5	0	1	15	1
Lettuce, crisp head, raw, head	1 head	539	70	5	1	0.1	0	0.5	0	11	102	2.7	49	178	21
Lettuce, crisp head, raw, wedge	1 wedge	135	20	1	0	0	0	0.1	0	3	26	0.7	12	45	5
Lettuce, crisp head, raw, pieces	1 cup	55	5	1	0	0	0	0.1	0	1	10	0.3	5	18	2
Lettuce, loose leaf	1 cup	56	10	1	0	0	0	0.1	0	2	38	0.8	5	106	10
Mushrooms, raw	1 cup	70	20	1	0	0	0	0.1	0	3	4	0.9	3	0	2
Mushrooms, cooked	1 cup	156	40	3	1	0.1	0	0.3	0	8	9	2.7	3	0	6
Mushrooms, canned	1 cup	156	35	3	0	0.1	0	0.2	0	8	17	1.2	663	0	0
Mustard greens, cooked	1 cup	140	20	3	0	0	0.2	0.1	0	3	104	1.0	22	424	35
Okra pods, cooked	8 pods	85	25	2	0	0	0	0	0	6	54	0.4	4	49	14
Onions, raw, chopped	1 cup	160	55	2	0	0.1	0.1	0.2	0	12	40	0.6	3	0	13
Onions, raw, sliced	1 cup	115	40	1	0	0.1	0	0.1	0	8	29	0.4	2	0	10
Onions, raw, cooked, drained	1 cup	210	60	2	0	0.1	0	0.1	0	13	57	0.4	17	0	12
Onions, spring, raw	6 onions	30	10	1	0	0	0	0	0	2	18	0.6	1	150	14
Onion rings, breaded, frozen	2 rings	20	80	1	5	1.7	2.2	1.0	0	8	6	0.3	75	5	0
Parsley, raw	10 sprigs	10	5	0	0	0	0	0	0	1	13	0.6	4	52	9
Parsley, freeze-dried	1 tbsp.	0.40	0	0	0	0	0	0	0	0	1	0.2	2	25	1
Parsnips, cooked	1 cup	156	125	2	0	0.1	0.2	0.1	0	30	58	0.9	16	0	20
Peas with edible pods, cooked	1 cup	160	65	5	0	0.1	0	0.2	0	11	67	3.2	6	21	77
Peas, green, canned	1 cup	170	115	8	1	0.1	0.1	0.3	0	21	34	1.6	372	131	16
Peas, green, cooked from frozen	1 cup	160	125	8	0	0.1	0	0.2	0	23	38	2.5	139	107	16
Peppers, hot chili, raw, red	1 pepper	45	20	1	0	0	0	0	0	4	8	0.5	3	484	109
Peppers, hot chili, raw, green	1 pepper	45	20	1	0	0	0	0	0	4	8	0.5	3	35	109
Peppers, sweet, raw, green	1 pepper	74	20	1	0	0	0	0.2	0	4	4	0.9	2	39	95
Peppers, sweet, raw, red	1 pepper	74	20	1	0	0	0	0.2	0	4	4	0.9	2	422	141
Peppers, sweet, cooked, green	1 pepper	73	15	0	0	0	0	0.1	0	3	3	0.6	1	28	81
Peppers, sweet, cooked, red	1 pepper	73	15	0	0	0	0	0.1	0	3	3	0.6	1	274	121
Potatoes, baked with skin	1 potato	202	220	5	0	0.1	0	0.1	0	51	20	2.7	16	0	26
Potatoes, baked flesh only	1 potato	156	145	3	0	0	0	0.1	0	34	8	0.5	8	0	20
Potatoes, boiled	1 potato	135	115	2	0	0	0	0.1	0	27	11	0.4	7	0	10
Potatoes, french-fries, frozen, baked	10 strips	50	110	2	4	2.1	1.8	0.3	0	17	5	0.7	16	0	5
Potatoes, french-fries, frozen, fried	10 strips	50	160	2	8	2.5	1.6	3.8	0	20	10	0.4	108	0	5
Potatoes, au gratin, mix	1 cup	245	230	6	10	6.3	2.9	0.3	12	31	203	0.8	1076	76	8
Potatoes, au gratin, home-made	1 cup	245	325	12	19	11.6	5.3	0.7	56	28	292	1.6	1061	93	24
Potatoes, hashed brown, frozen	1 cup	156	340	5	18	7.0	8.0	2.1	0	44	23	2.4	53	0	10
Potatoes, mashed, home-made	1 cup	210	160	4	1	0.7	0.3	0.1	4	37	55	0.6	636	12	14
Potatoes, mashed, from dehydrated mix	1 cup	210	235	4	12	7.2	3.3	0.5	29	32	103	0.5	697	44	20
Potato salad	1 cup	250	360	7	21	3.6	6.2	9.3	170	28	48	1.6	1323	83	25
Potatoes, scalloped, mix	1 cup	245	230	5	11	6.5	3.0	0.5	27	31	88	0.9	835	51	8
Potatoes, scalloped, home-made	1 cup	245	210	7	9	5.5	2.5	0.4	29	26	140	1.4	821	47	26

Food Item	Serving Size	Weight (g)	Calories	Protein (g)	Fat (g)	Saturated Fat (g)	Mono-unsaturated Fat (g)	Poly-unsaturated Fat (g)	Cholesterol (g)	Carbohydrate (g)	Calcium (mg)	Iron (mg)	Sodium (mg)	Vitamin A (µg)	Vitamin C (mg)
Potato chips	10 chips	20	105	1	7	1.8	1.2	3.6	0	10	5	0.2	94	0	8
Pumpkin, cooked from raw	1 cup	245	50	2	0	0.1	0	0	0	12	37	1.4	2	265	12
Pumpkin, canned	1 cup	245	85	3	1	0.4	0.1	0	0	20	64	3.4	12	5404	10
Radishes, raw	4 radishes	18	5	0	0	0	0	0	0	1	4	0.1	4	4	4
Sauerkraut, canned	1 cup	236	45	2	0	0.1	0	0.1	0	10	71	3.5	1560	4	35
Seaweed, kelp, raw	1 ounce	28.35	10	0	0	0.1	0	0	0	3	48	0.8	66	3	0
Seaweed, spirulina, dried	1 ounce	28.35	80	16	2	0.8	0.2	0.6	0	7	34	8.1	297	16	3
Spinach, raw	1 cup	55	10	2	0	0	0	0.1	0	2	54	1.5	43	369	15
Spinach, cooked from raw	1 cup	180	40	5	0	0.1	0	0.2	0	7	245	6.4	126	1474	18
Spinach, cooked from frozen	1 cup	190	55	6	0	0.1	0	0.2	0	10	277	2.9	163	1479	23
Spinach, canned	1 cup	214	50	6	1	0.2	0	0.4	0	7	272	4.9	683	1878	31
Spinach soufflé	1 cup	136	220	11	18	7.1	6.8	3.1	184	3	230	1.3	763	675	3
Squash, summer, cooked	1 cup	180	35	2	1	0.1	0	0.2	0	8	49	0.6	2	52	10
Squash, winter, baked	1 cup	205	80	2	1	0.3	0.1	0.5	0	18	29	0.7	2	729	20
Sweet potatoes, baked, peeled	1 potato	114	115	2	0	0	0	0.1	0	28	32	0.5	11	2488	28
Sweet potatoes, boiled	1 potato	151	160	2	0	0.1	0	0.2	0	37	32	0.8	20	2575	26
Sweet potatoes, candied	1 piece	105	145	1	3	1.4	0.7	0.2	8	29	27	1.2	74	440	7
Sweet potatoes, canned, mashed	1 cup	255	260	5	1	0.1	0	0.2	0	59	77	3.4	191	3857	13
Sweet potatoes, canned, vacuum packed	1 piece	40	35	1	0	0	0	0	0	8	9	0.4	21	319	11
Tomatoes, raw	1 tomato	123	25	1	0	0	0	0.1	0	5	9	0.6	10	139	22
Tomatoes, canned	1 cup	240	50	2	1	0.1	0.1	0.2	0	10	62	1.5	391	145	36
Tomato juice, canned	1 cup	244	40	2	0	0	0	0.1	0	10	22	1.4	881	136	45
Tomato paste, canned	1 cup	262	220	10	2	0.3	0.4	0.9	0	49	92	7.8	2070	647	111
Tomato puree, canned	1 cup	250	105	4	0	0	0	0.1	0	25	38	2.3	998	340	88
Tomato sauce, canned	1 cup	245	75	3	0	0.1	0	0.2	0	18	34	1.9	1482	240	32
Turnips, cooked, diced	1 cup	156	30	1	0	0	0.1	0.1	0	8	34	0.3	78	0	18
Turnip greens, cooked from raw	1 cup	144	30	2	0	0.1	0	0.1	0	6	197	1.2	42	792	39
Turnip greens, cooked from frozen	1 cup	164	50	5	1	0.2	0	0.3	0	8	249	3.2	25	1308	36
Vegetable juice cocktail, canned	1 cup	242	45	2	0	0	0	0.1	0	11	27	1.0	883	283	67
Vegetables, mixed, canned	1 cup	163	75	4	0	0.1	0.1	0.2	0	15	44	1.7	243	1899	8
Vegetables, mixed, cooked from frozen	1 cup	182	105	5	0	0.1	0	0.1	0	24	46	1.5	64	778	6
Water chestnuts, canned	1 cup	140	70	1	0	0	0	0	0	17	6	1.2	11	1	2
Miscellaneous Items															
Baking powder	1 tsp.	3	5	0	0	0	0	0	0	1	58	0	329	0	0
Baking powder, low sodium	1 tsp.	4	5	0	0	0	0	0	0	1	207	0	1	0	0
Gelatin, dry	1 envelope	7	25	6	0	0	0	0	0	0	1	0	6	0	0
Yeast, bakers, dry, active	1 package	7	20	3	0	0	0.1	0	0	3	3	1.1	4	0	0

Glossary

abdominal thrust. A technique that can help save a choking victim. (8)

acesulfamek. A type of sugar substitute sold in the United States. (3)

aged cheese. Cheese stored for a time before it is sold. (20)

al dente. Pasta that is cooked until it is tender but firm. (18)

all-purpose flour. The most common type of flour, which can be used in nearly all recipes. (18)

amino acids. The building blocks of proteins. (2)

anorexia nervosa. An eating disorder that causes people to starve themselves. (4)

antidote. A substance that works against a poison. (8)

appetite. The desire to eat certain foods and reject others. (1)

aquaculture. Raising fish like crops. (21)

aromatic seeds. Seeds that are tasty or scented. (16)

aspartame. A type of sugar substitute sold in the United States. (3)

bacteria. Tiny organisms that are found everywhere. A few types can cause food-borne illness. (9)

bake. To cook in hot air in an oven. (10)

bar cookies. Cookies made by spreading soft cookie dough in a pan. After baking, the cooled cookies are cut into bars. (23)

barbecue. To roast slowly over hot coals or in an oven and baste with a spicy sauce. (10)

baste. To moisten foods during baking or roasting with fat, juice, or sauce. Basting adds flavor and keeps the food moist. (10)

batter. A mixture containing flour and water that can be poured. (19)

beat. To stir quickly with a spoon, wire whisk, beater, or mixer until ingredients are smooth. (10)

beef. The meat from cattle that is over a year old. (21)

berries. Small, juicy fruits that contain many tiny seeds. (15)

binge eating. An eating disorder that involves the rapid eating (or chewing and spitting out) of thousands of calories in a short time. (4)

blanch. To put a food in boiling water for a very short time to precook it. (10)

blend. To mix ingredients until they are very smooth. (10)

blue plate style. A type of meal service in which the foods are placed on each person's plate in the kitchen and taken to the table. (13)

boil. To cook in hot liquid that has bubbles that rise and break on the surface of the liquid. (10)

botulism. A deadly foodborne illness. (9)

braise. To cook large pieces of meat or poultry slowly in a small amount of hot liquid. (10)

bran. The tough, outer coat of a kernel of grain. (18)

bread flour. A type of coarse flour used to make hearty, firm breads. (18)

broil. To cook directly under a very hot heating unit in an oven. (10)

brown. To make the surface of a food brown by baking, broiling, or toasting it. (10)

brown rice. The whole rice kernel. It contains more nutrients and fiber than other types of rice. (18)

browning pan. A pan made of materials that absorb microwave energy. This causes them to get so hot that foods become brown and crisp. (6)

buffet style. A type of meal service in which the serving dishes are placed together on a serving table. Diners pick up the tableware they need then walk around the serving table to serve themselves. (13)

built-in dishwasher. A type of dishwasher built into a cabinet with a permanent connection to hot water, a drain, and electricity. (5)

bulb. A short, rounded bud that has a very short stem covered with overlapping leaves. (16)

bulimia nervosa. An eating disorder that causes people to binge and purge themselves. (4)

butter. The fat found in milk. (20)

buttermilk. A cultured milk product made by adding bacteria to whole, lowfat, or fat free milk. (20)

C

cake flour. A smooth, silky flour used to make cakes that have a light and delicate texture. (18)

calcium. A nutrient needed to build bones and teeth, transmit nerve signals, and contract muscles. (2)

calorie. A measure of the energy value of food. (2)

calorie balance. Eating the same number of calories as you burn. (4)

campylobacter. Bacteria that are the most common cause of foodborne illness. (9)

candling. Shining a very bright light on eggs in order to judge their quality. (22)

carbohydrate. A nutrient that provides energy. It is found in every food of plant origin. Sugars, starch, and fiber are types of carbohydrates. (2)

carbon monoxide. A colorless, odorless deadly gas. (8)

cardiopulmonary resuscitation (CPR). A lifesaving technique that helps save a victim who isn't breathing and whose heart has stopped. (8)

career. The work in a certain field that a person does for a long period. (24)

career ladder. A series of jobs in the same field to which a person can advance. (24)

casing. A thin skin shaped like a tube; holds ground meats such as sausage. (21)

chalazae. Two white stringlike structures that hold the yolk in the middle of an egg. (22)

chest freezer. A freezer with the door on top. (5)

chiffon pies. Light, airy pies that contain gelatin and beaten eggs. (23)

chill. To put food in the refrigerator to make it cold. (10)

cholesterol. A fatlike substance that occurs naturally in the body. (2)

chop. To cut into small, uneven pieces. (10)

citrus fruit. A type of fruit that has a leathery skin, many segments filled with juicy pellets, and grows on trees. (15)

clostridium botulinum. Bacteria that cause botulism. (9)

clostridium perfringens. Bacteria that grow quickly at danger zone temperatures. (9)

cold pack cheese. A blend of cheeses. (20)

color additives. Additives that make foods look more appealing. (12)

complete protein. Food of animal origin that contains all the amino acids needed by the body. (2)

connective tissue. Long, thin tissue that holds muscles together. (21)

continuous cleaning oven. A type of oven with special coating on the inside walls. This coating causes spatters and spills to burn away during cooking. (5)

convection oven. A type of oven that cooks food with circulating hot air. (5)

convenience food. Food that has been partially or totally prepared when you buy it. (11)

convenience store. A type of store often located near or in residential areas that are usually open longer than most other food stores. (12)

conventional method. Mixing method used for shortened cakes in which fat and sugar are creamed together, the eggs added, and sifted dry ingredients are added alternately with the liquid ingredients. (23)

conventional oven. A type of oven that uses the hot air inside to cook food. (5)

converted rice. Rice made by steaming whole rice kernels. Steaming draws some of the nutrients from the bran and germ into the endosperm where they are trapped. After the kernels dry, the bran and germ are removed. (18)

cooked dressing. A dressing made with vinegar or fruit juice and flour, cornstarch, or egg yolks. Cooked dressings do not contain fat or oil. (17)

cooking and serving center. The space in a kitchen where food is cooked and placed in serving dishes; it can include a range, microwave oven, and convection oven. (5)

cool. To let heated food come to room temperature. (10)

corn oil. Oil made by squeezing the germ of corn kernels. (18)

corn syrup. Syrup made by changing the starch of the endosperm of the corn kernel into sugar. (18)

cornmeal. Meal ground from the whole corn kernel or just the endosperm. (18)

cornstarch. A fine, white powder made from the starch of corn endosperm. (18)

cover. The space needed on a table for one place setting. (13)

cream. To beat sugar and a solid fat, such as butter, together until they are smooth, light, and fluffy. (10)

cream pies. Pies that have a baked crust filled with pudding and topped with meringue or whipped cream. (23)

cross-contamination. Spreading bacteria to a clean food from contaminated work surfaces, utensils, hands, or food. (9)

cube. To cut food into cubes about ½-inch in size. Dice means the same thing as cube. (10)

culture. The knowledge, beliefs, religion, and traditions shared by a group of people. (1)

cultured milk products. Dairy products produced by adding certain helpful bacteria to milk. (20)

curds. The solid pieces in milk that can stick together to form lumps. (20)

custard pies. Pies that contain eggs and milk. (23)

custom. A practice a group of people do often; the usual way of doing things. (1)

customer service. Career area that involves working with customers. (24)

cut in. To combine solid fat, such as shortening, with a flour mixture by cutting the fat into tiny pieces with knives or a pastry blender. (10)

cuts. Animal carcasses cut into smaller portions. (21)

D

danger zone. Temperatures at which bacteria grow fastest (40° to 140°F or 5° to 60°C). (9)

deep-fry. To cook food by completely immersing it in hot fat. This is also called French frying. (10)

diet. All the foods a person eats. (1)

Dietary Guidelines for Americans. A set of statements that can help people choose nutritious diets. (3)

Dietary Reference Intakes (DRIs). A set of guidelines for the amounts of many nutrients needed each day. (2)

dietitian. A nutrition expert. (2)

discount food stores. A type of food store that offers food at lower prices because the store buys large amounts of food and offers few services. (12)

dough. A mixture containing flour and water that is thick and stiff enough to be handled or kneaded. (19)

dovetail. To do two or more tasks at the same time. (13)

drain. To remove liquid from a food by pouring off the liquid or drying the food with paper towels. (10)

drawn fish. A whole fish with only its inner organs removed. (21)

dressed fish. A drawn fish with its scales, head, tail, and fins removed. (21)

drop cookies. Cookies made by dropping spoonfuls of dough onto a cookie sheet. (23)

drop-in range. A range designed to fit between two counters. (5)

drupes. A type of fruit that has one large pit or seed and grows on trees. (15)

E

E. coli 0157:H7. One of the most dangerous types of bacteria, found in undercooked meat. (9)

eating center. Space in a kitchen where people can sit to eat a meal or snack. (5)

egg white. Part of the egg that is almost pure protein and is fat free. (22)

egg yolk. Part of the egg where most of the nutrients, fat, and cholesterol are found. (22)

electric range. A type of range that produces heat when electricity flows through coils of wire. (5)

emulsifier. An ingredient that causes oil to mix with water. (17)

emulsion. A mixture of oil and water. (17)

endosperm. The largest part of a grain kernel. It contains mostly starch. (18)

enriched. Foods that have nutrients that were lost during processing added back to them. (18)

environment. A person's surroundings and experiences. (1)

evaporated milk. Milk product made by removing half the water from fresh milk and canning it. (20)

exhaust fan. A fan used with a cooktop that helps remove smoke, odors, steam, and grease from the air. (5)

expiration date. The last date a food should be eaten. (12)

F

fad diet. A quick weight loss diet that doesn't usually work and can be harmful to health. (4)

family style. A type of meal service in which each person serves his or her own plate then passes the serving dish to the next person. (13)

farina. A coarsely ground flour. Most of the bran and germ are removed. It is cooked and served as a hot breakfast cereal. (18)

farmers' market. A marketplace where people can buy fresh fruits, vegetables, and eggs directly from the farm at lower prices. (12)

fat. A nutrient used to supply calories to the body. (2)

fat free milk. Milk that has the fat skimmed off before it is homogenized. (20)

fat-soluble vitamin. Vitamin that dissolves in fat. (2)

fat substitute. A product that makes foods moist and creamy without adding fat. (3)

finfish. Fish that has a backbone and fins. (21)

first aid. Treatment given right after an accident happens that helps relieve pain and prevent further injury. (8)

fish fillets. The sides of a dressed fish. They are cut along the backbone from behind the head to the tail. (21)

fish steaks. Crosswise slices of a dressed fish. (21)

fish sticks. Strips cut from fillets. Most fish sticks are breaded and sold frozen. (21)

flavor additives. Additives that make foods taste more appealing. (12)

flour. A fine powder ground from wheat kernels. (18)

foam cakes. Cakes that contain no fat; sometimes called unshortened cakes. (23)

folate. A B-vitamin that is used to build strong, healthy blood and fight infections. (2)

fold. To combine ingredients by sliding a spatula down through a mixture, gently lifting and turning the ingredients until the mixture is blended. (10)

food additive. Any substance added to foods. (12)

Food and Drug Administration (FDA). Federal organization that sets the standards for food labels for all foods except for meat and poultry. (12)

food cooperative. A discount food store that is formed when a group of people get together and buy large amounts of food. (12)

Food Guide Pyramid. An outline of the foods and amounts a person should eat each day for a nutritious diet and good health. (3)

food poisoning. Another name for foodborne illness. (9)

food preparation. A career area that involves preparing food to be sold. (24)

food science. The study of how foods change chemically through natural processes or when they are prepared or stored. (1)

foodborne illness. Disease caused by a pathogen in food. (9)

formal style. A type of meal service in which the kitchen staff serves one course at a time. After you eat the course, the tableware you have used is removed. Clean tableware is brought to the table with the next course. This process continues until the whole meal is served. (13)

free-standing range. A type range that has surface units on the top and an oven below. (5)

freeze. To lower the temperature of a food to its freezing point or below. (10)

freezer burn. Pale, dry, tough patches appearing on food that has been in the freezer too long. (21)

French dressing. A dressing made with salad oil, vinegar or lemon juice, mustard, and paprika. (17)

fresh cheese. Cheese that is ready to eat as soon as it is made. (20)

fresh cream. Milk product that contains much more fat than milk.(20)

fresh juice. The liquid from squeezed fresh fruit. (15)

freshness date. The date that indicates how long a food will be fresh and tasty.

frozen juice concentrate. Fresh juice with most of its water removed. Sometimes sugar is added. (15)

frozen milk concentrate. Milk product made by removing most of the water and fat from milk. (20)

fruit ade. A drink that contains water and sugar. Some contain juice; others only fruit flavoring. (15)

fruit drink. A drink that has natural juice flavor, but may not contain any real fruit juice. (15)

fruit juice drink. A drink made by adding water and sugar to small amounts of juice. (15)

fruit nectar. Fruit juice and pureed fruit. (15)

fruit pies. Pies made with fresh, frozen, or canned fruit blended with sugar and cornstarch or flour. (23)

full warranty. A warranty that covers an entire appliance. (5)

G

garnish. A decoration you can eat that adds color to meals. (11)

gas range. A type of range that produces heat when gas combines with oxygen in the air and burns. (5)

gelati. Ice cream. (18)

gelatin. A powdered protein substance that, when mixed with liquid, forms a firm, jellylike consistency. (17)

gelatinization. This process occurs when starch granules absorb water, swell, and cause a liquid to become thicker. (18)

generic products. Products that have plain labels and are not advertised. They are often the least expensive. (12)

germ. The smallest part of a grain kernel. It contains most of the kernel's nutrients. A new plant sprouts from the germ. (18)

gluten. A sticky, elastic protein that forms when flour is mixed with liquid. (19)

goals. Aims you want to achieve. (24)

grades. An evaluation system for beef based on the age of the animal, amount of marbling, and the color and texture of the muscle. (21)

gram. A measure of weight. (2)

grate. To cut food into small pieces using the small holes of a grater. (10)

gratuity. A sum of money given to restaurant staff to show thanks for good service; also called a tip. (14)

grease. To rub lightly with fat or oil. (10)

grind. To crush food into very tiny bits by putting it through a food grinder. (10)

grits. Coarsely ground hominy. Grits are served as a hot breakfast cereal. (18)

H

half-and-half. A mixture of milk and cream. It has the least fat of all creams. (20)

healthy weight. The weight that is right for a person's age and height. (4)

heat susceptor. A cooking tray or cover that works like a browning pan. (6)

hepatitis. Foodborne illness caused by a virus found in water contaminated with sewage. (9)

herbs. Leaves from certain shrubs used to add flavor to foods. (16)

hominy. Large, dried pieces of corn endosperm that are boiled and served as a side dish. (18)

homogenized. Milk or cream in which the fat has been broken into tiny pieces by a special process. This process keeps the fat and watery liquid in milk or cream from separating. (20)

hunger. The physical need for food. (1)

hydrogenation. The process that turns an unsaturated fat into a saturated one. (2)

I

impulse buying. Making an unplanned purchase. (12)

incomplete protein. Food of plant origin that contains most, but not all, of the amino acids needed by the body. (2)

infection. A disease resulting from the establishment of a pathogen in a host. (9)

injection oven. An oven that blasts hot air over food at high speeds, causing the food to cook very rapidly. (5)

instant flour. A special form of all-purpose flour. It is processed in a way that allows it to mix easily in cold liquids. (18)

interview. A planned meeting between a job applicant and an employer. (24)

iron. A nutrient found in red blood cells. Its job is to carry oxygen to body cells and remove carbon dioxide. (2)

iron deficiency anemia. A common disease caused by a low intake of iron. (2)

J

juice made from concentrate. Juice made by adding water to juice concentrate. The added water replaces the water that was removed to make the concentrate. (15)

julienne. To cut food into long, thin strips the size of matchsticks. (10)

K

knead. To press and fold a ball of dough with the heels of your hands until the dough is smooth and elastic. (10)

L

lamb. The meat from a sheep that is less than one year old. (21)

landfill. Large hole in the ground where trash is stored. (11)

leavened bread. Bread that contains baking soda, baking powder, or yeast, which causes it to rise. (19)

leavening agent. Ingredient added to baked goods that produces gas bubbles, which cause the baked goods to rise. (19)

legumes. High-protein seeds, such as dry peas, dry beans, lentils, and peanuts, that grow in a pod. (22)

lifestyle. The type of life a person leads based on energy and time use. (1)

light cream. Cream that has less fat than whipping cream. (20)

limited warranty. A warranty that states conditions under which an appliance will be serviced, repaired, or replaced. (5)

listeria. Bacteria that are found mostly in raw milk. (9)

long grain rice. A type of rice that is light and fluffy when it is cooked. (18)

lowfat milk. Milk that has some of the fat skimmed off. (20)

M

magnetron. A device that converts electricity into microwaves. (6)

major food groups. The five food groups shown in the three lower sections of the Food Guide Pyramid. (3)

malt. A sticky, sugary substance produced when barley sprouts. (18)

marbling. Streaks of fat running through lean meat. (21)

mayonnaise. A type of dressing made with oil, egg yolks, and vinegar or lemon juice. (17)

medium grain rice. A type of rice that sticks together when cooked. (18)

melons. Large, moist fruits that grow on vines and contain seeds. They have a thick skin that may be smooth or rough. (15)

microwaveable foods. Foods specially packaged for microwave cooking. (6)

microwaves. A type of electromagnetic energy. (6)

mince. To cut food into very small pieces. (10)

mineral. Inorganic substance that is needed for function, growth, and repair of the body. (2)

mix. To combine ingredients by stirring or beating them. (10)

moderation. A reasonable amount; not too little or too much. (3)

mold. Bacterial colonies that look like fuzzy growths on the surface of foods. (9)

molded cookies. Cookies shaped with the hands. (23)

Mr. Yuk symbol. A symbol that lets people, especially children, know that a product is poisonous. (8)

mutton. Meat from an older sheep. (21)

N

name brands. Brands that cost the most because they have fancy packages and are advertised. (12)

natural toxins. Poisons found in certain plants and animals. (9)

neighborhood grocery store. Small food store often owned and run by one family. (12)

nonfat dry milk. Milk product made by removing all the fat and water from whole milk. (20)

noodles. A type of pasta with egg added to the dough. (18)

nutrient additives. Vitamins and minerals added to foods to make them more nutritious. (12)

nutrient supplement. Product used to add nutrients to the diets of people who are sick, injured, or known to have a nutrient deficiency. (2)

nutrients. The materials found in foods that are needed to build and repair body tissues and provide energy. (1)

nutrition. The study of nutrients and how the body uses them. (1)

nutritious diet. A diet that includes energy and all the nutrients in the amounts needed. (1)

O

obese: Having an excessive amount of body fat. (4)

open dating. A system of putting dates on foods to help you to decide which package to buy and which to use first at home. (12)

organic foods. Crops grown on farmland that has not been treated with human-made pesticides or weed killers or fertilized with sewage sludge. Organic meats are from farm animals that received no drugs or hormones to speed their growth rate. (12)

osteoporosis. A disease resulting from a lack of calcium in the diet that causes bones to wear away, become brittle, and break easily. (2)

oven. Part of a range that uses hot air to cook food in pans on shelves. (5)

P

pan-broil. To cook meat in its own fat. (10)

parasite. An organism that lives inside or on a host. (9)

parboil. To boil until partly cooked. (10)

pare. To cut off outer skin with a knife or vegetable peeler. (10)

partially prepared food. Food that needs some preparation. Most need to be blended with other ingredients. (11)

pasta. A shaped dough made with wheat flour and water. (18)

pasteurized. Milk or cream that has been heated to a high temperature for a few seconds to kill harmful bacteria. (20)

pasteurized process cheese. A blend of two or more cheeses. (20)

pathogen. An organism or substance that invades the body and damages its cells. (9)

peel. To strip or pull off the outer skin using your fingers or a knife. (10)

perishable foods. Foods that spoil in a few days, such as fresh milk and meat. (12)

permanent emulsion. A type of emulsion in which the ingredients do not separate. They stay mixed. (17)

place setting. All the dinnerware, flatware, glassware, and table linen used by one person. (13)

planning and message center. Part of a kitchen with counter space for writing menus and making shopping lists and storage space for cookbooks. (5)

poach. To cook food gently in simmering liquid. (10)

polenta. A pudding made with cornmeal. (18)

polished rice. The endosperm of the rice kernel. It has less than half as many nutrients as brown rice. (18)

pome. A type of fruit that has a core that contains seeds and grows on trees. (15)

popcorn. A type of corn that contains a tiny drop of water inside each kernel. When it is heated, the water turns into steam. The pressure of the steam causes the kernel to explode. (18)

pork. The meat from pigs. (21)

portable dishwasher. A type of dishwasher that can be stored anywhere and is rolled to the sink to wash dishes. (5)

poultry. Any bird raised for meat. (21)

preheat. To heat an oven to the cooking temperature before putting food in the oven. (10)

preparation and storage center. The space in a kitchen where foods are prepared and stored, usually between the refrigerator and range. (5)

preservative. An additive that help keep foods fresh longer by preventing the growth of mold or bacteria. (12)

pressed cookies. Cookies made by pushing dough through a cookie press. (23)

prime. The top grade of beef and veal. (21)

processed meat. Any meats that have been prepared in some way other than cutting or grinding. (21)

produce. Fresh fruits and vegetables. (15)

protein. A type of nutrient needed for growth and repair of the body. Proteins are made of amino acids. (2)

pull date. The last day a food should be sold. (12)

purée. To grind or mash food until it becomes smooth and liquid. (10)

purge. To rid the body of food by vomiting or abusing laxatives. (4)

Q

quick-mix method. Mixing method used for shortened cakes in which dry ingredients are sifted into a mixing bowl, the fat and liquid are added, then the eggs are added. (23)

R

R.S.V.P. An abbreviation written on invitations that means " please reply." (13)

ready-to-eat food. Packaged food that doesn't need any preparation. (11)

recipe. A list of ingredients and directions for preparing a food. (10)

references. People an employer can call to ask about your abilities as a worker. (24)

refrigerator cookies. Cookies formed when dough is shaped into a roll. It is then wrapped tightly and refrigerated. Once it is well chilled, the dough is cut with a knife into thin slices and baked. (23)

resources. Ways and means, such as time and money, that are used to complete a task. (11)

roast. To bake meat, fish, or poultry uncovered in hot air in an oven or over hot coals. (10)

rolled cookies. Cookies made by rolling out the dough and cutting it into shapes. (23)

S

saccharin. A type of sugar substitute sold in the United States. (3)

salmonella. Type of bacteria found in raw poultry and eggs. (9)

salt substitute. A product that contains the mineral potassium instead of sodium; used to help people reduce their sodium intake. (3)

sanitation. The study and use of methods that create a clean, healthy environment. (9)

saturated fat. A type of fat that causes the level of cholesterol in the blood to rise higher than normal. (2)

sauté. To brown or cook lightly and quickly in a small amount of hot fat; also is called panfrying. (10)

scald. To heat milk just until tiny bubbles form at the edge of the pan. (10)

scrape. To remove a very thin layer of outer skin by rubbing it with a knife or vegetable peeler. (10)

seasoners. Substances that add fragrance and flavor to foods. (16)

seasoning. A blend of two or more spices, herbs, or seeds. (16)

self-cleaning oven. A type of oven that, when set on "clean," becomes very hot and burns food spills to ashes. (5)

self-rising flour. All-purpose flour that has salt and baking powder added to it. (18)

sell date. The last day a food should be sold. (12)

serrated. Having a sawtooth edge. (7)

shellfish. Fish that have a hard shell. (21)

shopping plan. A plan that helps you save time, energy, and money. It also helps you reach your food shopping goal of getting what you need at the best price. (12)

short grain rice. A type of rice that sticks together when cooked. (18)

shortened cakes. Cakes that contain fat such as butter or shortening. (23)

shred. To cut food into long, very thin strips using a knife or the large holes of a grater. (10)

sift. To put dry ingredients through a flour sifter or fine sieve. (10)

simmer. To cook in liquid that is almost boiling, but is not hot enough to bubble. (10)

slice. To cut food into flat pieces. The pieces may be thick or thin. (10)

slide-in range. A range designed to slide in between two counters. (5)

small appliances. Electrical tools that can be moved easily from one place to another. (7)

sodium. A mineral that performs many vital functions, such as maintaining the body's water balance, helping muscles relax, and helping nerves transmit messages to the brain. (2)

sodium nitrite. An ingredient added to cured meats. It gives them a pink color and helps to preserve them. (21)

sour cream. Product made by adding bacteria to light cream. (20)

specialty shop. A store that features one type of food. (12)

spices. Bits of bark, fruits, flowers, and roots used to add flavor to foods. (16)

standing time. The period of time that occurs right after cooking time in a microwave oven. During this time, the heat inside the food causes it to finish cooking. It also helps to evenly distribute heat inside the food. (6)

staphylococci. Bacteria that are found in protein-rich foods, cream filled pastries, and moist salads made with chopped foods (such as potato salad, macaroni salad, and ham salad). (9)

staple foods. Foods that stay fresh for a long time, such as flour and sugar. (12)

starch. A type of carbohydrate stored in plants. It must be broken down by the body before it can be used as an energy source. (2)

steam. To cook in a pan using steam that rises from boiling liquid. (10)

stew. To slowly cook small pieces of food in moderate amounts of liquid. (10)

stir. To slowly move a spoon in a circle to combine ingredients. (10)

stir-fry. To cook small pieces of food by stirring quickly in a very small amount of hot fat. (10)

store brands. Brands sold by the supermarket chain. (12)

sucralose. A type of sugar substitute sold in the United States. (3)

sugar. A type of carbohydrate that furnishes calories but no other nutrient. It is used by the body as an energy source. (2)

sugar substitute. A product that sweetens foods without adding calories. (3)

supermarket. A type of large food store that offers special services and also sells nonfood items. (12)

surface unit. Part of a range that is used to cook food in pots. (5)

sweetened condensed milk. Milk product made by adding a very large amount of sugar to evaporated milk and canning it. (20)

T

tarts. Small pies. (23)

temporary emulsion. Type of emulsion in which the ingredients mix when shaken, but separate again in a few minutes. (17)

texture food additives. Additives that help ingredients blend well or improve the texture of foods. (12)

tip. A sum of money given to restaurant staff to show thanks for good service. (14)

toast. To brown foods using dry heat, usually in an oven or toaster. (10)

tofu. A soft, custardlike food made from soybeans. (22)

toxin. Poison. (9)

trichina. Roundworms found in raw or partly cooked pork or bear meat. (9)

trichinosis. A disease caused by roundworms. (9)

tropical fruit. A type of fruit that grows only in warm, sunny climates. (15)

tuber. The swollen portion of a plant's underground stem. (16)

turnovers. Pockets of pastry dough filled with any food used in a pie filling. (23)

U

U.S. Department of Agriculture (USDA). Federal organization that sets the standards for meat and poultry labels. (12)

UHT milk. A form of milk that is pasteurized at a higher temperature than normally used. The higher temperature preserves the milk, which stays fresh for several months when stored in a cool, dry place. (20)

underweight. A body weight that is much lower than a healthy weight. (4)

Underwriters Laboratories (UL). Association that tests electrical appliances. (5)

unit price. The cost per unit of an item. (12)

universal product code (UPC). A series of black lines, bars, and numbers printed on food labels to identify the product and its manufacturer, size, and style or form for a computer programmed to reflect the current price of that item. (12)

unleavened bread. Bread that does not contain leavening agents, so it does not rise. (19)

unsaturated fat. A type of fat that does not cause blood cholesterol levels to rise. (2)

upright freezer. A type of freezer with a door that swings outward. (5)

V

values. Beliefs and ideas that are important to you. (24)

variety meats. The organs of an animal. (21)

veal. The meat from cattle that is a few weeks old. (21)

vegetable spices. Strongly flavored vegetables. (16)

vegetarian. Person who does not eat meat, fish, or poultry. (22)

virus. An agent of infectious disease. (9)

vital functions. Body processes that keep you alive. (4)

vitamin. An organic substance needed by the body for function, growth, and repair. (2)

vitamin C. A vitamin that helps the body heal wounds and keeps gums healthy.

volume. The space an ingredient occupies. (10)

W

warranty. A seller's guarantee that a product will perform as specified and will be replaced or repaired if it fails within a certain time. (5)

water-soluble vitamin. Vitamin that dissolves in water. (2)

weight. A unit of mass. (10)

weight control. Keeping your body at a healthy weight. (4)

wheat bran. The outer covering of a kernel of grain. It is high in fiber. (18)

wheat germ. The germ of the wheat kernel. (18)

whey. The liquid portion of milk that is left after curds form. (20)

whip. To beat rapidly with a wire whisk, beater, or mixer in order to make a mixture smooth and fluffy. (10)

white flour. A flour made by grinding only the endosperm. The bran and germ are removed. (18)

whole fish. Fish that is sold just as it was when it was caught. (21)

whole grain foods. Cereal foods that include all three parts of the grain kernel. (18)

whole milk. Milk that contains the most fat. (20)

whole wheat flour. A flour made by grinding the entire wheat kernel. (18)

wild rice. The seeds of a water plant. (18)

work center. Area in the kitchen where a certain type of task is done and the equipment needed for the task is stored. (5)

work schedule. A plan that lists the time needed to prepare a meal, eat, and clean up. (13)

Y

yeast. A tiny plant that is the leavening agent used in breads. (19)

yield. The number and size of portions a recipe will make. (10)

yogurt. Product made by adding bacteria to fat free, lowfat, or whole milk. (20)

Z

zinc. A mineral needed for normal body growth and repair. (2)

Index